Advanced Statistics in Regulatory Critical Clinical Initiatives

Chapman & Hall/CRC Biostatistics Series
Series Editors
Shein-Chung Chow, *Duke University School of Medicine*, USA
Byron Jones, *Novartis Pharma AG*, Switzerland
Jen-pei Liu, *National Taiwan University*, Taiwan
Karl E. Peace, *Georgia Southern University*, USA
Bruce W. Turnbull, *Cornell University*, USA

For more information about this series, please visit: https://www.routledge.com/Chapman–Hall-CRC-Biostatistics-Series/book-series/CHBIOSTATIS

Advanced Statistics in Regulatory Critical Clinical Initiatives

Edited by
WEI ZHANG, FANGRONG YAN, FENG CHEN
AND SHEIN-CHUNG CHOW

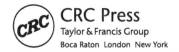

CRC Press
Taylor & Francis Group
Boca Raton London New York

CRC Press is an imprint of the
Taylor & Francis Group, an **informa** business

A CHAPMAN & HALL BOOK

First edition published in 2022
by CRC Press
6000 Broken Sound Parkway NW, Suite 300, Boca Raton, FL 33487-2742
and by CRC Press

4 Park Square, Milton Park, Abingdon, Oxon, OX14 4RN

CRC Press is an imprint of Taylor & Francis Group, LLC

Library of Congress Cataloging-in-Publication Data

Names: Zhang, Wei (Biometrician), editor. | Yan, Fangrong, editor. | Chen, Feng (Professor of biostatistics), editor. | Chow, Shein-Chung, 1955- editor.
Title: Advanced statistics in regulatory critical clinical initiatives /
edited by Wei Zhang, Fangrong Yan, Feng Chen and Shein-Chung Chow.
Description: First edition. | Boca Raton : CRC Press, 2022. |
Series: Statistics | Includes bibliographical references and index.
Identifiers: LCCN 2021048220 (print) | LCCN 2021048221 (ebook) |
ISBN 9780367561789 (hardback) | ISBN 9780367609955 (paperback) |
ISBN 9781003107323 (ebook)
Subjects: LCSH: United States. 21st Century Cures Act. |
Drugs--Testing--Statistical methods. | Clinical trials--Statistical
methods. | Biometry. | Drugs--Standards--United States. | Clinical
trials--Law and legislation--United States.
Classification: LCC RM301.27 .A38 2022 (print) | LCC RM301.27 (ebook) |
DDC 615.1072/4--dc23/eng/20211220
LC record available at https://lccn.loc.gov/2021048220
LC ebook record available at https://lccn.loc.gov/2021048221

ISBN: 978-0-367-56178-9 (hbk)
ISBN: 978-0-367-60995-5 (pbk)
ISBN: 978-1-003-10732-3 (ebk)

DOI: 10.1201/9781003107323

Typeset in Palatino
by KnowledgeWorks Global Ltd.

Contents

About the Editors

Wei Zhang, PhD, is Vice President, Head of Biometrics at AffaMed Therapeutics, New York, NY. Dr. Zhang has over a decade of experience working at the United States Food and Drug Administration (FDA) as a master statistical reviewer and supervisory mathematical statistician. Dr. Zhang was the president of the FDA Statistical Association in 2014. She is a member of the Executive Committee of the American Statistical Association Biopharmaceutical Section and has led the Distance Learning Committee since 2016. She has also served on multiple data monitoring committees.

Fangrong Yan, PhD, is a professor of biostatistics at the School of Science and Director of Biostatistics and Computational Pharmacy Research Center at the China Pharmaceutical University (CPU). Dr. Yan is a visiting scholar in the Department of Biostatistics, MD Anderson Cancer Research Center, USA. His professional research focused mainly on biostatistical problems in clinical trials, adaptive design, survival analysis and precision cancer therapy, cancer genomics analysis, population pharmacokinetic analysis, pharmaceutical experimental data modeling and analysis, biomedical big data, and medical big data analysis theory and application. In recent years, Dr. Yan has published more than 70 papers in journals with the highest impact factor. He was honored as part of the "Six Big Talent" in the Peak Project in Jiangsu Province and the "Blue Project" Middle-Aged and Young Academic Leaders in Jiangsu Province. Now he maintains part of the National Natural Science Fund Project, National Social Science Fund Project, Province Departmental Level Topic, and many latitudinal topics. He has also charged for many clinical trials, built many clinical databases, and developed a series of clinical trials and practical software. Dr. Yan published a monograph on Cancer Clinical Trial (CCT) methodology: Bayesian Design Method for CCT. As the chief editor and deputy chief editor, he has edited many textbooks.

Feng Chen, PhD, is a professor of biostatistics in the School of Public Health, Nanjing Medical University (NJMU). Dr. Chen received his BSc in mathematics from Sun Yat-Sen University (Guangzhou), and PhD in biostatistics from West China University of Medical Sciences. Dr. Chen is currently the chairperson of the China Association of Biostatistics (CABS), chairperson of the China Clinical Trial Statistics (CCTS) working group, and vice-chair of IBS-China. He is a member of the Drafting Committee of China Statistical Principles for Clinical Trials. As an external review expert of the Drug Evaluation Center, NMPA, Dr. Chen dedicated himself to the drafting of dozens of guidelines for clinical trials, as well as statistical theory and methodologies in medical research, especially in the analysis of non-independent data, high-dimensional data, and clinical trials. He studied multilevel models in London University in 1996 and as a Visiting Scholar, he was engaged in the Genome-Wide Association Study (GWAS) at the School of Public Health, Harvard University from 2008–2010. As a statistician, he was involved in dozens of grants, in charge of design, data management, and statistical analysis. Dr. Chen has over 200 publications, and 18 textbooks and monographs published.

Shein-Chung Chow, PhD, is currently a professor in the Department of Biostatistics and Bioinformatics, Duke University School of Medicine, Durham, North Carolina. Dr. Chow is also a Special Government Employee (SGE) appointed by the FDA as an Oncologic Drug Advisory Committee (ODAC) voting member and Statistical Advisor to the FDA. Dr. Chow was editor-in-chief of the *Journal of Biopharmaceutical Statistics* (1992–2020) and of the Biostatistics Book Series, Chapman & Hall/CRC Press of Taylor & Francis Group. He was elected Fellow of the American Statistical Association in 1995 and was elected member of the ISI (International Statistical Institute) in 1999. Dr. Chow is the author or co-author of over 330 methodology papers and 33 books including *Design and Analysis of Clinical Trials, Adaptive Design Methods in Clinical Trials,* and *Innovative Methods for Rare Diseases Drug Development.*

Contributors

Xiuyu Julie Cong
Everest Medicines
Shanghai, China

Haoda Fu
Advanced Analytics and Data Sciences
Eli Lilly and Company
Lilly Corporate Center
Indianapolis, IN, USA

Vivian Gu
PPC China
Shanghai, China

Beibei Guo
Department of Experimental Statistics
Louisiana State University
Baton Rouge, LA, USA

Xiang Guo
BeiGene
Beijing, China

Yan Hou
Peking University
Bejing, China

Kang Li
Harbin Medical University
Harbin City
Heilongjiang Province, China

Meijuan Li
Foundation Medicine, Inc.
Cambridge, MA, USA

Xiao Lin
BeiGene
Beijing, China

Haochen Liu
China Pharmaceutical University
Nanjing, China

Amir Nikooienejad
Advanced Analytics and Data Sciences
Eli Lilly and Company
Lilly Corporate Center
Indianapolis, IN, USA

Xin Sun
Chinese Evidence-Based Medicine Center
West China Hospital
Sichuan University
NMPA Key Laboratory for Real World
    Data Research and Evaluation in
    Hainan
Sichuan Center of Technology
    Innovation for Real World Data
Chengdu, China

Fan Xia
CSPC Pharmaceutical Group Limited
Shanghai, China

Xiaoyan Yan
Peking University Clinical
    Research Institute
Beijing, China

Chen Yao
Peking University Clinical
    Research Institute
Beijing China

Yongpei Yu
Peking University Clinical
    Research Institute
Beijing, China

Ying Yuan
Department of Biostatistics
The University of Texas
MD Anderson Cancer Center
Houston, TX, USA

Yafei Zhang
PPC China
    Shanghai, China

Shutian Zhang
National Clinical Research Center for
    Digestive Disease
Beijing Friendship Hospital
Capital Medical University
Beijing, China

1

Introduction

Wei Zhang[1], Fangrong Yan[2], Feng Chen[3], and Shein-Chung Chow[4]

[1] *AffaMed Therapeutics, New York, NY, USA*

[2] *China Pharmaceutical University School of Science, China*

[3] *School of Public Health, Nanjing Medical University, China*

[4] *Duke University School of Medicine, Durham, North Carolina, USA*

CONTENTS

1.1 The 21st Century Cure Act

The 21st Century Cures Act is a United States (US) law enacted by the 114th US Congress on 13 December 2016. It authorized $6.3 billion in funding, mostly for the National Institutes of Health (NIH) (Park, 2016). The Act was supported especially by large pharmaceutical manufacturers and was opposed especially by some consumer organizations (Mukherjee, 2016).

The goal of the 21st Century Cures Act is to decrease the administrative burdens, encourage innovation and enhance America's healthcare field. Along this line, the 21st Century Cures Act is designed to help accelerate medical product development and bring innovations and advances to patients who need them faster and more efficiently. Thus, the 21st Century Cures Act builds on Food and Drug Administration's (FDA's) ongoing work to incorporate the perspectives of patients into the development of drugs, biological products and devices in FDA's decision-making process. Cures enhance the ability to modernize clinical trial designs, including the use of RWD/RWE, and clinical outcome assessments, which will speed or shorten the development and review of novel medical products. The 21st Century Cures Act also provides new authority to help FDA improve its ability not only to recruit and retain scientific, technical and professional experts, but also to establish new expedited product development programs, including (i) the regenerative medicine advanced therapy (RMAT) that offers a new expedited option for certain eligible biologics products, and (ii) the breakthrough devices program, designed to speed or shorten the review of certain innovative medical devices. In addition, the 21st Century Cures Act directs FDA to create one or more inter-center institutes to help coordinate activities in major disease areas between the drug, biologics and device centers which improves the regulation of combination products.

The 21st Century Cures Act includes 18 titles: (i) Title I – Innovation Projects and States Responses to Opioid Abuse, (ii) Title II – Discovery, (iii) Title III – Development, (iv) Title IV – Delivery, (v) Title V – Savings, (vi) Title VI – Strengthening Leadership and Accountability, (vii) Title VIII – Supporting State Prevention Activities and Responses to Mental Health and Substance Use Disorder Needs, (ix) Title IX –Promoting Access to Mental Health and Substance Use Disorder Care, (x) Title X – Strengthening Mental and Substance Use Disorder Care for Children and Adolescents, (xi) Title XI – Compassionate Communication on (Health Insurance Portability and Accountability Act) HIPAA, (xii) Title XII – Medicaid Mental Health Coverage, (xiv) Title XIII – Mental Health Parity, (xv) Title XIV – Mental Health and Safe Communities, (xv) Title XV – Provisions Relating to Medicare Part A, (xvi) Title XVI – Provisions Relating to Medicare part B, (xvii) Title XVII – Other Medicare Provisions, and (xviii) Title XVIII – Other Provisions.

It is worth mentioning that Title III, development focuses on (i) patient-focused drug development, (ii) advancing new drug therapies, (iii) modern trial design and evidence development, (iv) patient access to therapies and information, (v) antimicrobial innovation and stewardship, (vi) medical device innovations, (vii) improving scientific expertise and outreach at FDA, and (viii) medical countermeasures innovation which will assist the sponsors in increasing the efficiency and the probability of success in pharmaceutical research and development.

Following the 21st Century Cures Act, the Secretary of the US Department of Health and Human Services (HHS) was authorized to establish a Tick-Borne Disease Working Group to serve as a Federal Advisory Committee. The Working Group is to comprise Federal and public members with diverse disciplines and views pertaining to Tick-Borne Diseases. The Act charges the Working Group to provide a report to the Congress and the HHS Secretary on its findings and any recommendations every two years. Working Group responsibilities include a review of ongoing research and resulting advances, Federal epidemiological and research efforts, and identification of research gaps.

1.2 FDA User Fee Programs

The FDA User Fee programs for prescription drugs, generic drugs, biosimilar products and medical devices primarily include (i) prescription drug user fee, (ii) generic drug user fee, (iii) biosimilar user fee and (iv) medical device user fee. The User Fee programs help the FDA to fulfill its mission of protecting public health and accelerating innovation in the pharmaceutical industry. The Office of Financial Management (OFM) is responsible for the financial management of the user fee programs. OFM maintains accounts receivable system used for user fee invoicing, collections, reporting and data maintenance. As indicated in Josephson (2020), the process for reauthorizing human medical product user fee programs at the FDA for another 5-year period is getting started this year. Below we highlight some changes made to the programs when they were last reauthorized through the 2017 Food and Drug Administration Reauthorization Act (FDARA) (P.L. 115-52) and consider what could be included in the upcoming user fee reauthorization package.

1.2.1 The Prescription Drug User Fee Act (PDUFA)

PDUFA was first enacted in 1992 and authorizes FDA to collect fees from companies that manufacture certain human drugs and biological products in exchange for FDA improving the review process for New Drug Applications (NDAs) and Biologics License Applications (BLAs). The PDUFA authorizes FDA (specifically the Center for Drug Evaluation and Research (CDER) and the Center for Biologics Evaluation and Research (CBER)) to assess and collect fees for prescription drug products. FDA dedicates these fees toward expediting the drug development process and the process for the review of human drug applications, including post-market drug safety activities.

With the most recent reauthorization, known as PDUFA VI, Congress and FDA created two new fee types: an application fee and an annual prescription drug program fee, which replaced the previously authorized supplemental application fee and annual establishment fee. The new fee types are assessed based on each "prescription drug product," which is defined as an approved drug with specific strength or potency in its final dosage form that is dispensed only with a valid prescription. Because a single NDA or BLA can cover dozens of prescription drug products, PDUFA VI also limits prescription drug program fees to five fees (i.e., five prescription drug products) per NDA or BLA.

Additionally, FDA committed in PDUFA VI, under the Breakthrough Therapy Program that had been created as part of the 2012 PDUFA cycle, to expedite the development and review of drug and biological products for serious or life-threatening diseases or conditions when preliminary clinical evidence indicates that the drug may demonstrate substantial improvement over existing therapies. PDUFA VI provides funding and resources to this program to enable FDA to continue to work closely with sponsors throughout the designation, development, and review process for breakthrough therapies, which has been considered wildly successful. At the same time, however, PDUFA VI has some shortcomings that we expect to be addressed by the FDA and Congress as part of the next reauthorization. FDA has said that it requires additional funding to better regulate regenerative medicine products and manufacturing facilities. That industry has grown significantly in just the last few years and may seek, in exchange for fees to support a more predictable premarket review process, clarification from FDA on manufacturing standards and marketing exclusivity for non-traditional product types.

1.2.2 The Generic Drug User Fee Act (GDUFA)

GDUFA was originally enacted in 2012 following negotiations between FDA and the generic drug industry to improve access to generic drugs, making it a very young program in comparison to PDUFA. The first iteration of GDUFA provided FDA with resources to expedite the review of Abbreviated New Drug Applications (ANDAs), including significant resources to eliminate a substantial backlog of ANDAs that had built up over several years and were awaiting a final FDA decision of approvability. GDUFA II, included as part of FDARA in 2017, changed the structure of the generic drug user fee program by adding a program fee for all approved ANDA holders. User fees under GDUFA II include application fees, facility fees and Drug Master File fees. In addition, ANDA holders will pay a fixed annual ANDA Sponsor Program fee, which depends on the number of ANDAs owned by companies (ANDA fees are divided into three tiers: small, medium and large). Although the application fees have increased compared to the program's first iteration, the fees associated with ANDA supplements have been removed. GDUFA II also brought relief to small businesses without any approved ANDAs by postponing the payment of the sponsor's facility fee until the ANDA is approved. Similarly, GDUFA II brought relief to Contact Manufacturing Organizations (CMOs) that manufacture the product for another ANDA sponsor.

In addition to those specific fee changes, GDUFA II attempts to quicken the time for approval of certain generic product candidates for which the reference product has limited competition. FDARA requires the FDA to prioritize review of ANDAs that rely upon a reference product that has fewer than three approved generics and ANDAs for products on the drug shortages list. This provision was not part of the GDUFA II agreement negotiated between FDA and the generics industry; rather, it is an example of how Congress can supplement the negotiated agreements with legislative riders that can be quite significant for the industry.

Despite those changes, GDUFA II has also faced significant challenges that we expect will be addressed in the next reauthorization cycle as well. According to the FDA, many ANDAs are not lawfully approvable at the time they are submitted because the reference product still has market exclusivity. Therefore, the ANDA has to undergo several review cycles before it achieves final agency approval. FDA, industry and Congress may have to think creatively to come up with potential solutions to address this particular challenge.

1.2.3 The Biosimilar User Fee Act (BsUFA)

Like GDUFA, it was first enacted in 2012 to enable FDA to collect fees from biosimilar companies to aid in the assessment of development programs and applications for marketing approval. A biosimilar is to a reference biological product what a generic is to a brand drug, often referred to as the reference listed drug. BsUFA authorizes FDA (specifically the Center for Drug Evaluation and Research (CDER) and the Center for Biologics Evaluation and Research (CBER)) to assess and collect fees for biosimilar biological products. FDA dedicates these fees toward expediting the review process for biosimilar biological products. BsUFA facilitates the development of safe and effective biosimilar products for the American public.

BsUFA II aims to improve the predictability of funding levels and the management of resources allocated to the agency's biosimilars program. BsUFA II copies several elements from PDUFA from a financial and programmatic standpoint. Additionally, as part of BsUFA II, FDA committed to devoting more user fee resources to educating health care professionals and patients about the benefits of biosimilars. In particular, FDA is establishing dedicated staff capacity for key functions such as internal training and educational outreach and communication in order to deliver information to the public and to improve public understanding of biosimilarity and interchangeability.

However, BsUFA II has also run into challenges. For instance, "Type 2" meetings between sponsors and the agency – which are meetings designed to discuss a specific issue or question in which FDA can provide targeted advice regarding the Biosimilar Product Development program – continue to suffer from timely scheduling. BsUFA I required the scheduling of Type 2 meetings to occur within 75 days of the request, which was modified in BsUFA II to be within 90 days of the request. Despite the change, however, FDA is still not meeting that performance goal. The agency also has not provided existing staff with enough resources to research and review biosimilar applications for approval. Further, FDA has struggled to hire highly educated, experienced and talented employees, which is a problem that is unfortunately not unique to the biosimilars program.

1.2.4 The Medical Device User Fee Act (MDUFA)

MDUFA was enacted in 2002 and is on deck to be reauthorized for the fourth time (known as MDUFA V). The 2017-enacted MDUFA IV created new goals for pre-submissions and introduced performance goals and a fee for De Novo device classification requests. MDUFA IV also included funding for the nascent digital health, patient input and quality management programs housed within the Center for Devices and Radiological Health, as well as funding for the National Evaluation System for health Technology (NEST), a public-private partnership whose goals include improving the quality and quantity of Real-World Evidence (RWE) available for regulatory uses.

Because of the novelty of the NEST and sensitivity about industry funding a post-market surveillance tool (due, in part, to the way the user fee law is written), the industry limited its investment and the scope of related activities. For example, the MDUFA IV Commitment Letter requires that NEST investigate using RWE to support expanding the indications for use of existing devices and clearances and approvals of new devices, but it said nothing about improving post-market surveillance (despite FDA touting such functionality as a key benefit of NEST). Further, the Commitment Letter states that NEST management will seek to make the enterprise financially self-sustaining, signaling the industry's reluctance to provide funding for the program in perpetuity.

Congress, unsatisfied with the MDUFA IV agreement's limitations on the use of NEST for premarket-focused activities, included a rider in FDARA mandating that NEST be used to conduct one or more post-market surveillance studies. Like the GDUFA legislative rider mentioned earlier, this is a good example of how Congress can supplement the user fee agreement between industry and FDA with a separate mandate. Unfortunately, however, as was the case for the mandatory NEST post-market studies, Congress does not always provide additional funding to fulfill its mandates.

We expect to see NEST as a subject of continued discussion in the MDUFA V negotiations. Further, we expect the agency's De Novo and pre-submission performance goals will be refined based on experience and data gathered during the MDUFA IV period. We also anticipate a rider about an issue that has remained unresolved despite Congressional interest during the last user fee reauthorization cycle: medical device servicing. We have covered this topic extensively over the past several years; in short, there continues to be concerns raised about the safety of devices serviced without appropriate regulatory oversight, but defining and getting servicers and Original Equipment Manufacturers (OEMs) to agree on what level of regulatory oversight is appropriate remains a challenge.

1.3 FDA Critical Clinical Initiatives

In the past several decades, it has been recognized that increasing spending on biomedical research does not reflect an increase in the success rate of pharmaceutical/clinical research and development. The low success rate of pharmaceutical/clinical development could be due to the following factors: (i) there is a diminished margin for improvement that escalates the level of difficulty in proving drug benefits, (ii) genomics and other new sciences have not yet reached their full potential, (iii) mergers and other business arrangements have decreased candidates, (iv) easy targets are the focus as chronic diseases are harder to study, (v) failure rates have not improved and (vi) rapidly escalating costs and complexity decreases the willingness/ability to bring many candidates forward into the clinic (Woodcock, 2004).

1.3.1 FDA Critical Path Initiative

In March 2004, the FDA kicked off the *Critical Path Initiative* with the release of FDA's landmark report *Innovation/Stagnation: Challenge and Opportunity on the Critical Path to New Medical Products*. The purpose of the Critical Path Initiative is to assist the sponsors in (i) identifying possible causes, (ii) providing resolutions and (iii) increasing the efficiency and the probability of success in pharmaceutical research and development. In its 2004 Critical Path Report, the FDA presented its diagnosis of the scientific challenges underlying the medical product pipeline problems. The landmark report diagnosed the reasons for the widening gap between scientific discoveries that have unlocked the potential to prevent and cure some of today's biggest killers, such as diabetes, cancer and Alzheimer's, and their translation into innovative medical treatments. Sounding the alarm on the increasing difficulty and unpredictability of medical product development, the report concluded that collective action was needed to modernize scientific and technical tools as well as harness information technology to evaluate and predict the safety, effectiveness and manufacturability of medical products. The Critical Path Initiative is considered as FDA's national strategy for transforming the way FDA-regulated medical products are developed, evaluated and manufactured.

On 16 March 2006, the FDA released a Critical Path Opportunities List that outlines 76 initial projects to bridge the gap between the quick pace of new biomedical discoveries and the slower pace at which those discoveries are currently developed into therapies. (See, e.g., http://www.fda.gov/oc/initiatives/criticalpath.) The Critical Path Opportunities List consists of six broad topic areas of (i) development of biomarkers, (ii) clinical trial designs, (iii) bioinformatics, (iv) manufacturing, (v) public health needs and (iv) pediatrics. As indicated in the Critical Path Opportunities Report, biomarker development and streamlining clinical trials are the two most important areas for improving medical product development. The streamlining clinical trials call for advancing innovative trial designs such as adaptive designs to improve innovation in clinical development. Many researchers interpret it as the encouragement of using innovative adaptive design methods in clinical trials, while some researchers believe it is the recommendation for the use of the Bayesian approach for assessment of treatment effect in pharmaceutical/clinical development (Chang and Chow, 2005). The purpose of adaptive design methods in clinical trials is to provide flexibility to the investigator for identifying the best (optimal) clinical benefit of the test treatment under study in a timely and efficient fashion without undermining the validity and integrity of the intended study.

1.3.2 FDA Critical Clinical Initiatives

For the implementation of the 21st Century Cures Act, the FDA has kicked off several critical clinical initiatives to accelerate medical product development and bring innovations and advances to patients who need them faster and more efficiently. These critical clinical initiatives include, but are not limited to, (i) complex innovative design (CID), (ii) biomarker-development, (iii) model-informed drug development (MIDD), (iv) real-world data (RWD) and real world evidence (RWE), (v) artificial intelligence (AI) and machine learning (ML) (for imaging medicine and mobile individualized medicine), (vi) flexible and efficient assessment of biosimilar products, (vii) statistical methods for complex generic drug products, (viii) rare diseases drug development. These critical clinical initiatives are briefly outlined below.

1.3.2.1 Complex Innovative Design (CID)

As indicated in PDUFA VI, CIDs include designs involving complex adaptations, Bayesian methods, or other features requiring simulations to determine operating characteristics. Thus, CIDs include (i) n-of-1 trial design, (ii) adaptive trial design, (iii) master protocol induced study designs such as umbrella, basket and platform designs and (iv) Bayesian sequential design.

An n-of-1 trial design is defined as a clinical trial design in which a single patient is the entire trial, a single case study. Thus, in an n-of-1 trial, n is the number of treatments and one is the single patient. An n-of-1 trial in which random allocation can be used to determine the order in which an experimental and a control are given to a patient. An n-of-1 trial is a multiple crossover study in a single participant.

Depending upon adaptations applied, Chow and Chang (2012) classified adaptive designs into the following categories: (i) adaptive randomization design, (ii) adaptive group sequential design, (iii) sample size re-estimation design, (iv) drop-the-losers design, (v) adaptive dose-finding design, (vi) adaptive treatment-switching design, (vii) biomarker-adaptive design, (viii) hypothesis-adaptive design, (ix) adaptive seamless design (e.g., two-stage phase I/II adaptive trial design) and (x) multiple adaptive designs.

In clinical trials, a master protocol is defined as a protocol designed with multiple sub-studies, which may have different objectives and involves coordinated efforts to evaluate one or more investigational drugs in one or more disease sub-types within the overall trial structure (Woodcock and LaVange, 2017). Clinical trials utilizing the concept of the master protocol are usually referred to as platform trials, which are to test multiple therapies in one indication, one therapy for multiple indications or both. Thus, master protocols may involve one or more interventions in multiple diseases or a single disease, as defined by current disease classification, with multiple interventions, each targeting a particular biomarker-defined population or disease subtype. Under this broad definition, a master protocol consists of three distinct entities: umbrella, basket and platform trials.

Under the assumption that historical data (e.g., previous studies or experience) are available, Bayesian methods for borrowing information from different data sources may be useful. These data sources could include, but are not limited to, natural history studies and expert's opinion regarding prior distribution about the relationship between endpoints and clinical outcomes. The impact of borrowing on results can be assessed through the conduct of sensitivity analysis. One of the key questions of particular interest to the investigator and regulatory reviewer is that how much to borrow in order to (i) achieve desired statistical assurance for substantial evidence, and (ii) maintain the quality, validity and integrity of the study.

1.3.2.2 Model-Informed Drug Development (MIDD)

There are many new topic areas that should be addressed since the publication of FDA 2003 guidance entitled "*Exposure-Response Relationships – Study Design, Data Analysis, and Regulatory Application.*" These new topic areas include the use of innovative trial design (e.g., adaptive dose-finding design) and the Bayesian approach. The use of innovative adaptive trial design in conjunction with the Bayesian approach for adaptive dose-finding is commonly considered in the early stage of drug development (see, e.g., Chow and Chang, 2012). Chang and Chow (2005) proposed a hybrid Bayesian adaptive design for a dose-response trial based on *safety* endpoint under a toxicity model in cancer research. Ivanova et al. (2009), on the other hand, considered an adaptive design for identifying the dose with the best *efficacy/tolerability* profile under a crossover design. Most recently, the assessment of generalizability of the results of exposure-response analysis also receives much attention (Lu et al. 2017). The generalizability is referred to the generalizability of the analysis results from one patient population (e.g., adults) to another (e.g., elderly or pediatrics) or from a geographical location (e.g., study site or medical center) to another.

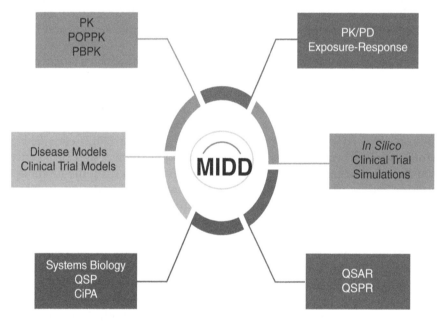

FIGURE 1.1
Model-informed drug development

1.3.2.3 Biomarker Development

With the surge in advanced technology especially in the "OMICS" space (e.g., Genomics, proteomics, etc.), the adaptive clinical trial designs that incorporate biomarker information for interim decisions have attracted significant attention.

The biomarker, which usually is a short-term endpoint that is indicative of the behavior of the primary endpoint, has the potential to provide substantial added value to interim study population selection (biomarker-enrichment designs) and interim treatment selection (biomarker-informed adaptive designs).

Jiang et al. (2007) proposed a biomarker-adaptive threshold design for settings in which a putative biomarker to identify patients who were sensitive to the new agent was measured on a continuous or graded scale. The design combined a test for the overall treatment effect in all randomly assigned patients with the establishment and validation of a cut point for a pre-specified biomarker of the sensitive subpopulation. Freidlin et al. (2010) proposed a cross-validation extension of the adaptive signature design that optimizes the efficiency of both the classifier development and the validation components of the design. Zhou et al. (2008) proposed Bayesian adaptive randomization enrichment designs for targeted agent development.

Shun et al. (2008) studied a biomarker-informed two-stage winner design with normal endpoints. Wang et al. (2014) showed that the bivariate normal model that only considers the individual-level correlation between biomarker and primary endpoint is inappropriate when little is known about how the means of the two endpoints are related. Wang et al. (2014) further proposed a two-level correlation (individual-level correlation and mean level correlation) model to describe the relationship between biomarker and primary endpoint. The two-level correlation model incorporates a new variable that describes the mean level correlation between the two endpoints. The new variable, together with its distribution, reflects the uncertainty about the mean-level relationship between the two endpoints due to a small sample size of historical data. It was shown that the two-level correlation model is a better choice for modeling the two endpoints.

1.3.2.4 Real-World Data (RWD) and Real-World Evidence (RWE)

The 21st Century Cures Act passed by the US Congress in December 2016 requires the US FDA shall establish a program to evaluate the potential use of RWE which is derived from RWD to (i) support approval of new indication for a drug approved under section 505 (c) and (ii) satisfy post-approval study requirements. RWE offers the opportunities to develop robust evidence using high-quality data and sophisticated methods for producing causal-effect estimates regardless randomization is feasible. In this article, we have demonstrated that the assessment of treatment effect (RWE) based on RWD could be biased due to the potential selection and information biases of RWD. Although fit-for-purpose RWE may meet regulatory standards under certain assumptions, it is not the same as substantial evidence (current regulatory standard in support of approval of regulatory submission). In practice, it is then suggested that when there are gaps between fit-for-purpose RWE and substantial evidence, we should make efforts to fill the gaps for an accurate and reliable assessment of the treatment effect.

1.3.2.5 Artificial Intelligence (AI) and Machine Learning

For implementation of the 21st Century Cures Act, the FDA has kicked off several critical clinical initiatives to accelerate medical product development and bring innovations and advances to patients. Among these, AI and ML are one of the most important pieces. In recent years, AI/ML has brought significant impacts for the drug discovery, development, manufacture and commercialization. Target identification and molecule designs are the two key topics in drug discovery. Machine learning methods have shown to be efficient to identify a new drug target, such as identifying Baricitinib as a potential treatment for COVID-19 in early pandemic and end up with an FDA-approved indication (Richardson et al. 2020). Recently, DeepMind released AlphaFold 2 has significantly improved protein structure prediction and achieved experimental level accuracy (Tunyasuvunakool et al. 2021). The solutions will have a profound impact on how molecules will be designed and optimized. Beyond drug discovery space, AI/ML methods also have had significant impacts on drug development, such as speeding up clinical enrollment through identifying promising sites, identifying the right sub population for precision medicine. Digital health, by leveraging digital device, has achieved significant attention recently. Apple, Eli Lilly and Evidation have demonstrated that digital device can identify Alzheimer's disease and cognitive impairment (e.g., https://cacm.acm.org/news/238766-apple-eli-lilly-evidation-present-first-results-from-digital-alzheimers-study/fulltext). Drug formulation and manufacturing also start to leverage AI/ML solutions to better manufacturing drugs and optimize supply chains. Among all the new technology in AI/ML, reinforcement learning and deep learning are the two key themes to drive innovations. We are going to provide additional details in Chapter 6.

1.3.2.6 *Flexible and Efficient Assessment of Biosimilar Products*

For assessment of biosimilar products, FDA recommended a stepwise approach for obtaining totality-of-the-evidence in support of regulatory approval of a proposed biosimilar product. The stepwise approach starts with the assessment of analytical similarity followed by Pharmacokinetic (PK) and Pharmacodynamics (PD) similarity and clinical similarity including immunogenicity. For analytical similarity assessment of a given Critical Quality Attribute (CQA) between a proposed biosimilar (test) product and an innovative (reference) biological product, FDA recommended an equivalence test with an Equivalence Acceptance Criteria (EAC), a margin of $1.5\sigma_R$ (standard deviation of the reference product) be performed (FDA, 2017; FDA, 2019). This EAC, however, has been criticized due to its inflexibility (Shutter, 2017). As a result, FDA is seeking a more flexible and efficient statistical test for analytical similarity assessment.

As current equivalent test is data-dependent, which EAC depends upon an estimate of σ_R. In practice, an estimate of σ_R can be considered as any values from a 95% confidence interval of σ_R, $(\hat{\sigma}_L, \hat{\sigma}_U)$. Following this idea, Lee et al. (2019) proposed a statistical test with a flexible margin. Let f be a flexible index such as $\hat{\sigma}_R^* = f \times \hat{\sigma}_R$. Then the flexible margin becomes $\delta = 1.5 \times \hat{\sigma}_R^* = 1.5 f \times \hat{\sigma}_R$. One idea is to select f achieving the maximum power for testing the following interval hypotheses for equivalence or similarity,

$$H_0 : |\varepsilon| \geq \delta \text{ versus } H_a : |\varepsilon| < \delta,$$

where $\varepsilon = \mu_T - \mu_R$ and $\delta = 1.5 f \hat{\sigma}_R$.

For $n = 6,7,8,9$, and 10, the optimal f maximizing power can be found in Tables 1.5 and 1.6 of Lee et al. (2019).

1.3.2.7 *Statistical Methods for Complex Generic Drug Products*

As described in the GDUFA II Commitment Letter, a complex generic drug product generally means the following (i) a product with a complex active ingredient(s) (e.g., peptides, polymeric compounds, complex mixtures of Active Pharmaceutical Ingredient(APIs), naturally sourced ingredients); a complex formulation (e.g., liposomes, colloids); a complex route of delivery (e.g., locally acting drugs such as dermatological products and complex ophthalmological products and otic dosage forms that are formulated as suspensions, emulsions or gels); a complex dosage form (e.g., transdermals, metered-dose inhalers, extended-release injectables); (ii) complex drug-device combination products (e.g., auto-injectors, metered dose inhalers); and (iii) other products where complexity or uncertainty concerning the approval pathway or possible alternative approaches would benefit from early scientific engagement. For complex generic drug products, standard methods for assessment of bioequivalence may not be appropriate and hence should not be applied directly.

For complex generic drug products, such as nasal spray products, *in vitro* bioequivalence testing is often conducted for bioequivalence assessment. In this case, standard cross-over design is not feasible. Alternatively, the Assessment Of Population Bioequivalence (PBE) under a parallel-group design is often considered (see, e.g., Chow, Shao and Wang, 2003a,b). For other complex generic drug products, the search for other statistical methods is needed.

1.3.2.8 Rare Disease Drug Development

A rare disease is defined by the Orphan Drug Act of 1983 as a disorder or condition that affects less than 200,000 persons in the United States. Most rare diseases are genetic related, and thus are present throughout the person's entire life, even if symptoms do not immediately appear. Many rare diseases appear early in life, and about 30%of children with rare diseases will die before reaching their fifth birthday. FDA is to advance the evaluation and development of products including drugs, biologics and devices that demonstrate promise for the diagnosis and/or treatment of rare diseases or conditions. Along this line, FDA evaluates scientific and clinical data submissions from sponsors to identify and designate products as promising for rare diseases and to further advance the scientific development of such promising medical products. Following the Orphan Drug Act, FDA also provides incentives for sponsors to develop products for rare diseases. The program has successfully enabled the development and marketing of over 600 drugs and biological products for rare diseases since 1983.

To encourage the development of rare disease drug products, FDA provides several incentive (expedited) programs including (i) fast track designation, (ii) breakthrough therapy designation, (iii) priority review designation and (iv) accelerated approval for approval of rare disease drug products. In its recent guidance, however, FDA emphasizes that FDA will not create a statutory standard for approval of orphan drugs that are different from the standard for approval of drugs in common conditions (FDA, 2015). For the approval of drug products, FDA requires that substantial evidence regarding the effectiveness and safety of the drug products be provided. Substantial evidence is based on the results of adequate and well-controlled investigations (21 CFR 314.126(a)).

As most rare diseases may affect far fewer persons, one of the major concerns of rare disease clinical trials is that often there are only a small number of subjects available. With the limited number of subjects available, it is expected that there may not have sufficient power for detecting a clinically meaningful difference (treatment effect). In rare disease clinical trials, power calculation for the required sample size may not be feasible for rare disease clinical trials. In this case, alternative methods such as precision analysis, reproducibility analysis, or probability monitoring approach may be considered for providing substantial evidence with certain statistical assurance. In practice, however, a small patient population is a challenge to rare disease clinical trials for obtaining substantial evidence through the conduct of adequate and well-controlled investigations.

For the development of drug products for rare disease development, data collection from an adequate and well-controlled clinical investigation is essential for obtaining substantial evidence for approval of the drug products. Data collection is a key to the success of the intended trial. Thus, utilizing innovative trial designs and statistical methods in rare disease setting is extremely important to the success of rare diseases drug development.

1.4 Innovative Thinking for Challenging Statistical Issues

Endpoint Selection – In clinical trials, the selection of appropriate study endpoints is critical for an accurate and reliable evaluation of the safety and effectiveness of a test treatment under investigation. In practice, however, there are usually multiple endpoints available for measurement of disease status and/or therapeutic effect of the test treatment under study. For example, in cancer clinical trials, overall survival, response rate and/or time to disease progression are usually considered as primary clinical endpoints for the evaluation of the safety and effectiveness of the test treatment under investigation. Once the study endpoints have been selected, the sample size required for achieving the study objective with a desired power is then determined. It, however, should be noted that different study endpoints may result in different sample sizes. In practice, it is usually not clear which study endpoint can best inform the disease status and measure the treatment effect. Moreover, different study endpoints may not translate one another although they may be highly correlated with one another. In practice, it is very likely that one study endpoint may achieve the study objective while the others may not. In this case, it is an interesting question that which endpoint is telling the truth.

To address these questions, Chow and Huang (2019) proposed developing an innovative endpoint namely therapeutic index based on a utility function to combine and utilize information collected from all study endpoints. Statistical properties and performances of the proposed therapeutic index are evaluated both theoretically and via clinical trial simulations. The results showed that the developed therapeutic index outperforms individual endpoints in terms of both false-positive and false-negative rates.

1.4.1 Margin Selection

The selection of margin (e.g., non-inferiority or equivalence/similarity) has always been a challenging problem in clinical research. It plays a critical role in the testing of non-inferiority or equivalence/similarity between a test product and its innovative (reference) drug product. For comparative clinical studies, a scientific justification based on clinical knowledge about the reference product, usually obtained from historical studies, is commonly considered to establish an appropriate non-inferiority or equivalence/similarity margin in support of a demonstration that there are no clinically meaningful differences between the test product and the reference product with respect to the study endpoints. FDA and ICH E10 have both published guidelines to assist the sponsors for the selection of an appropriate non-inferiority margin, but little was mentioned for evaluating the effect of different margins on the testing of equivalence/similarity which directly influences the approval rate of drugs. In practice, different equivalence/similarity margins in clinical trials are often proposed by the sponsors. In this case, the sponsors are usually asked to provide scientific rationale or justification for the wider margin. Nie et al. (2020) proposed conducting a risk and benefit analysis to facilitate the communication between the sponsor and the FDA in making the final decision for margin selection. The performance of the proposed strategy by Nie et al. (2020) is evaluated via extensive clinical trial simulations for various scenarios.

Based on risk assessment using the four proposed criteria given in Nie et al. (2020), the proposed strategy cannot only close up the gap between the sponsor proposed margin and the FDA recommended margin, but also select an appropriate margin by taking clinical judgement, statistical rationale and regulatory feasibility into consideration. In this book, for simplicity, we focus on a continuous endpoint. The proposed strategy with the four criteria can be applied to other data types such as discrete endpoints (e.g., binary response) and time-to-event data. In addition to the evaluation of the risk of sponsor's proposed margin, we can also assess the risk of the FDA-recommended margin assuming that the margin proposed by the sponsor is the true margin.

1.4.2 Sample Size

Chow (2011) indicated that sample size calculation based on the estimate of $\theta = \sigma^2 / \delta^2$ is rather unstable. The asymptotic bias of $E(\hat{\theta} = s^2 / \hat{\delta}^2)$ is given by

$$E(\hat{\theta}) - \theta = N^{-1}(3\theta^2 - \theta) = 3N^{-1}\theta^2 \{1 + o(1)\}.$$

Alternatively, it is suggested that the median of $s^2 / \hat{\delta}^2$, i.e., $P(s^2 / \hat{\delta}^2 \leq \eta_{0.5}) = 0.5$ be considered. It can be shown that the asymptotic bias of the median of $s^2 / \hat{\delta}^2$ is given by

$$\eta_{0.5} - \theta = -1.5N^{-1}\theta \{1 + o(1)\},$$

Whose leading term is linear in θ. As it can be seen that bias of the median approach can be substantially smaller than the mean approach for a small sample size and/or small effect size. However, in practice, we usually do not know the exact value of the median of $s^2 / \hat{\delta}^2$. In this case, a bootstrap approach in conjunction with a Bayesian approach may be useful.

In practice, it is not uncommon that there is a shift in the target patient population due to protocol amendments. In this case, the sample size is necessarily adjusted for achieving a desired power for correctly detecting a clinically meaningful difference with respect to the original target patient population. One of the most commonly employed approaches is to consider adjusting the sample size based on the change in effect size.

$$N_1 = \min\left\{N_{\max}, \max\left(N_{\min}, sign(E_0 E_1)\left|\frac{E_0}{E_1}\right|^a N_0\right)\right\},$$

where N_0 and N_1 are the required original sample size before population shift and the adjusted sample size after population shift, respectively, $N_{\max}$ and $N_{\min}$ are the maximum and minimum sample sizes, a is a constant that is usually selected so that the sensitivity index Δ is within an acceptable range, and sign(x)=1 for $x > 0$; otherwise sign(x) = –1.

1.5 Aim and Scope of the Book

This book is intended to be the first book entirely devoted to the discussion of regulatory critical clinical initiatives for drug research and development. The scope of this book will focus on the critical clinical initiatives described in the previous section (Section 1.3). This book consists of 10 chapters concerning regulatory requirements, innovative design and analysis for rare diseases drug development. Chapter 1 provides some background regarding regulatory critical clinical initiatives as the follow-up of the 21st Century Cures Act and User Fee programs (PDUFA, GDUFA, BsUFA and MDUFA). Some complex innovative designs including adaptive trial design, the n-of-1 design, master protocols and

Bayesian sequential design are discussed in Chapter 2. Chapter 3 focuses on biomarker development for precision/personalized medicine. Chapter 4 describes the concept of model-informed drug development. Also included in this chapter is the study of various statistical models for exposure-response relationships. The potential use of RWD and RWE in support of regulatory submission are given in Chapter 5. Chapter 6 introduces ML for imaging medicine by focusing on deep learning and neural networks, statistical algorithm and model, and decision trees and model selection. Some challenging issues that are commonly encountered in cancer clinical trials such as analysis and interpretation of Progression-Free Survival (PFS) with Non-Proportional Hazard (NPH) are given in Chapter 7. Chapters 8–9 cover statistical methods for the assessment of biosimilar products and complex generic drug products, respectively. Chapter 10 provides innovative thinking and approach for rare diseases drug development.

References

Chang, M. and Chow, S.C. (2005) A hybrid Bayesian adaptive design for dose response trials. *J Biopharm Stat.*, 15(4):677–91.

Chow, S.C. (2011). *Controversial Issues in Clinical Trials*. Chapman and Hall/CRC Press, Taylor & Francis, New York, New York.

Chow, S.C. and Chang, M. (2012). *Adaptive Design Methods in Clinical Trials*. 2nd edition, Chapman and Hall/CRC Press, Taylor & Francis, New York, New York.

Chow, S.C. and Huang, Z. (2019). Innovative thinking on endpoint selection in clinical trials. *Journal of Biopharmaceutical Statistics*, 29, 941–951.

Chow, S.C., Shao, J., and Wang, H. (2003a). *In vitro* bioequivalence testing. *Statistics in Medicine*, 22, 55–68.

FDA (2017). *Guidance for Industry – Statistical Approaches to Evaluate Analytical Similarity*. Center for Drug Evaluation and Research (CDER) and Center for Biologics Evaluation and Research (CBER), the United States Food and Drug Administration, Silver Spring, Maryland, September 2017.

FDA (2019). *Guidance for Industry – Development of Therapeutic Protein Biosimilars: Comparative Analytical Assessment and Other Quality-Related Considerations*. Center for Drug Evaluation and Research (CDER) and Center for Biologics Evaluation and Research, the United States Food and Drug Administrations, Silver Spring, Maryland.

Freidlin, B., Jiang, W., and Simon, R. (2010). The cross-validated adaptive signature design. *Clinical Cancer Research*, 16(2), 691–698.

Ivanova, A., Liu, K., Snyder, E.S., and Snavely, D.B. (2009). An adaptive design for identifying the dose with the best efficacy/tolerability profile with application to a crossover dose-finding study. *Statistics in medicine*, 28(24), 2941–51.

Jiang, W., Freidlin, B., and Simon, R. (2007). Biomarker-adaptive threshold design: a procedure for evaluating treatment with possible biomarker-defined subset effect. *Journal of the National Cancer Institute*, 99(13), 1036–1043.

Josephson, A.J. (2020). FDA User Fees: Highlights from FDARA & Our Forecast for the Next Round. https://www.mintz.com/insights-center/viewpoints/2146/2020-02-fda-user-fees-highlights-fdara-our-forecast-next-round.

Lee, S.J., Oh, M., and Chow, S.C. (2019). Equivalent test with flexible margin in analytical similarity assessment. *Enliven: Biosimilars Bioavailability*, 3(2), 1–11.

Lu Y., Kong Y.Y., Chow, S.C. (2017). Analysis of sensitivity index for assessing generalizability in clinical research. *Jacobs J Biostat.* 2(1):009.

Mukherjee, S. (2016). Everything you need to know about the massive health reform law that just passed Congress Fortune. Retrieved 14 December 2016. Congress Passes 21st Century Cures Act, But Critics Sound a Sour Note | Fortune

Nie, L., Niu, Y., Yuan, M., Gwise, T., Levin, G., and Chow, S.C. (2020). Strategy for similarity margin selection in comparative clinical biosimilar studies. Submitted.

Park, A. (2016). Learn from Cures Act bipartisanship. Editorial. Asbury Park Press, Asbury Park, NJ. Gannett. 17 December 2016. Retrieved 31 December 2016. https://www.app.com/story/opinion/editorials/2016/12/17/st-century-cures-act-obama/95567222/

Richardson, P., Griffin, I., Tucker, C., Smith, D., Oechsle, O., Phelan, A., Rawling, M., Savory, E., and Stebbing, J. (2020). Baricitinib as potential treatment for 2019-nCoV acute respiratory disease. *Lancet (London, England)*, 395(10223), e30.

Shun, Z., Lan, K.K., and Soo, Y. (2008). Interim treatment selection using the normal approximation approach in clinical trials. *Statistics in Medicine*, 27(4), 597–618.

Shutter, S. (2017). Biosimilar sponsors seek statistical flexibility when reference product change. FDA Pink Sheet, 21 December 2017.

Tunyasuvunakool, K., Adler, J., Wu, Z., Green, T., Zielinski, M., Žídek, A., Bridgland, A., Cowie, A., Meyer, C., Laydon, A. and Velankar, S., (2021). Highly accurate protein structure prediction for the human proteome. *Nature*, 596(7873), 590–596.

Wang, J., Chang, M., and Menon, S. (2014). *Clinical and Statistical Considerations in Personalized Medicine; Biomarker-Informed Adaptive Design*. Chapman and Hall/CRC, Taylor & Francis Group, New York. 129–148.

Woodcock, J. (2004). FDA's Critical Path Initiative. FDA website: http://www.fda.gov/oc/initiatives/criticalpath/woodcock0602/woodcock0602.html

Woodcock, J. and LaVange, L.M. (2017). Master protocols to study multiple therapies, multiple diseases, or both. *New England Journal of Medicine*, 377, 62–70.

Zhou, X., Liu, S., Kim, E.S, Herbst, R.S., and Lee, J. (2008). Bayesian adaptive design for targeted therapy development in lung cancer - a step toward personalized medicine. *Clinical Trials*, 5(3), 181–193.

2

Complex Innovative Design

Beibei Guo[1] and Ying Yuan[2]

[1]*Department of Experimental Statistics, Louisiana State University, Baton Rouge, LA, USA*

[2]*Department of Biostatistics, The University of Texas MD Anderson Cancer Center, Houston, TX, USA*

CONTENTS

DOI: 10.1201/9781003107323-2

2.1 Complex Innovative Design

As described in Chapter 1, the 21st Century Cures Act (Cures Act), signed into law on 13 December 2016, is designed to accelerate medical product development and bring innovations and advances to patients faster and more efficiently. One important approach to achieving this goal is the use of innovative clinical trial designs, as set forth in Section 3021 of the Cures Act. In accordance with this mandate, US Food and Drug Administration (FDA) released the draft guidance on master protocols in 2018, the guidance on Adaptive Designs for Clinical Trials of Drugs and Biologics in 2019, and guidance on Interacting with the FDA on Complex Innovative Clinical Trial Designs for Drugs and Biological Products in 2020. Although Complex Innovative Design (CID) is often used to refer to complex adaptive, Bayesian, and other novel clinical trial designs, there is no accurate definition of CID because what is considered innovative or novel can change over time, and also the scope of CID may be too broad to be accurately defined. Actually, the topic of Bayesian adaptive design alone requires several books for coverage, see for example Berry et al. (2010); Yin (2011); Yuan, Nguyen and Thall (2016) and Yan, Wang and Yuan (2021). In this chapter, we will use several Bayesian adaptive design examples to illustrate some essential elements of CID, while noting that CID is broader and not necessarily restricted to Bayesian design. In what follows, we will describe:

- (Section 2) A Bayesian adaptive design to optimize the dose for immunotherapy. This example illustrates some essence of CID: consideration of the risk-benefit tradeoff of the treatment based on multiple endpoints, and the use of complex Bayesian statistical model to guide adaptive decisions based on accumulative trial data.

- (Section 3) Bayesian adaptive designs for basket trials to illustrate the use of Bayesian hierarchical models to borrow information, an important topic of CID.

- (Section 4) Bayesian platform designs to illustrate the use of master protocol as an efficient CID strategy to accelerate drug development.

- (Section 5) A Bayesian adaptive enrichment design to illustrate how to simultaneously and adaptively identify the target subpopulation, based on biomarkers and evaluate the treatment effect, another important topic of CID.

2.2 A Bayesian Adaptive Design to Optimize the Dose for Immunotherapy

Cancer immunotherapy—treatments that harness and enhance the innate power of the immune system to fight cancer—represents the most promising new cancer treatment approach since the first chemotherapies were developed in the late 1940s (Couzin-Frankel, 2013; Makkouk and Weiner, 2015; Topalian, Weiner, and Pardoll, 2011). Immunotherapeutic approaches include the use of antitumor monoclonal antibodies, cancer vaccines and nonspecific immunotherapies. These approaches have revolutionized the treatment of almost every kind of cancer (Couzin-Frankel, 2013; Kaufman, 2015).

Because of a vastly different functional mechanism, immunotherapy behaves differently from conventional chemotherapies. For conventional chemotherapies, it is reasonable to assume that efficacy and toxicity monotonically increase with the dose; however, this assumption may not hold for Immunotherapy Agents (IAs). As a result, traditional dose-finding designs that aim to identify the Maximum Tolerated Dose (MTD) are not suitable for immunotherapy. To achieve optimal treatment effects, IAs are not necessarily administered at the MTD. In addition, immunotherapy often involves multiple endpoints (Brody et al., 2011; Cha and Fong, 2011; Topalian, Weiner, and Pardoll, 2011). Besides toxicity and efficacy (i.e., tumor response) outcomes, immune response is a unique and important outcome that is essential for the assessment of immunotherapy. Immune response measures the biological efficacy of IAs in activating the immune system, manifested by the proliferation of CD8+ T-cells, CD4+ T-cells and various cytokines (e.g., IFN-α, IL-1β, IL-6, IL-8). As immunotherapy achieves its therapeutic effect by activating the immune system, it is critical to incorporate the immune response in the trial design and leverage its close relationship with clinical endpoints (i.e., efficacy and toxicity) for efficient and practical decision making. Pardoll (2012) described several studies that showed that post-treatment immune responses correlate with clinical outcomes.

In this section, we describe a phase I/II trial design described in Liu, Guo, and Yuan (2018) to find the Biologically Optimal Dose (BOD) for immunotherapy. The innovative design strategies proposed in this design are general, including the consideration of multiple endpoints, the risk benefit tradeoff, adaptive randomization and adaptive decision rule. These strategies can be combined with other statistical and design methods to address a variety of clinical trial challenges.

2.2.1 Probability Models

Consider a phase I-II trial with J prespecified doses, $d_1 < \cdots < d_J$, under investigation. Let Y_T denote the binary toxicity outcome, with $Y_T = 1$ indicating toxicity (or severe adverse events), and = 0 otherwise. Let Y_E denote the tumor response, which is often classified as CR, PR, SD, or PD. Although CR and PR are generally more desirable, in immunotherapy, SD is often regarded as a positive response because some immunotherapies prolong survival by achieving durable SD without notable tumor shrinkage. Thus, Y_E is defined as a trinary ordinal outcome, with $Y_E = 0$, 1, and 2 indicating PD, SD and PR/CR, respectively. As described previously, besides Y_T and Y_E, an essential endpoint for immunotherapy is immune response. Let Y_I denote a measure of the immune response (e.g., the count of CD8+ T-cells or the concentration of cytokine), which takes a real value after appropriate transformation. More generally, Y_I can be any relevant pharmacodynamics or biomarker endpoints. The outcome used for dose finding in this section is a trinary vector $\boldsymbol{Y} = (Y_I, Y_T, Y_E)$.

Adaptive decisions in the trial (e.g., dose assignment and selection) are based on the behavior of $\boldsymbol{Y}$ as a function of dose d. To reflect the fact that in immunotherapy, clinical responses rely on the activation of the immune system, we factorize the joint distribution $[Y_I, Y_T, Y_E \,|\, d]$ into the product of the marginal distribution of Y_I and the conditional distributions of Y_T and Y_E as follows,

$$\left[Y_I, Y_T, Y_E \mid d, \boldsymbol{\theta} \right] = \left[Y_I \mid d, \boldsymbol{\theta}_1 \right] \left[Y_T, Y_E \mid d, Y_I, \boldsymbol{\theta}_2 \right],$$

where $\boldsymbol{\theta}$ is the vector of the parameters, and $\boldsymbol{\theta}_1$ and $\boldsymbol{\theta}_2$ are subvectors of $\boldsymbol{\theta}$. For notational brevity, we suppress arguments $\boldsymbol{\theta}_1$ and $\boldsymbol{\theta}_2$ when it will not cause confusion.

We model the marginal distribution $[Y_I \,|\, d]$ using an Emax model,

$$Y_I \mid d = \alpha_0 + \frac{\alpha_1 d^{\alpha_3}}{\alpha_2^{\alpha_3} + d^{\alpha_3}} + \varepsilon, \tag{2.1}$$

where α_0 is the baseline immune activity in the absence of the IA; α_1 is the maximum immune activity that is possibly achieved by the IA above the baseline activity, often known as E_{max}; α_2 is the dose that produces half of the maximum immune activity (i.e., ED_{50}); α_3 is the Hill factor that controls the steepness of the dose-response curve; and ε is the random error, which is normally distributed with a mean of 0 and variance σ^2, i.e., $\varepsilon \sim N(0, \sigma^2)$.

Modeling the joint distribution of $[Y_T, Y_E \mid d, Y_I]$ is more complicated because Y_T and Y_E are different types of variables, i.e., Y_T is a binary variable whereas Y_E is an ordinal variable, and they are correlated. To this end, we take the latent variable approach. Specifically, let Z_T and Z_E denote two continuous latent variables that are related to Y_T and Y_E, respectively, as follows,

$$Y_T = \begin{cases} 0, & Z_T < \varsigma_1 \\ 1, & Z_T \geq \varsigma_1 \end{cases} \quad \text{and} \quad Y_E = \begin{cases} 0 & Z_E < \xi_1 \\ 1 & \xi_1 \leq Z_E < \xi_2, \\ 2 & Z_E \geq \xi_2 \end{cases}$$

where ς_1, ξ_1 and ξ_2 are unknown cutpoints. Z_T and Z_E can be interpreted as the patient's latent traits, and Y_T and Y_E are the clinical manifestations of unobserved Z_T and Z_E. When Z_T and Z_E pass certain thresholds, certain clinical outcomes (e. g., toxicity, CR/PR) are observed.

We assume that $[Z_T, Z_E \mid d, Y_I]$ follows a bivariate normal distribution

$$\begin{pmatrix} Z_T \\ Z_E \end{pmatrix} \Big| Y_I, \; d \sim N_2 \left(\begin{pmatrix} \mu_T(Y_I, d) \\ \mu_E(Y_I, d) \end{pmatrix}, \; \begin{pmatrix} \sigma_{11} & \sigma_{12} \\ \sigma_{12} & \sigma_{22} \end{pmatrix} \right),$$

where $\mu_k(Y_I, d) = E(Z_k \mid Y_I, d)$, $k = E$ or T, is the conditional mean of Z_k. Specification of $\mu_T(Y_I, d)$ and $\mu_E(Y_I, d)$ requires some consideration. Immune activity is a normal biological phenomenon consistently occurring in the human body; thus, it is typically expected that a low or normal level of immune activity will not cause any immune-related toxicity and that severe immune-related toxicity will occur only when the therapy-induced immune response exceeds a certain threshold. To account for such a threshold effect, we model the relationship between $\mu_T(Y_I, d)$ and Y_I and d as

$$\mu_T(Y_I, d) = \beta_0 + \beta_1 d + I(Y_I > \beta_3)\beta_2 Y_I, \tag{2.2}$$

where β_0, β_1, β_2 and β_3 are unknown parameters, and the indicator function $I(Y_I > \beta_3) = 1$ when $Y_I > \beta_3$, and 0 otherwise. Under this model, Y_I induces toxicity only when it passes threshold β_3. Because we do not expect the immune response to be the sole cause of toxicity, in (2), we include dose d as a covariate to capture other possible treatment-related toxicity.

To model the mean structure $\mu_E(Y_I, d)$ for efficacy, we assume a quadratic model,

$$\mu_E(Y_I, d) = \gamma_0 + \gamma_1 Y_I + \gamma_2 Y_I^2, \tag{2.3}$$

where the quadratic term is used to accommodate the possibility that efficacy may not monotonically increase with the immune response. In practice, $\mu_E(Y_I, d)$ may first increase with Y_I and then plateau after Y_I reaches a certain value. Although the quadratic model cannot directly take an increasing-then-plateau shape, it works reasonably well in that case in numerical studies (Liu, Guo, and Yuan, 2018). This is because the goal here is not to accurately estimate the whole immune-response curve, but to use (2.3) as a "working" model to obtain a reasonable local fit to guide the dose escalation and de-escalation. As the quadratic model can provide good approximation to the plateau (e.g., by taking a slowly increasing shape) locally around the current dose, it leads to appropriate dose transition and selection. In addition, as the Emax model (2.1) allows Y_I to plateau with the dose d, the efficacy model (2.3) indeed accommodates the case that efficacy Y_E plateaus with d.

In equation (2.3), we assume that conditional on Y_I, Y_E is independent of dose d to reflect the consideration that the treatment effect of immunotherapy is mostly mediated by the immune response. For cases in which such an assumption may not be true, we can add d as a covariate in the model. Because latent variables Z_T and Z_E are never observed, to identify the model, we set $\varsigma_1 = \xi_1 = 0$, $\sigma_{11} = \sigma_{22} = 1$ and accordingly constrain $0 \leq \sigma_{12} \leq 1$.

The joint model for $[Y_I, Y_T, Y_E \mid d]$ involves many parameters. Given the limited sample size of early phase trials, it is important to specify appropriate prior distributions for the model parameters to ensure robust inference and operating characteristics. The details can be found in Liu, Guo, and Yuan (2018).

2.2.2 Desirability Based on Risk-Benefit Tradeoff

For each individual endpoint Y_I, Y_T or Y_E, the evaluation of the desirability of a dose is straightfoward. We prefer a dose that has low toxicity, strong immune response and high objective response. However, when we consider (Y_I, Y_T, Y_E) simultaneously, the evaluation of the desirability of a dose becomes more complicated. We need to consider the risk-benefit tradeoffs between the undesirable and desirable clinical outcomes, as physicians routinely do in almost all medical decisions when selecting a treatment for a patient. A convenient tool to formalize such a process is to use a utility function $U(Y_I, Y_T, Y_E)$ to map the multi-dimensional outcomes into a single index to measure the desirability of a dose in terms of the risk-benefit tradeoffs. The utility should be elicited from physicians and/or patients to reflect medical practice.

A convenient way of eliciting $U(Y_I, Y_T, Y_E)$ that works well in practice is as follows: we first dichotomize the immune response Y_I as desirable ($\tilde{Y}_I = 1$) or undesirable ($\tilde{Y}_I = 0$) based on a cutoff C_I specified by clinicians (i.e., $\tilde{Y}_I = 1$ if $Y_I \geq C_I$, and 0 otherwise), and fix the score of the most desirable outcome (i.e., desirable immune response, no toxicity and CR/PR) as $U(\tilde{Y}_I = 1, Y_T = 0, Y_E = 2) = 100$ and the least desirable outcome (i.e., undesirable immune response, toxicity and PD) as $U(\tilde{Y}_I = 0, Y_T = 1, Y_E = 0) = 0$. Using these two boundary cases as the reference, we then elicit the scores for other possible outcomes from clinicians, which must be located between 0 and 100. An example of elicited utility is given in Table 2.1. Note that the purpose of dichotomizing Y_I here is to simplify the elicitation of utilities from clinicians. Our model and inference are based on the original scale of Y_I. If desirable, Y_I can

TABLE 2.1

Utility Based on Toxicity, Efficacy and Immune Response

Toxicity	Immune Response	Efficacy		
		PD ($Y_E = 0$)	SD ($Y_E = 1$)	CR/PR ($Y_E = 2$)
No ($Y_T = 0$)	Desirable ($\tilde{Y}_I = 1$)	5	75	100
	Undesirable ($\tilde{Y}_I = 0$)	0	50	80
Yes ($Y_T = 1$)	Desirable ($\tilde{Y}_I = 1$)	0	20	40
	Undesirable ($\tilde{Y}_I = 0$)	0	10	35

be categorized into more than two levels, which allows us to account for the desirability of Y_I at a finer scale, but at the cost of slightly increasing the logistic burden for utility elicitation. For example, if we categorize Y_I into three levels (e.g., low, median, or high), a total of 18 utility values are required to be elicited from clinicians.

Although Y_I and Y_E are generally positively correlated, there are several benefits to considering both of them when constructing the utility. First, immunotherapy achieves its therapeutic effect of killing cancer cells by activating the immune response, and the tumor response Y_E (i.e., a short-term endpoint) may not be a perfect surrogate of the long-term treatment effect of the immunotherapy, e.g., Progression-Free Survival (PFS) or overall survival time. Thus, when two doses have similar Y_T and Y_E, we often prefer the dose that has higher potency to activate the immune response, which is potentially translated into better long-term treatment efficacy. Second, using Y_I and Y_E simultaneously improves the power to identify the optimal dose. For example, given two doses with $\left(\Pr(Y_E > 0) = 0.3, E(Y_I) = 20\right)$ and $\left(\Pr(Y_E > 0) = 0.4, E(Y_I) = 60\right)$, respectively, the second dose is more likely to be identified as more desirable when we use Y_I and Y_E rather than Y_E only, because the difference in the value of Y_I is much larger than that of Y_E between the two doses.

Constructing the utility requires close collaboration between statisticians and clinicians, and should be customized for each trial to best reflect the clinical needs and practice. For example, if Y_E is the long-term efficacy endpoint of interest (e.g., PFS) or Y_I is believed to have little impact on the clinical desirability of the dose (after considering Y_E), we may prefer to define the utility using only (Y_E, Y_T), while ignoring Y_I. Although the elicitation of utility seems rather involved, in our experience, the process actually is quite natural and straightforward. For many trials, this may be done by simply explaining what the utilities represent to the Principal Investigator (PI) during the design process, and asking the PI to specify all necessary values of $U(Y_I, Y_T, Y_E)$ after fixing the scores for the best and worst elementary outcomes as described previously. After the initial values of utility are specified, comparing outcomes that have the same or similar numerical utilities often motivates the PI to modify the initial specification. In our experience, clinicians quickly understand what the utilities mean, since they reflect actual clinical practice. After completing this process and simulating the trial design, it then may be examined by the PI. In some cases, the simulation results may motivate slight modification of some of the numerical utility values, although such modification typically has little or no effect on the design's operating characteristics. One possible criticism for using the utility values is that they require subjective input. However, we are inclined to view this as a strength rather than a weakness. This is because the utilities must be elicited from the physicians planning the trial, and thus their numerical values are based on the physician's experience in treating the disease and observing the good and bad effects that the treatment has on the patients. The process of specifying the utility requires physicians to carefully consider the potential risks and benefits of the treatment that underlie their clinical decision making in a more formal way and incorporate that into the trial.

For a given dose d, its true utility is given by

$$E\big(U(d)\mid \boldsymbol{\theta}\big) = \int U(\tilde{Y}_I, Y_T, Y_E) f(\tilde{Y}_I, Y_T, Y_E \mid d, \boldsymbol{\theta}) \, d\tilde{Y}_I \, dY_T \, dY_E.$$

Since $\boldsymbol{\theta}$ is not known, the utility of dose d must be estimated. Given interim data $\mathcal{D}_n$ collected from the first n patients at a decision-making point in the trial, the utility of dose d is estimated by its posterior mean

$$E\big(U(d)\mid \mathcal{D}_n\big) = \int E\big(U(d)\mid \boldsymbol{\theta}\big) p(\boldsymbol{\theta}\mid \mathcal{D}_n) d\boldsymbol{\theta}.$$

This posterior mean utility will be used to measure the desirability of a dose and guide dose escalation and selection.

Let $\pi_T = \Pr(Y_T = 1 | d)$ denote the toxicity rate and $\pi_E = \Pr(Y_E > 0 | d)$ denote the response rate of SD/PR/CR. Let ϕ_T denote the upper limit of the toxicity rate, and ϕ_E denote the lower limit of the response rate, specified by physicians. We define the BOD as the dose with the highest utility while satisfying $\pi_T < \phi_T$ and $\pi_E > \phi_E$.

2.2.3 Dose Admissibility Criteria

A practical issue is that a dose that is "optimal" in terms of the utility alone may be unacceptable in terms of either safety or the response rate. To ensure that any administered dose has both an acceptably high success rate and an acceptably low adverse event rate, based on interim data $\mathcal{D}_n$, we define a dose d as admissible if it satisfies both the safety requirement

$$\Pr\left(\pi_T < \phi_T | \mathcal{D}_n\right) > C_T, \tag{2.4}$$

and the efficacy requirement

$$\Pr\left(\pi_E > \phi_E | \mathcal{D}_n\right) > C_E, \tag{2.5}$$

where C_T and C_E are prespecified toxicity and efficacy cutoffs. We denote the set of admissible doses by $\mathcal{A}_n$. Because the objective of the admissible rules (2.4) and (2.5) is to rule out doses that are excessively toxic or inefficacious, in practice we should set C_T and C_E at small values, such as $C_T = C_E = 0.05$, which could be further calibrated through simulation. To see this point, it is useful to state the two rules in the following equivalent forms: a dose is unacceptable or inadmissible if $\Pr(\pi_T > \phi_T | \mathcal{D}_n) > 1 - C_T = 0.95$ or $\Pr(\pi_E < \phi_E | \mathcal{D}_n) > 1 - C_E = 0.95$. This says that the dose is unacceptable if it is either very likely to be inefficacious or very likely to be too toxic. If we set C_T and C_E at large values, then the design is very likely to stop the trial early with all doses declared inadmissible due to the large estimation uncertainty at the beginning of the trial; see page 62 of the book by Yuan, Nguyen and Thall (2016) for more discussion on this issue.

2.2.4 Adaptive Dose-Finding Algorithm

Based on the above considerations, the dose-finding algorithm is described formally as follows. Assume that patients are treated in cohorts of size m with the maximum sample size of $N = m \times R$. We allow $m = 1$ such that patients are treated one by one. The first cohort of patients is treated at the lowest dose d_1. Assume that r cohort(s) of patients have been enrolled in the trial, where $r = 1, \ldots, R - 1$. Let d_h denote the current highest tried dose, C_{es} denote the probability cutoff for escalation based on toxicity, and $n = m \times r$. To assign a dose to the $(r + 1)$th cohort of patients:

1. If the posterior probability of toxicity at d_h satisfies $\Pr(\pi_T(d_h) < \phi_T | \mathcal{D}_n) > C_{es}$ and $d_h \neq d_J$, then we treat the $(r + 1)$th cohort of patients at d_{h+1}. In other words, if the current data show that the highest tried dose is safe, we want to continue to explore the dose space by treating the next cohort of patients at the next higher new dose.

2. Otherwise, we identify the admissible set $\mathcal{A}_n$ and adaptively randomize the $(r + 1)$th patient or cohort of patients to dose $d_j \in \mathcal{A}_n$ with probability

$$\psi_{j,n} = \Pr\left[U\left(d_j\right) = max\left\{U\left(d_{j'}\right),\ j' \in \mathcal{A}_n\right\} \middle| D_n\right],$$

which is the posterior probability that dose j is the optimal dose having the highest posterior mean utility. We restrict the randomization in admissible dose set $\mathcal{A}_n$ to avoid treating patients at doses that are futile or overly toxic. If $\mathcal{A}_n$ is empty, the trial is terminated.

3. Once the maximum sample size of N is exhausted, the dose in $\mathcal{A}_N$ with the largest posterior mean utility $E(U(d)|\mathcal{D}_N)$ is recommended.

In step 2, to assign a patient to a dose, we use adaptive randomization rather than the greedy algorithm that always assigns the patient to the dose with the currently highest estimate of utility. This is because the latter method tends to become stuck at the local optima and leads to poor precision for identifying the BOD. Adaptive randomization provides a coherent mechanism to avoid that issue and improve the operating characteristics of the design (Yuan, Nguyen, and Thall, 2016).

Liu, Guo, and Yuan (2018) show that by leveraging novel CID strategies (e.g., consideration of multiple endpoints, the risk benefit tradeoff, adaptive randomization, and Bayesian adaptive updating and decision rule), the resulting design has desirable operating characteristics. It better reflects the clinical practice, and substantially improves the accuracy and reliability of finding the BOD and subsequent phase III trials.

2.3 Bayesian Adaptive Designs for Basket Trials

Basket trial is an important type of master protocol and an essential element of CID. Per FDA guidance, the basket trial is defined as a master protocol designed to test a single investigational drug or drug combination in different populations defined by disease stage, histology, number of prior therapies, genetic or other biomarkers, or demographic characteristics. For ease of exposition, we here focus on the case that "different populations" are defined by cancer types, i.e., the basket trials evaluating the treatment effect of a targeted therapy in different cancer types with the same genetic or molecular aberration.

Evaluating targeted therapies in basket trial is challenging. Although the patients enrolled in a basket trial have the same genetic or molecular aberration, that does not necessarily mean that they will respond homogeneously to a targeted agent regardless of the primary tumor site. Cancer type often has profound effects on the treatment effect, and it is not uncommon for a targeted agent to be effective for some cancer types, but not others. As a result, when evaluating the treatment effect in basket trials, an analysis that simply pools the data across cancer types is often problematic. It leads to large biases and inflated type I error rates if the treatment effect actually is heterogeneous across different cancer types. The independent approach, which evaluates the treatment effect in each cancer type independently, avoids these issues, but is less efficient and often lacks power to detect the treatment effect due to the limited sample size in each cancer type.

In this section, we will focus on the use of Bayesian Hierarchical Models (BHM) to borrow information across cancer types. The methodology can be combined with other methods described in other sections to build more complex innovative designs. A related topic of great interest for CID is to borrow information from historical data or Real World Data (RWD). Interested readers can refer to the work of Ibrahim and Chen (2000; power prior),

Hobbs et al. (2011; commensurate prior), Schmidli et al. (2014; meta-analytic-predictive prior), and Jiang et al. (2020; elastic prior).

2.3.1 Bayesian Hierarchical Model

To overcome the drawbacks of pooled and independent approaches, Thall et al. (2003) proposed using a BHM to adaptively borrow information across different tumor subgroups, and Berry et al. (2013) applied it to basket trials. Consider a phase II tissue-agnostic trial that evaluates the treatment effect of a new antitumor drug in J different cancer types. Let p_j denote the response rate in cancer type j. The objective of the trial is to test whether the new drug is effective in each cancer type, with null and alternative hypotheses:

$$H_0: p_j \le p_{0,j} \text{ versus } H_1: p_j \ge p_{1,j} \quad j = 1, \cdots, J,$$

where $p_{0,j}$ is the null response rate that is deemed futile, and $p_{1,j}$ is the target response rate that is deemed promising for cancer type j.

Suppose at an interim analysis time, for cancer type j, n_j patients are enrolled, and among them x_j patients responded to the treatment. BHM can be used to model p_j's as follows,

$$x_j \mid p_j \sim Binomial\,(n_j, p_j),$$

$$\theta_j = log\left(\frac{p_j}{1-p_j}\right) - log\left(\frac{p_{0,j}}{1-p_{0,j}}\right),$$

$$\theta_j \mid \theta, \sigma^2 \sim N(\theta, \sigma^2),$$

$$\theta \sim N\left(\alpha_0, \tau_0^2\right),$$

(2.6)

where α_0, τ_0^2 are hyperparameters, such as $\alpha_0 = 0, \tau_0^2 = 100$. In the second equation, we use $log(\frac{p_{0,j}}{1-p_{0,j}})$ as the offset to account for different null (or baseline) value $p_{0,j}$ across cancer types, making the exchangeability assumption of θ_j more plausible. If the deviation from the targeted value $p_{1,j}$ is more likely to be exchangeable across cancer types, $log(\frac{p_{1,j}}{1-p_{1,j}})$ can be used as the offset. When estimating p_j, BHM borrows information across J cancer types by shrinking the cancer-type-specific mean θ_j toward the common mean θ. Shrinkage parameter σ^2 controls the degree of information borrowing. A small value of σ^2 induces strong information borrowing across cancer types, with the extreme case that $\sigma^2 = 0$ is identical to directly pooling data across cancer types. A large value of σ^2 induces little information borrowing, with the extreme case that $\sigma^2 = \infty$ is identical to an independent analysis approach, which evaluates the treatment in each cancer type independently without any information borrowing.

Borrowing information can be beneficial or detrimental, depending on whether the treatment effect is homogeneous or heterogeneous across cancer types. When the treatment effect θ_j is homogenous across cancer types (e.g., the treatment is effective for all cancer types), borrowing information significantly improves power. However, when the treatment effect θ_j is heterogeneous (i.e., the treatment is effective for some cancer types and not effective for other cancer types), borrowing information may substantially inflate the type I error for insensitive cancer types and reduce the power for sensitive cancer types. Thus, it is desirable to borrow information when θ_j is homogenous, and refrain from borrowing information when θ_j is heterogeneous.

To achieve such adaptive information borrowing, a natural approach is to assign the shrinkage parameter σ^2 a vague prior with a large variance, e.g., IG(0.0005, 0.000005) as suggested by Berry et al. (2013), and let the trial data determine how much information to borrow, with the intent that BHM induces strong shrinkage when the treatment effect is homogenous, and little shrinkage when the treatment effect is heterogeneous across cancer types (i.e., adaptive information borrowing).

Unfortunately, BHM does not work well when the number of cancer types $J < 10$. It may still induce strong shrinkage when the treatment effect is heterogeneous, resulting in an inflated type I error for insensitive cancer types and reduced power for sensitive cancer types (Freidlin and Korn, 2013; Chu and Yuan, 2018a). Simulation study shows that BHM with an IG(0.0005, 0.000005) prior can inflate the type I error rate from the nominal level of 10% to over 50% in some scenarios. The fundamental reason for this issue is that σ^2 represents the between-cancer-type variance, and thus the observation unit contributing to the estimation of σ^2 is cancer types, rather than patients. When the number of cancer types J is small, the observed data are insufficient to estimate σ^2 reliably, even when the number of patients in each cancer type is large.

2.3.2 Calibrated BHM (CA-BHM) Design

To address this issue, Chu and Yuan (2018a) described a CA-BHM approach to adaptively borrow information across cancer subgroups for phase II basket trials. Unlike the BHM approach, which assigns a prior to σ^2 and estimates it from the data, this approach defines σ^2 as a function of the measure of homogeneity among the cancer subgroups. The key is that the function is prespecified and calibrated in a way such that when the treatment effects in the cancer subgroups are homogeneous, strong information borrowing occurs and thus improves power, and when the treatment effects in the cancer subgroups are heterogeneous, little or no borrowing across groups occurs, thereby controlling the type I error rate. In what follows, we first describe a homogeneity measure and then describe a procedure to determine and calibrate the function that links the homogeneity measure and shrinkage parameter σ^2. For simplicity, in this section, we assume the null response rate and target response rate are both the same across cancer types, i.e., $p_{0,1} = \cdots = p_{0,J} \equiv q_0$ and $p_{1,1} = \cdots = p_{1,J} \equiv q_1$. The method can be readily applied to the case with different null and target values across cancer types by using an offset as described in model (2.6).

A natural measure of homogeneity is the chi-squared test statistic of homogeneity, given by

$$T = \sum_{j=1}^{J} \frac{(O_{0j} - E_{0j})^2}{E_{0j}} + \sum_{j=1}^{J} \frac{(O_{1j} - E_{1j})^2}{E_{1j}},$$

where O_{0j} and O_{1j} denote the observed counts of failures and responses for subgroup j (i.e., $n_j - x_j$ and x_j); and E_{0j} and E_{1j} are the expected counts of failures and responses, given by

$$E_{0j} = n_j \frac{\sum_j n_j - \sum_j x_j}{\sum_j n_j} \text{ and } E_{1j} = n_j \frac{\sum_j x_j}{\sum_j n_j}.$$

A smaller value of T indicates higher homogeneity in the treatment effect across subgroups. Note that the chi-squared test statistic T is used here for measuring the strength of homogeneity, not conducting hypothesis testing. Therefore, when some cell counts (i.e., O_{0j} and O_{1j}) are small, it does not cause any issue because the described procedure does not rely on the large-sample distribution of T.

CA-BHM links the shrinkage parameter σ^2 with T through

$$\sigma^2 = g(T),$$

where $g(.)$ is a monotonically increasing function. Although different choices of $g(.)$ are certainly possible, numerical studies show that the following two-parameter exponential model yields good and robust operating characteristics,

$$\sigma^2 = g(T) = exp\{a + b \times \log(T)\}, \tag{2.7}$$

where a and b are tuning parameters that characterize the relationship between σ^2 and T. We require $b > 0$ such that greater homogeneity (i.e., a small value of T) leads to stronger shrinkage (i.e., a small value of σ^2).

The key to the CA-BHM approach is that the values of a and b are calibrated such that strong shrinkage occurs when the treatment effect is homogeneous across the cancer subgroups; and no or little shrinkage occurs when the treatment effect is heterogeneous. This can be done using the following 3-step simulation-based procedure.

1. Simulate the case in which the treatment is effective for all cancer subgroups; thus, we should borrow information across cancer subgroups. Specifically, we generate R replicates of data by simulating $x = (x_1, \cdots, x_J)$ from $Bin(N, q_1)$, where $N = (N_1, \cdots, N_J)$ and $q_1 = (q_1, \cdots, q_1)$, and then calculate T for each simulated dataset. Let H_B denote the median of T from R simulated datasets.

2. Simulate the cases in which the treatment effect is heterogeneous across cancer subgroups; thus, we should not borrow information across cancer subgroups. Let $q(j) = (q_1, \cdots, q_1, q_0, \cdots, q_0)$ denote the scenario in which the treatment is effective for the first j subgroups with the response rate of q_1, but not effective for subgroups $j+1$ to J with the response rate of q_0. Given a value of j, we generate R replicates of data by simulating x from $Bin(N, q(j))$, calculate T for each simulated dataset, and then obtain its median $H_{\bar{B}j}$. We repeat this for $j=1, \ldots, J-1$, and define

$$H_{\bar{B}} = \min_j H_{\bar{B}j}. \tag{2.8}$$

3. Let σ_B^2 denote a prespecified small value (e.g., 1) for shrinkage parameter σ^2 under which strong shrinkage or information borrowing occurs under the hierarchical model, and let $\sigma_{\bar{B}}^2$ denote a prespecified large value (e.g., 80) of shrinkage parameter σ^2, under which little shrinkage or information borrowing occurs. Solve a and b in (7) based on the following two equations:

$$\sigma_B^2 = g(H_B; a, b), \tag{2.9}$$

$$\sigma_{\bar{B}}^2 = g(H_{\bar{B}}; a, b), \tag{2.10}$$

where the first equation enforces strong shrinkage (i.e., information borrowing) when the treatment is effective for all subgroups, and the second equation enforces little shrinkage (i.e., weak information borrowing) when the treatment effect is heterogeneous across all subgroups. The solution of the equations is given by

$$a = \log(\sigma_B^2) - \frac{\log(\sigma_{\bar{B}}^2) - \log(\sigma_B^2)}{\log(H_{\bar{B}}) - \log(H_B)} \log(H_B), \tag{2.11}$$

$$b = \frac{\log(\sigma_{\bar{B}}^2) - \log(\sigma_{B}^2)}{\log(H_{\bar{B}}) - \log(H_B)}. \tag{2.12}$$

Remarks: In step 2, $H_{\bar{B}}$ is defined as the minimum value of the $\{H_{\bar{B}j}\}$, i.e., equation (2.8), and impose that little shrinkage occurs when $T = H_{\bar{B}}$, as dictated by equation (2.10) in step 3. This is to reflect that when the treatment is effective for some subgroups, but not effective for the other subgroup(s), the treatment effect is regarded as heterogeneous and no information should be borrowed across subgroups. For example, in a basket trial with four tumor subgroups, if the treatment is effective for three subgroups, but not effective for one subgroup, the treatment effect is regarded as heterogeneous and no information should be borrowed across subgroups. Such "strong" definition of heterogeneity and "strong" control of borrowing is necessary for controlling type I error, and any information borrowing will inflate the type I error of the ineffective subgroup due to the shrinkage of that subgroup's treatment effect towards the effective subgroups, i.e., overestimating the treatment effect for the ineffective subgroup. Because the shrinkage parameter σ^2 is a monotonically increasing function of T, as long as we control that little shrinkage occurs when $T = H_{\bar{B}}$, we automatically ensure that little shrinkage occurs for cases with larger values of $H_{\bar{B}j}$ (i.e., higher levels of heterogeneity), for example when the treatment is effective for two subgroups but not effective in the other two subgroups. In some situations, for example, when the majority of subgroups are responsive and only one subgroup is not responsive, it may be debatable whether controlling type I error for each of subgroups is the best strategy. We might be willing to tolerate a certain type I error inflation in one subgroup in exchange for power gain in the majority of subgroups. This can be conveniently done by relaxing the "strong" definition of heterogeneity. For example, rather than defining $H_{\bar{B}} = \min_j H_{\bar{B}j}$, we can define $H_{\bar{B}}$ as the minimal value of $H_{\bar{B}j}$ when the treatment is not effective in at least two subgroups. That is, if the treatment is not effective for only one subgroup, we do not treat the treatment effect as heterogenous. Consequently, information can be borrowed across subgroups, but at the expense of some inflated type I error for the ineffective subgroup. Actually, this is one of important advantages of the proposed CA-BHM over the standard BHM. The CA-BHM provides us abundant flexibility to control the degree of borrowing in an intuitive and straightforward way.

Another advantage of the CA-BHM is that the calibration procedure relies only on the null response rate q_0, alternative response rate q_1 and sample size of tumor groups N_j, which are known before the trial is conducted. This is an important and very desirable property because it allows the investigator to determine the values of a and b and to include them in the study protocol before the onset of the study. This avoids the common concern about the method for borrowing information; that is, the method could be abused by choosing the degree of borrowing to favor a certain result, e.g., statistical significance. When the true response rates of some subgroups are between q_0 and q_1, the CA-BHM induces partial information borrowing, depending on the actual value of homogeneity measure T. In addition, the resulting CA-BHM has the following desirable large-sample property.

Theorem 1: When the sample size in each subgroup is large, the CA-BHM achieves full information borrowing when the treatment effect is homogeneous across subgroups, and no information borrowing when the treatment effect is heterogeneous across subgroups.

In contrast, to achieve the above asymptotic property, the standard BHM requires an additional assumption that the number of subgroups is large because the shrinkage parameter σ^2 represents the inter-subgroup variance. To precisely estimate σ^2 and ensure appropriate shrinkage behavior, we must increase the number of subgroups. This extra requirement, unfortunately, is restrictive and often unrealistic in practice because the number of tumor subgroups with a certain genetic or molecular aberration is often fixed and cannot be manipulated within the trial design.

2.3.2.1 Trial Design

The phase II basket trial design has a total of K interim looks, with the kth interim observation occurring when the sample size of the jth subgroup reaches n_{jk}. Let $\mathcal{D}_k = \{(n_{jk}, x_{jk}), j = 1, \cdots, J, k = 1, \cdots, K\}$ denote the data from the kth interim look, where x_{jk} is the number of responses from n_{jk} patients. The phase II basket trial design with K interim looks is described as follows.

1. Enroll n_{j1} patients in the jth subgroup, $j = 1, \cdots, J$.
2. Given the data $\mathcal{D}_k$ from the kth interim look,
   a. (Futility stopping) if $Pr(p_j > (q_0 + q_1)/2 \mid \mathcal{D}_k) < C_f$, suspend the accrual for the jth subgroup, where $(q_0 + q_1)/2$ denotes the rate halfway between the null and target response rate and C_f is a probability cutoff for futility stopping;
   b. otherwise, continue to enroll patients until reaching the next interim analysis.
3. Once the maximum sample size is reached or the treatment of all subgroups is stopped early due to futility, evaluate the efficacy for each subgroup based on all the observed data. If $Pr(p_j > q_0 \mid \mathcal{D}) > C$, then the treatment for the jth group will be declared effective; otherwise, the treatment for that group will be declared ineffective, where C is a probability cutoff.

In step 2a, we use $(q_0 + q_1)/2$ as the boundary for assessing futility to be consistent with the BHM design (Berry et al., 2013). Another natural boundary is q_0, that is, if there is a high posterior probability that p_j is less than q_0, we stop the accrual for the jth subgroup for futility. To ensure good operating characteristics, the probability cutoffs C_f and C should be calibrated through simulations to achieve a desired type I error rate and early stopping rate for each subgroup.

2.3.3 Clustered BHM Design

One important assumption of BHM and CA-BHM is an exchangeable treatment effect across cancer types. This assumption, however, is not always appropriate, and it is not uncommon that some cancer types are responsive to the treatment, while others are not. For example, BRAF-mutant melanoma and hairy-cell leukemia are associated with a high response rate to the BRAF inhibitor PLX4032(vemurafenib), whereas BRAF-mutant colon cancer is not (Flaherty et al., 2010; Tiacci et al., 2011; Prahallad et al., 2012). Trastuzumab is effective for treating human epidermal growth factor receptor 2 (HER2)-positive breast cancer, but shows little clinical benefit for HER2-positive recurrent endometrial cancer (Fleming et al., 2010) or HER2-positive non-small-cell lung cancer (Gatzemeier et al., 2004). In this case, using the BHM will lead to inflated type I errors. CA-BHM has a better control of type I errors. However, due to its "strong" control of type I error, it will prevent information borrowing when the response rate of one cancer type is different from the others, missing the opportunity to borrow information between a subset of cancer types that actually have similar response rates.

To improve the performance of BHM and CA-BHM, Jiang et al. (2021) propose a precision information-borrowing approach, called clustered BHM (CL-BHM). The basic idea is, based on the interim data, we first cluster the cancer types into responsive (sensitive) and non-responsive (insensitive) subgroups; and we then apply BHM to borrow information within each subgroup. We allow a subgroup to be empty to accommodate the homogeneous case that all cancer types are responsive or non-responsive. We here focus on the two subgroups based on the practical consideration that targeted therapy is often either effective (i.e., hit the target) or ineffective (i.e., miss the target), and the number of cancer types is typically small (2–6), and thus it is not practical to form more than two subgroups. Nevertheless, the method can be readily extended to more than two subgroups.

Jiang et al. (2021) used the following Bayesian rule to cluster cancer types: a cancer type is allocated to the responsive cluster $\mathcal{R}$ if it satisfies

$$\Pr\left(p_j > \frac{p_{0,j} + p_{1,j}}{2} \,\bigg|\, x_j, n_j\right) > \psi \left(\frac{n_j}{N_j}\right)^\omega,$$

otherwise allocated to the non-responsive cluster $\bar{\mathcal{R}}$, where N_j is the prespecified maximum sample size of cancer type j, and ψ and ω are positive tuning parameters. We recommend default values $\psi = 0.5$ and $\omega = 2$ or 3, which can be further calibrated to fit a specific trial requirement in operating characteristics. One important feature of this clustering rule is that its probability cutoff is adaptive and depends on the subgroup interim sample size n_j. At the early stage of the trial, where n_j is small, we prefer to use a more relaxed (i.e., smaller) cutoff to keep a cancer type in the responsive subgroup to avoid inadvertent stopping due to sparse data and to encourage collecting more data on the cancer type. When a trial proceeds, we should use a more strict (i.e., larger) cutoff to avoid incorrectly classify non-responsive cancer types to a responsive subgroup. In the above Bayesian clustering rule, the posterior probability $\Pr(p_j > \frac{p_{0,j}+p_{1,j}}{2} | x_j, n_j)$ is evaluated based on the Beta-Binomial model,

$$x_j | p_j \sim Binomial\,(n_j, p_j),$$

$$p_j \sim Beta\,(a_1, b_1),$$

(2.13)

where a_1 and b_1 are hyperparameters, typically set at small values (e.g., $a_1 = b_1 = 0.1$) to obtain a vague prior. As a result, the posterior distribution of p_j is given by $Beta\,(x_j + a_1, n_j - x_j + b_1)$. The described method is certainly not the only way to cluster the cancer types. Other clustering methods (e.g., K-means or hierarchical clustering methods) can also be entertained. However, because the number of cancer types is often small and the interim data are sparse, we found that using these alternative (often more complicated) methods often worsens, rather than improves performance.

After clustering, we apply the BHM (2.6) to subgroups $\mathcal{R}$ and $\bar{\mathcal{R}}$ independently with $\sigma^2 \sim IG(a_0, b_0)$, where IG(.) denotes inverse-gamma distribution and a_0, b_0 are hyperparameters. Typically, we set $\mu_0 = 0$ and τ_0^2 at a large value (e.g, $\tau_0^2 = 10^6$), and a_0 and b_0 at small values (e.g., $a_0 = b_0 = 10^{-6}$), which is known to favor borrowing information (Chu and Yuan, 2018a).

If subgroup $\mathcal{R}$ or $\bar{\mathcal{R}}$ only has one member, we replace the above BHM with the Beta-Binomial model (2.13). As cancer types within subgroup $\mathcal{R}$ and $\bar{\mathcal{R}}$ are relatively homogenous, the exchangeable assumption required by BHM is more likely to hold. As a result, CL-BHM yields better performance, as shown by simulation in Jiang et al. (2021). Because that the treatment effect θ_j in $\mathcal{R}$ should be better than that in $\bar{\mathcal{R}}$, one might consider imposing this order constraint when fitting the BHM for $\mathcal{R}$ and $\bar{\mathcal{R}}$. This, however, is not necessary and does not improve the estimation of θ_j. This is because the order on θ_j has been (implicitly) incorporated by the clustering procedure, that is, the cancer types showing high treatment effect (i.e., large θ_j) are clustered into the responsive cluster, whereas cancer types showing low treatment effect (i.e., low θ_j) are clustered into the non-responsive cluster.

2.3.4 Bayesian Model Averaging Approach

An alternative, statistically more sophisticated approach to do cluster-then-borrow is to use the Bayesian model averaging (BMA), along the line of Hobbs and Landin (2018). With J cancer types, there are a total of $L = 2^J$ ways to partition the cancer types into $\mathcal{R}$ and $\bar{\mathcal{R}}$. Let M_l denote the lth partition, $l = 1, \cdots, L$. Given the interim data D, the posterior probability of M_l is given by

$$\Pr(M_l | D) = \frac{L(D| M_l)\Pr(M_l)}{\sum_{i=1}^{L} L(D| M_i)\Pr(M_i)},$$

where $\Pr(M_l)$ is the prior probability of M_l. In general, we apply the non-informative prior, i.e., $\Pr(M_l) = 1/L$, when there is no preference for any specific partition. $L(D| M_l)$ is the likelihood of M_l, given by

$$L(D| M_l) = \prod_{j=1}^{J} \binom{n_j}{x_j} p_{[l]j}^{x_j} \left(1 - p_{[l]j}\right)^{n_j - x_j},$$

where $p_{[l]j}$ is the response rate for cancer type j given the lth partition, i.e., $p_{[l]j} = p_{1,j}$ if $j \in \mathcal{R}$ and $p_{[l]j} = p_{0,j}$ if $j \in \bar{\mathcal{R}}$.

Given the lth partition (i.e., M_l), the members of $\mathcal{R}$ and $\bar{\mathcal{R}}$ are known, and we apply the BHM (2.6) to $\mathcal{R}$ and $\bar{\mathcal{R}}$ independently to calculate $\Pr(p_j > (p_{0,j} + p_{1,j})/2 | D, M_l)$, $j = 1, \cdots, J$ and $l = 1, \cdots, L$. Then, the futility go/no-go rule can be calculated as follows:

$$\Pr\left(p_j > (p_{0,j} + p_{1,j})/2 | D\right) = \sum_{l=1}^{L} \Pr\left(p_j > (p_{0,j} + p_{1,j})/2 | D, M_l\right)\Pr(M_l | D).$$

The BMA approach is statistically sophisticated and computationally intensive, but the simulation shows that it has similar performance as the CL-BHM with the simple Bayesian clustering rule described above. The reason is that given the small number of cancer types and the limited interim (binary) data in each cancer type, the complicated BMA method introduces more noise (e.g., accounting for 2^J possible partitions or models) and thus often fails to improve the performance.

2.3.5 Bayesian Latent Subgroup Trial (BLAST) Design for Basket Trials

In most basket trials, biomarkers are routinely measured longitudinally to evaluate the biological activity of the targeted agent, i.e., measure how well the targeted agent hits its molecular target and triggers the downstream biological activities (e.g., expression of a certain gene, proliferation of certain cells, or increase in enzyme activity). For example, in immunotherapy, the number of CD8+ T-cells, CD4+ T-cells or the concentration of cytokines (e.g., IFN-α, IL-6, IL-8) are routinely measured to assess the biological activity (i.e., immunogenicity) of immune checkpoint inhibitors.

The BLAST design (Chu and Yuan, 2018b) leverages this rich information to achieve more accurate information borrowing. It aggregates different cancer types into subgroups (e.g., sensitive or insensitive subgroups) based on both response and longitudinal biomarker data via a latent-class modeling approach. Within each subgroup, the treatment effect is similar and approximately exchangeable such that information borrowing can be carried out using a BHM.

The differences between BLAST and CL-BHM are (i) BLAST performs information borrowing (based on BHM) and clustering jointly, while CL-BHM is a two-stage approach (i.e., cluster and then borrow information); (ii) BLAST utilizes both outcome data and biomarkers data, whereas CL-BHM is based only on the outcome data. Therefore, BLAST can achieve more accurate information borrowing, but requires more complicated statistical modelling and estimation.

2.3.5.1 Probability Model

For simplicity, we assume the null response rate and target response rate are both the same across cancer types, i.e., $p_{0,1} = \cdots = p_{0,J} \equiv q_0$ and $p_{1,1} = \cdots = p_{1,J} \equiv q_1$. Generalization to different values is straightforward.

Assume at an interim go/no-go treatment decision time, n_j patients with the jth cancer type have been enrolled. Let Y_{ij} denote a binary variable for the treatment response of the ith patient in the jth cancer type, with $Y_{ij} = 1$ denoting the favorable treatment response (e.g., CR/PR). Let Z_{ijl} denote the biomarker measurement for the ith patient in the jth cancer type at the time t_l, for $l = 1, \cdots, L$. For notational brevity, we assume that the biomarker is measured according to the same time schedule across patients, but the method allows different patients to have different numbers of measurements taken on different time schedules.

We assume that J cancer types can be classified into K subgroups, $1 \le K \le J$, such that within each subgroup, patients respond similarly to the treatment. A simple but practically important case is $K = 2$ like in CL-BHM, with a sensitive subgroup consisting of cancer types that are sensitive to the targeted agent, and an insensitive subgroup consisting of cancer types that are not sensitive to the targeted agent. The methodology here is not limited to two subgroups (sensitive/insensitive), but allows for multiple subgroups with varying levels of sensitivity, for example $K = 3$ subgroups representing insensitive, somewhat sensitive, and highly sensitive. We temporarily assume that the number of subgroups K is known, and discuss how to determine the value of K later. Let C_j denote the latent subgroup membership indicator, with $C_j = k$ denoting that the jth cancer type belongs to the kth subgroup, $k = 1, \cdots, K$. We assume that C_j follows a multinomial distribution

$$C_j \sim Multinomial\,(\pi_1, \cdots, \pi_K),$$

where $\pi_k = \Pr(C_j = k)$, $k = 1, \cdots, K$, is the probability of the jth cancer type belonging to the kth subgroup, with $\sum_{k=1}^{K} \pi_k = 1$. As C_j is latent, its value is never observed and is estimated jointly with other model parameters using the Markov chain Monte Carlo (MCMC) method (see Chu and Yuan, 2018b for details).

Conditional on C_j, we model the joint distribution of (Y, Z) by first specifying a model for Y and then a model for Z conditional on Y. Specifically, we assume that treatment response Y_{ij} follows a latent-subgroup hierarchical model

$$Y_{ij} \mid p_j \sim Ber(p_j),$$

$$\theta_j = log\left(\frac{p_j}{1-p_j}\right), \tag{2.14}$$

$$\theta_j \mid C_j = k \sim N\left(\theta_{(k)}, \tau_{(k)}^2\right),$$

where $Ber(.)$ denotes a Bernoulli distribution, $N(.)$ denotes a normal distribution, θ_j is the logit transformation of response rate p_j, and $\theta_{(k)}$ is the mean of θ_j in the kth subgroup. We assume that θ_j is random and follows a normal distribution to accommodate that although the response rates of the cancer types in the kth subgroup are generally similar, they may deviate from the subgroup mean $\theta_{(k)}$. A more parsimonious but slightly more restrictive model is to treat θ_j as a fixed effect by setting $\theta_j = \theta_{(k)}$, or equivalently $\tau_{(k)}^2 = 0$, which indicates that all cancer types in the kth subgroup have the same response rate $\theta_{(k)}$. Here, we focus on the case in which Y_{ij} is a binary response variable. Our approach can be easily extended to accommodate a continuous outcome Y_{ij} as follows,

$$Y_{ij} \sim N\left(\theta_j, \sigma_y^2\right),$$

$$\theta_j \mid C_j = k \sim N\left(\theta_{(k)}, \tau_{(k)}^2\right).$$

Conditional on C_j and Y_{ij}, we model the longitudinal biomarker measures Z_{ijl} using a semi-parametric mixed model as follows,

$$Z_{ijl} \mid (Y_{ij}, C_j = k) = \mu_{(k)}(t_l) + \upsilon_j + \omega_{ij} + \beta Y_{ij} + \epsilon_{ijl},$$

$$\upsilon_j \sim N\left(0, \sigma_\upsilon^2\right),$$

$$\omega_{ij} \sim N\left(0, \sigma_\omega^2\right),$$

which reflects the unique data structure of the basket trial: patients are nested in a cancer type, and cancer types are nested in a subgroup. Specifically, $\mu_{(k)}(t_l)$ is a nonparametric function of time t_l that specifies the mean trajectory of the biomarker for the kth subgroup; υ_j is the cancer-type-specific random effect accounting for the fact that the mean biomarker trajectory for a cancer type may deviate from the mean trajectory for its subgroup; and ω_{ij} is a subject-specific random effect to allow the biomarker trajectory for an individual patient to deviate from the mean trajectory for his/her cancer type. Regression parameter β captures the relationship between the biomarker Z and treatment response Y. We assume residuals $\epsilon_{ijl} \sim N(0, \sigma_\epsilon^2)$. When appropriate, a more complicated model can be entertained, for example, letting the cancer-type-level random variation υ_j and patient-level random variation ω_{ij} be time dependent, i.e., $\upsilon_j(t)$ and $\omega_{ij}(t)$.

We model the nonparametric function $\mu_{(k)}(t_l)$ using the penalized spline (Eilers and Marx, 1996; and Ruppert et al., 2003) because of its flexibility and close ties to the BHM. Other smoothing methods, such as smoothing splines (Green and Silverman, 1993) and the local polynomial (Fan and Gijbels, 1996) can also be used. Let $\kappa_1 < \kappa_2 < \cdots < \kappa_S$ denote S prespecified knots that partition the time interval $[t_1, t_L]$ into $S+1$ subintervals, and define the truncated power function as

$$(t_l - \kappa_s)_+^d = \begin{cases} (t_l - \kappa_s)^d & \text{if } t_l > \kappa_s \\ 0 \ \textit{otherwise} \end{cases}.$$

The penalized spline with the d-th degree truncated power basis function for $\mu_{(k)}(t_l)$ can be expressed as

$$\mu_{(k)}(t_l) = \gamma_{0(k)} + \gamma_{1(k)}t_l + \gamma_{2(k)}t_l^2 + \cdots + \gamma_{d(k)}t_l^d + \sum_{s=1}^{s} a_{s(k)}\left(t_l - \kappa_s\right)_+^d ,$$

$$a_{s(k)} \sim N\left(0, \sigma_{a(k)}^2\right),$$

where $\gamma_{0(k)}, \cdots, \gamma_{d(k)}$ are unknown parameters; $a_{1(k)}, \cdots, a_{S(k)}$ are random effects that follow a normal distribution with mean 0 and variance $\sigma_{a(k)}^2$. The smoothness of $\mu_{(k)}(t_l)$ is controlled by the smoothing parameter $\sigma_{a(k)}^2$. One advantage of the Bayesian approach is that by treating $\sigma_{a(k)}^2$ as a variance parameter, it can be estimated simultaneously with other model parameters. Ruppert et al. (2003) showed that the penalized spline is generally robust to the choice of knots and basis functions. In practice, different basis functions with reasonably spaced knots often provide similar results.

We now discuss how to choose the number of latent subgroups. We choose the value of K such that the corresponding model has the best goodness-of-fit according to a certain model selection statistic, such as the deviance information criterion (DIC; Spiegelhalter et al., 2002). In principle, the selection of K can be done by fitting the model with $K = 1, \cdots, J$, and then selecting the value of K that yields the smallest value of DIC as the number of latent subgroups. However, because the number of cancer types included in a basket trial is typically small (e.g., 4 to 15) and all enrolled patients carry the same genetic or molecular aberration, in practice, it is often adequate to restrict the search space of K to {1, 2, 3}. This also facilitates the interpretation of the results. For example, $K = 1$ means that all cancer types are sensitive or insensitive to the treatment; $K = 2$ accommodates the most common case in which some cancer types are sensitive to the treatment (i.e., sensitive subgroup) while the others are insensitive to the treatment (i.e., insensitive subgroup). During the trial, the value of K will be updated in the light of accumulating data. As a result, the value of K may differ from one interim evaluation to another, depending on the observed data. Instead of using the DIC to choose the value of K, an alternative approach is to treat K as an unknown parameter, and estimate it together with the other parameters. This can be done using the reversible jump Markov Chain Monte Carlo (MCMC) algorithm (Green, 1995).

2.3.5.2 Trial Design

The BLAST design has a total of M planned interim looks. Let $\mathcal{D}_m = \{(Z_{ij}, Y_{ijl}),\ j = 1, \cdots, J, i = 1, \cdots, n_{j,m}, l = 1, \cdots, L\}$ denote the interim data at the mth look, where $n_{j,m}$ is the sample size for the jth cancer type at the mth interim look, $m = 1, \cdots, M$. The BLAST design is described as follows,

1. Enroll $n_{j,1}$ patients with the jth cancer type for $j = 1, \cdots, J$.
2. Given the mth interim data $\mathcal{D}_m, m = 1, \cdots, M$, fit the proposed model.
   a. (Futility stopping) If $\Pr\left(p_j > \frac{q_0 + q_1}{2} \mid \mathcal{D}_m\right) < Q_f$, suspend the accrual for the jth cancer type, where $\frac{q_0 + q_1}{2}$ denotes the rate halfway between the null and target response rate,
   b. Otherwise, continue to enroll patients until the next interim analysis is reached.

3. Once the maximum sample size is reached or the accrual is stopped for all cancer types due to futility, evaluate the treatment efficacy based on the final data D as follows: if $\Pr(p_j > q_0 | D) > Q$, declare that the treatment is effective for the jth cancer type; otherwise, declare that the treatment is not effective for the jth cancer type, where Q is a probability cutoff.

In the design, the probability cutoffs Q_f and Q should be calibrated through simulation to achieve a desired type I error rate and power for each cancer type.

2.4 Bayesian Adaptive Designs for Platform Trials

The platform design is another important emerging type of master protocol (Woodcock and LaVange, 2017) and CID. According to FDA guidance, platform design may be loosely defined as designs that evaluate multiple investigational drugs and/or drug combination regimens across multiple tumor types. This is in contrast to the traditional clinical trials that focus on evaluating a single treatment in a single population. Clinical trials, such as BATTLE (Zhou et al, 2008) and I-SPY2 (Barker et al, 2009), provide early examples of adaptively investigating multiple agents in a trial.

Traditional phase II clinical trial designs were developed mainly for evaluating candidate treatments in a one treatment at a time fashion, e.g., Simon's two-stage design (Simon, 1989) and its extensions (Chen, 1997; Jung, Carey, and Kim, 2001; Lin and Shih, 2004}. This paradigm is cumbersome and grossly inefficient when the number of agents to be tested is large and increases over time, due to several reasons. First, the traditional approach requires the separate development of a research protocol, regulatory compliance, funding, and related infrastructure for each trial, which results in excessive "time-to-clinical use", overhead and overlap of infrastructure. In addition, the "white" space between trials slows down the process of testing candidate agents. Using the traditional approach in multiple randomized trials of different single agents requires the repeated use of the control arm (i.e., the standard therapy), which wastes patient and medical resources. Furthermore, differences among trials (e.g., different patient populations, different treatment procedures, and possibly different treatments as the control) make it difficult, if not impossible, to compare candidate agents across trials without bias. Traditional multi-arm trials can alleviate some of these issues, but still face significant logistic and statistical difficulties. For example, the inherent challenges associated with conducting a large multi-center, multi-agent clinical trial, limit the feasibility of conducting a single multi-arm trial that includes all the candidate agents. Even when such a design is possible, during the course of the trial emerging clinical data on the agents being tested is likely to change the equipoise between the arms and may even make some agents irrelevant. Thus, several independent multiple-arm trials are still needed, resulting in difficulties already described. Finally, standard multi-arm trials do not have a built-in mechanism to allow researchers to adaptively add new agents to the ongoing trial. The ability to accommodate the addition of new agents during a trial is important in the current, rapidly evolving research environment where new agents are developed at unprecedented speeds.

In what follows, we present two platform designs, the Multi-candidate Iterative Design with Adaptive Selection (MIDAS) and the ComPAS designs, to illustrate this type of CID to address the limitations of the traditional paradigm.

2.4.1 MIDAS Design

Yuan et al. (2016) presented a Bayesian phase II trial design called the MIDAS. This design allows investigators to continuously screen a large number of candidate agents in an efficient and seamless fashion. MIDAS requires only one master protocol (and hence a single regulatory and contractual approval) and one control arm, which streamlines the trial conduct, decreases the overhead, saves resources, and provides a straightforward comparison of the experimental agents. MIDAS consists of one control arm, which contains a standard therapy as the control, and an adjustable number of experimental arms, which contain the experimental agents. Patients are adaptively randomized to the control and experimental agents based on their estimated efficacy. During the trial, we adaptively drop inefficacious or overly toxic agents from the trial and graduate the promising agents to the next stage of development. Whenever an experimental agent graduates or is dropped from the trial, the corresponding arm opens immediately for testing the next available new agent. In principle, MIDAS allows for an unending screening process that can efficiently select promising agents or combinations for further clinical development.

2.4.1.1 Probability Model

We assume that the efficacy endpoint is the progression-free survival T (i.e., PFS), and toxicity is measured by a binary variable Y, with $Y = 1$ indicating that a patient experienced dose-limiting toxicity. We choose to measure efficacy using the PFS rather than a simpler binary outcome (tumor response/no response) because the PFS is a better surrogate for the Overall Survival (OS), which is the endpoint of ultimate interest. This is especially true for immunotherapy and other targeted agents, which often delay cancer progression and prolong patient survival without substantially shrinking the tumor.

MIDAS evaluates multiple treatments simultaneously. We model each treatment independently without imposing any specific structure across treatments. Specifically, we assume that the time to disease progression, T, follows an exponential distribution with hazard θ,

$$T \sim Exp(\theta).$$

Let n denote the number of patients who have been assigned to a treatment arm at the time of any given interim decision. For the ith patient, where $i = 1, \cdots, n$, let T_i^o denote the observed time of failure or administrative right censoring, and let $\delta_i = I(T_i^o = T_i)$ denote the censoring indicator. Let $S(t) = Pr(T > t)$ denote the survival function, which takes the form of $S(t) = e^{-t\theta}$ under the exponential model. Given the interim data $\mathcal{D}_n = \{(T_i^o, \delta_i), i = 1, \cdots, n\}$, let $m = \sum_{i=1}^{n} \delta_i$ denote the total number of failures and $\tilde{T} = \sum_{i=1}^{n} T_i^o$ denote the total observation time. The likelihood is given by

$$L(\mathcal{D}_n \mid \theta) = \prod_{i=1}^{n} f(T_i^o \mid \theta)^{\delta_i} S(T_i^o \mid \theta)^{1-\delta_i} = \theta^m \exp(-\tilde{T}\theta).$$

We assign θ a conjugate gamma prior, $\theta \sim Ga(a, b)$, where $a, b > 0$ are fixed hyperparameters.

The posterior distribution of θ follows a gamma distribution,

$$\theta \mid D_n \sim Ga(a + m, b + \tilde{T}).$$

Caution is needed when choosing hyperparameters a and b. The straightforward approach of setting a and b at very small values (e.g., 0.001) is not appropriate here. This is because at the early stage of the trial, we may not observe any event (i.e., disease progression) in the control arm, i.e., $m=0$. The resulting posterior distribution of θ, i.e., $Ga(a+m, b+\tilde{T})$, has substantial mass at the values close to 0, which causes highly unstable posterior estimate of the hazard ratio of the experimental agent versus the control because the denominator (i.e., the hazard of control) is extremely close to zero. We suggest the following procedure to set hyperparameters a and b. We first elicit from clinicians the prior estimate of median survival time η and its lower limit $\tilde{\eta}$, which correspond to hazards $\log(2)/\eta$ and $\log(2)/\tilde{\eta}$, respectively, under the exponential distribution. We choose the values of a and b such that the median of $Ga(a, b)$ matches $\log(2)/\eta$ and the prior probability of $\theta > \log(2)/\tilde{\eta}$ is small (e.g., 5%).

The assumption that the time to disease progression T follows an exponential distribution is a strong parametric assumption, but well serves design purposes. The goal is not to precisely estimate the whole survival curve, but to identify the agents that have excessively low or high efficacy based on the median PFS. Thall, Wooten, and Tannir (2005) showed that the exponential model is remarkably robust for monitoring efficacy based on the median survival time. In the case that tumor response is an appropriate (binary) efficacy endpoint, the gamma-exponential model can be simply replaced by a beta-binomial model.

We assume a standard beta-binomial model for toxicity. Let z denote the number of patients who have experienced toxicity out of the n patients at the time of an interim decision. We assume that z follows a binomial distribution,

$$z \sim Binomial(n, p),$$

where p is the toxicity probability. Assigning a conjugate beta prior to p, say $p \sim Beta(a_T, b_T)$, the posterior distribution of p is given by

$$p|z, n \sim Beta(a_T + z, b_T + n - z).$$

To set hyperparameters a_T and b_T, we elicit an estimate of toxicity from clinicians, and then choose the values of a_T, b_T such that the prior mean of p matches that elicited estimate, while controlling the prior effective sample size $a_T + b_T$ equal a small value, like $a_T + b_T = 1$.

2.4.1.2 Trial Design

As illustrated in Figure 2.1, the MIDAS trial includes one control slot/arm and K experimental slots/arms. The control slot contains the standard therapy, which serves as the control arm. Each of the K experimental slots contains a new agent for testing, resulting in K experimental arms. Let arm 0 denote the control arm, and arm k denote the kth experimental arm, with λ_k denoting the true hazard ratio between the kth experimental arm, $k = 1, \cdots, K$, versus the control. By definition, $\lambda_0 \equiv 1$ for the control. Let p_k denote the toxicity probability for the agent tested in the kth experimental arm, and ϕ_T denote the upper limit of acceptable toxicity. The MIDAS trial can be described as follows:

1. The trial starts by assigning the standard treatment to the control slot and K new experimental agents to K experimental slots.
2. As a burn-in, the first $(K+1)N_{min}$ enrolled patients are equally randomized to $K+1$ treatment arms, i.e., each treatment arm receives N_{min} patients.
3. For patients enrolled subsequently, the general strategy is to adaptively randomize them to arm k with probability π_k that is proportional to

$$\alpha_k = Pr\{\lambda_k = min(\lambda_0, \cdots, \lambda_K)| data\}, k = 0, 1, \cdots, K,$$

which is the posterior probability that arm k is the best treatment that is associated with the lowest hazard. By doing so, we are more likely to randomize patients to efficacious treatments. To accommodate practical considerations, we include the following three adjustments for π_k.

a. *Catch-up rule*: One important feature of the MIDAS trial is its ability to continuously test experimental agents. Once an experimental agent is removed from the trial due to findings of superiority, excessive toxicity, or futility, the slot that contained that agent immediately opens for testing another new agent (details are provided in steps 4 and 5 below). It is desirable to skew the randomization probability for the newly added agent such that the new agent has a higher chance of receiving patients and its sample size thereby catches up with those of the agents that have been studied in the trial for a certain period of time. Let n_k denote the number of patients that have been assigned to arm k, and define $C = \{k, n_k < N_{min}\}$ as the set of experimental arms that need to catch up. We use N_{min} as the cutoff because that is the number of patients initially treated by each of the first K experimental arms after equal randomization. For an experimental arm $k \in C$, we set the randomization probability as

$$\pi_k = max\left(\frac{\alpha_k}{\sum_{i=0}^{K} \alpha_i}, \frac{1}{K+1} \right), k \in C.$$

This catch-up rule ensures that the treatment arms with fewer than N_{min} patients have a probability of receiving new patients that is at least $\frac{1}{K+1}$. As $\pi_k \geq \frac{1}{K+1}$, it is possible, although very rare, $\sum_{k \in C} \pi_k > 1$. When that occurs, we normalize them to have a sum of one. We use $\bar{C} = \{k, n_k \geq N_{min}\}$ to denote the experimental arms that do not need to catch up in terms of sample size.

b. *Curtail rule*: Under MIDAS, the control arm remains active until the trial is terminated. As a result, it is likely that a large number of patients will be assigned to the control arm after several rounds of screening new agents. This is not desirable because treating an excessive number of patients on the control arm wastes precious medical resources and contributes little to learning the efficacy of the experimental agents. In addition, it reduces the chance that patients receive the new treatments that are potentially more effective. Thus, we impose the following rule to curtail π_0, the probability of a patient being randomized to the control arm:

$$\pi_0 = \begin{cases} \left(1 - \sum_{k \in C} \pi_k\right) \dfrac{\alpha_0}{\alpha_0 + \sum_{k \in \bar{C}} \alpha_k} & \text{if } n_0 < \beta N_{max} \\[3ex] \left(1 - \sum_{k \in C} \pi_k\right) \dfrac{\alpha_0}{\alpha_0 + \sum_{k \in \bar{C}} \alpha_k} \left(\dfrac{\beta N_{max}}{n_0}\right)^{\gamma} & \text{if } n_0 \geq \beta N_{max} \end{cases},$$

where $0 < \beta < 1$ is a constant, N_{max} is the prespecified maximum sample size for each of the experimental arms, and the term $(1 - \sum_{k \in C} \pi_k)$ reflects that we have "spent" some randomization probabilities, i.e., $(\sum_{k \in C} \pi_k)$, for the agents that need to catch up. The first equation of this rule says that before the number of patients treated on the control arm (i.e., n_0) reaches a certain threshold, βN_{max}, we randomize patients to the control with the probability proportional to the posterior probability that the control is the best treatment (i.e., α_0). However, once n_0 reaches βN_{max}, as defined by the second equation, we tune down the randomization probability π_0 to assign fewer patients to the control via the term $(\frac{\beta N_{max}}{n_0})^\gamma$, where γ controls how quickly we tune down the randomization probability. We note that this is not the only way to tune down π_0; other approaches are certainly possible. A numerical study shows that $(\frac{\beta N_{max}}{n_0})^\gamma$ serves its purpose and controls the possibility of assigning too many patients to the control arm.

c. After applying the above two rules, the randomization probability for each of the remaining experimental arms, i.e., $k \in \bar{\mathcal{C}}$, is proportional to the posterior probability that arm k is associated with the lowest hazard,

$$\pi_k = \left(1 - \pi_0 - \sum_{k \in \mathcal{C}} \pi_k\right) \frac{\alpha_k}{\sum_{k \in \bar{\mathcal{C}}} \alpha_k}, \ k \in \bar{\mathcal{C}}.$$

4. During the trial, we conduct the following interim monitoring after each patient or each cohort of patients is randomized.

a. Drop the agent from slot k if either of the following two conditions is true:

$$(\text{stopping for futility}) \ \Pr(\lambda_k < \phi_E | data) < C_{E1},$$

$$(\text{stopping for toxicity}) \ \Pr(p_k > \phi_T | data) > C_T,$$

where ϕ_E (≤ 1) represents the upper limit of the hazard ratio for the experimental agent to be regarded as promising, ϕ_T represents the upper limit of the toxicity, and C_{E1} and C_T are prespecified cutoffs, which should be calibrated through simulations for good design operating characteristics. The first condition says that, conditional on the observed data, the agent has a small chance to have a hazard ratio lower than ϕ_E, and the second condition says that the agent has a high (posterior) probability of being overly toxic.

b. Graduate the agent from slot k if one of the following two conditions is true:

$$(\text{graduate for superiority}) \ \Pr(\lambda_k < \phi_E | data) > C_{E2},$$

$$(\text{graduate for saturation}) \ n_k \geq N_{max},$$

where C_{E2} is a prespecified cutoff. The first condition says that, conditional on the observed data, the agent has a high probability of having a hazard ratio lower than ϕ_E, thus the agent should graduate from the trial and move forward to further development (e.g., a large confirmative trial). The second condition reflects the practical consideration that when a certain number of patients have been treated with an experimental agent and that agent has not been dropped for being overly toxic or futile, the agent may be worth developing further and should graduate from the current trial. The agents that graduate can be prioritized on the basis of various clinical considerations for further development in large-scale confirmatory trials. For an arm with none of the stopping and graduation rules being satisfied, we will continue to randomize patients to that arm.

To reduce sampling variation, we add a minimum sample size requirement that an agent must be used to treat at least N_{min} patients before it graduates for superiority or is dropped for futility. In addition, we require that the last patient treated by an experimental agent be followed at least τ months before that agent is dropped for futility. In other words, when the futility stopping rule is satisfied, we do not immediately drop the agent, but continue to follow the patients in that arm for at least τ months to confirm its futility. During this confirmation period, no new patients will be enrolled into that arm. If it turns out that the agent does not satisfy the futility stopping rule, the arm will be reopened for enrolling new patients.

When we evaluate the stopping and graduation rules, all control patients are used to calculate hazard ratio λ_k. This approach is efficient, but may introduce biases for the experimental agent introduced later in the trial if patient characteristics change during recruitment. If that is a concern, we may restrict the comparison to the concurrent controls that are enrolled in the same time frame as the experimental arm. In that case, we may set $\gamma = 0$ in the curtail rule such that a reasonable number of patients will be concurrently randomized to the control arm.

5. Whenever an experimental agent is dropped or graduates, the corresponding slot immediately opens for testing a new agent. If needed, a phase I lead-in can be used to confirm the safety of the candidate agent before it enters the trial. We use the Bayesian optimal interval (BOIN) design (Liu and Yuan, 2015) as the phase I lead-in because of its simplicity and superior performance.

6. Continue steps 3 to 5 until all experimental agents in the candidate pool have been tested.

As MIDAS continuously screens a large number of candidate agents, one may concern about the multiplicity or type I/II rate. Since MIDAS is intended for phase II trials and aims to fast screen a large number of candidate agents, strictly controlling the type I/II error rate may not be necessary. The multiplicity or type I/II error rate can be empirically controlled by calibrating the design parameters to obtain desirable operating characteristics (e.g., reasonably low false positive and false negative).

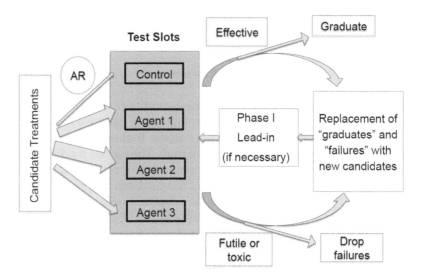

FIGURE 2.1
Diagram of the MIDAS trial.

2.4.2 ComPASS Design

Drug combination therapy has become commonplace for treating cancer and other complex diseases. Cancer is difficult to treat because it often involves multiple altered molecular pathways and can develop diverse mechanisms of resistance to the treatment regimen (Humphrey et al., 2011; Khamsi, 2011). Combining different treatment regimens provides an effective way to induce a synergistic treatment effect and overcome resistance to monotherapy. With the success of immune checkpoint inhibitors (e.g., nivolumab and pembrolizumab), more oncology trials are exploring combination therapy with immune-oncology drugs (Yuan and Yin, 2011; Bryan and Gordon, 2015). Given that hundreds of drugs have been approved by the FDA for the treatment of cancer, the number of possible combinations is huge. In addition, new potentially more efficacious compounds may become available at any time during drug development. Ideally, these new agents should be incorporated into the ongoing drug development pipeline in a seamless and timely fashion.

The ComPAS (Combination Platform design with Adaptive Shrinkage) design proposed by Tang, Shen, and Yuan (2018) provides a flexible Bayesian platform design to efficiently screen a set of drug combinations. The proposed design allows for dropping ineffective drug combinations and adding new combinations to the ongoing clinical pipeline in an adaptive and seamless way based on the accumulating trial data. A novel adaptive shrinkage method is developed to adaptively borrow information across different combinations to improve trial efficiency, using Bayesian model selection and hierarchical models.

2.4.2.1 Bayesian Hierarchical Model

Consider a phase II platform trial combining compound j, $j = 1, \ldots, J$, with a set of backbone regimens $k = 1, \ldots, K_j$, where the backbone regimens might be compound-specific. Let (j, k) denote the combination of compound j with backbone k. Suppose that n_{jk} patients have been treated with (j, k), and y_{jk} of them responded to the treatment. Let p_{jk} denote the true response rate associated with (j, k). We model y_{jk} using the BHM:

$$y_{jk} \,|\, n_{jk}, p_{jk} \sim Binom(n_{jk}, p_{jk}),$$

$$\text{logit}\,(p_{jk}) = \mu_{jk}, \tag{2.15}$$

$$\mu_{jk} \sim N(\mu_j, \sigma^2), \ k = 1, 2, \ldots, K_j,$$

$$\mu_j \sim N(0, 10^6), \ j = 1, 2, \ldots, J, \tag{2.16}$$

where *Binom*(.) denotes the binomial distribution. In the motivating trial in Tang, Shen and Yuan (2018), it is expected that the treatment effect may be rather heterogeneous across compounds, but relatively similar across backbones. That is, the treatment effect may be substantially heterogeneous between (j, k) and (j', k), but similar between (j, k) and (j, k') for $j \neq j'$ and $k \neq k'$. Therefore, in equation (2.16), we shrink the combination-specific response rate p_{jk} toward the compound-specific mean response rate μ_j, which renders information borrowing across combinations that share the same compound j. Depending on the clinical setting and application, other forms of shrinkage can be assumed in the BHM. For example, if it is expected that the treatment effect is similar across compound j rather than backbone k, we can shrink μ_{jk} toward the (logit-transformed) backbone-specific mean response rate, say φ_k, by assuming $\mu_{jk} \sim N(\varphi_k, \sigma^2)$. Alternatively, if the treatment effect of (j, k) is approximately exchangeable, we can shrink μ_{jk} toward the common (logit-transformed) mean response rate by assuming $\mu_{jk} \sim N(\mu, \sigma^2)$.

2.4.2.2 Adaptive Shrinkage via Bayesian Model Selection

The degree of shrinkage or information borrowing across combinations is controlled by the shrinkage parameter σ^2. As mentioned in previous sections, assigning a vague prior distribution to σ^2 doesn't work well when the number of second-level units (i.e., k's or the number of backbones in our example) is moderate. The ComPAS design uses an adaptive shrinkage method to circumvent this issue. The key is that rather than estimating the value of σ^2, we specify L discrete values of σ^2, $\sigma_1^2 < \ldots < \sigma_L^2$, where σ_1^2 is a small value that induces strong shrinkage and information borrowing, while σ_L^2 is a large value that induces little shrinkage and information borrowing. Each specification of σ^2 leads to a BHM. We then use Bayesian model selection to select the best-fitted model for statistical inference and decision making. By discretizing the space of σ^2 into L point masses, rather than assuming that it can take any value in the real line as in the Fully BHM (FBHM) approach, we reduce the domain of σ^2 and thus increase the power to determine the appropriate shrinkage and information borrowing. A practical procedure for specifying $\sigma_1^2 \ldots \sigma_L^2$ is provided later.

Specifically, let M_l denote the lth BHM with $\sigma^2 = \sigma_l^2$, $l = 1, \ldots, L$, and $\Pr(M_l)$ be the prior probability that model M_l is true. When there is no prior information on which model (i.e., the value of σ^2) is more likely, we can assign equal prior probabilities to L candidate models by simply setting $\Pr(M_l) = 1/L$, for $l = 1, \ldots, L$. Our experience is that $L = 3$ to 5 all work well and are adequate for practical use. Suppose at a certain stage of the trial, given the observed interim data $D = \{(n_{jk}, y_{jk}), j = 1, \ldots, J, k = 1, \ldots, K_j\}$, the posterior probability of M_l is given by

$$\Pr(M_l|D) = \frac{\Pr(M_l)L(D|M_l)}{\sum_{q=1}^{L} \Pr(M_q)L(D|M_q)},$$

where $L(D|M_l)$ is the marginal likelihood function under model M_l, given by

$$L(D|M_l) = \int \int f(y_i| n_{jk}, p_{jk}) f\left(\text{logit}(p_{jk}) \mid \mu_j, \sigma_l^2\right) f(\mu_j) dp_{jk} d\mu_j$$

$$= \int \int \binom{n_{jk}}{y_{jk}} p_{jk}^{y_{jk}-1}(1-p_{jk})^{n_{jk}-y_{jk}-1} \frac{1}{\sigma_l\sqrt{2\pi}} e^{-\frac{\left(\text{logit}(p_{jk})-\mu_j\right)^2}{2\sigma_l^2}} \frac{1}{10^3\sqrt{2\pi}} e^{-\frac{\mu_j^2}{2\times10^6}} dp_{jk} d\mu_j.$$

We select the optimal model (denoted as M_{opt}) as the model with the highest posterior probability,

$$M_{opt} = \text{argmax}_{\{M_l\}}\left(\Pr(M_l|D), l = 1, \ldots, L\right),$$

and use M_{opt} to make the adaptive decisions of dropping or graduating combinations during the course of the trial, as described later.

We now discuss how to specify the value of σ_l^2. Although it is generally true that a small value of σ^2 results in strong shrinkage and a large value of σ^2 induces little shrinkage, it is not immediately clear what value small or large is. In the BHM, the degree of shrinkage is determined by the ratio of the first-level to second-level variances, i.e., the variances associated with equations (2.15) and (2.16), respectively. To determine the appropriate value of σ_l^2, let $\bar{y}_{jk} = y_{jk}/n_{jk}$, we apply normal approximation to equation (2.15), resulting in

$$\bar{y}_{jk} \mid p_{jk} \sim N(p_{jk}, \ p_{jk}(1-p_{jk})/n_{jk}).$$

That is, the first-level variance is approximately $p_{jk}(1-p_{jk})/n_{jk}$. To obtain the second-level variance, we apply the Delta method to equation (2.16):

$$Var(p_{jk}) = \left\{ \frac{e^{\mu_{jk}}}{\left(1+e^{\mu_{jk}}\right)^2} \right\}^2 Var(\mu_{jk})$$

$$= \left\{ p_{jk}(1-p_{jk}) \right\}^2 \sigma^2$$

Therefore, the degree of shrinkage is determined by the relative variance between the first level and second level of the model, given by

$$w = \frac{\dfrac{p_{jk}(1-p_{jk})}{n_{jk}}}{\dfrac{p_{jk}(1-p_{jk})}{n_{jk}} + \left\{ p_{jk}(1-p_{jk}) \right\}^2 \sigma^2} = \frac{1}{1+n_{jk}p_{jk}(1-p_{jk})\sigma^2}.$$

The value of w can be interpreted as the relative contribution (or weight) of the prior of p_{jk} to the posterior estimate of p_{jk}, with respect to observed data y_{jk}. For example, $w = 0.001$ means that the prior of p_{jk} contributes 0.1% to the estimate of p_{jk}, inducing little shrinkage and the estimate of p_{jk} is essentially driven by the observed data y_{jk}; while $w = 0.999$ means that the prior of p_{jk} contributes 99.9% to the estimate of p_{jk} and thus induces strong shrinkage. Therefore, we propose to specify several values of w, say $w = (0.001, 0.25, 0.5, 0.75, 0.999)$, to represent weak, medium and strong shrinkage. Letting w_l denote the lth pre-specified weight, the value of σ_l^2 is determined as

$$\sigma_l^2 = \frac{1-w_l}{n_{jk}p_{jk}(1-p_{jk})w_l}, \tag{2.17}$$

where p_{jk} can be replaced with a reasonable estimate. Although in principle we could let σ_l^2 vary during the course of the trial, as σ_l^2 is a function of n_{jk} and p_{jk}, our experience is that it is not necessary and has little impact on the operating characteristics of the design. We can simply choose a set of values of w to represent the final weights we aim to target at the end of the trial, then set p_{jk} as the response rate under the alternative hypothesis and n_{jk} as the maximum sample size for each combination arm for calculating σ_l^2 using formula (2.17). For example, in the simulation described in Tang, Shen and Yuan (2018), we set $w = (0.999, 0.75, 0.5, 0.25, 0.001)$ with alternative response rate $p_{jk} = 0.7$ and the maximum sample size (for each combination arm) $n_{jk} = 22$, resulting in $\sigma_l^2 = (0.0002, 0.072, 0.216, 0.649, 216.2)$. Actually, this approach is preferred in practice because the values of σ_l^2, and thus candidate models, are prespecified and can be included in the trial protocol before the trial starts. This avoids potential biases due to choosing design parameters based on ongoing observed data.

2.4.2.3 Trial Design

ComPAS with R experimental arms and S interim analyses is described as follows. For notational brevity, the last (i.e., Sth) interim analysis denotes the final analysis.

Step 1: Equally randomize the first $n_1 R$ patients to R experimental arms. Each arm contains an experimental combination therapy.

Step 2: At the sth interim, $s=1, \ldots, S$, given the observed interim data D_s,

i. fit the L candidate BHMs $M_1, \ldots, M_L$, and identify M_{opt}, i.e., the model with the highest posterior probability.

ii. Conditional on M_{opt}, apply the futility stopping and superiority graduation rules to each of the R arms as follows:

a. *Futility stopping rule*: drop the combination therapy (j, k) if $\Pr(p_{jk} > p_0 | D_s, M_{opt}) < c_f$, where p_0 is the null response rate specified by clinicians, and c_f is a pre-specified probability cutoff. This futility stopping rule says that if the observed data suggest there is a small probability $(< c_f)$ that the response rate of combination therapy (j, k) is higher than the null p_0, we stop and drop that combination. The probability cutoff c_f can be easily calibrated by simulation as follows: specify a scenario where some combinations are efficacious and some combinations are futile, and use it as a basis to calibrate the value of c_f such that the probability of dropping the futile combinations is reasonably high, and the probability of dropping the efficacious combinations is reasonably low.

b. *Superiority graduation rule*: if $\Pr(p_{jk} > p_0 | D_s, M_{opt}) > c_g$, "graduate" the combination (j, k) for the next phase (e.g., phase III) development. The probability cutoff c_g is chosen as follows: specify the null scenario that all combinations are futile, and use it as a basis to calibrate the value of c_g such that the probability of graduating the futile combinations is controlled at a prespecified type I error rate.

iii. When a combination is dropped or graduated, a new combination, if available, is added to the trial.

iv. Stop the trial if (a) all combinations are dropped or graduated and no new combination is available for testing, or (b) the maximum sample size is reached. When the trial is stopped, depending on the trial objective, we select all or a subset of graduated combinations or simply the most efficacious combination as the optimal combination(s) for the next phase (i.e., phase III) development.

Step 3: Continue to randomize patients into the R arms until reaching the next planned interim analysis and repeat Step 2.

The above algorithm should be customized to fit trial requirements and considerations at hand. For example, in the above algorithm, we drop futile combinations by comparing them with a prespecified null response rate p_0. In some applications, it may be desirable to drop a combination by comparing it with other combinations: drop combination (j, k) if $\Pr(p_{jk} = \max(p_{11}, \ldots, p_{JK_J}) | D_s, M_{opt}) < c_{f2}$, where c_{f2} is a probability cutoff. That is, if the interim data suggest that there is little chance that (j, k) is to be the winner, we drop that combination early. For the trial requiring a control arm, we can make the interim drop/ graduation decision by comparing experimental combinations with the control, which can be done by simply replacing p_0 with the response rate of the control (denoted as p_{ctr}) in the futility dropping and superiority graduation rules. For example, the futility stopping rule in step 2(ii) becomes: drop the combination therapy $\Pr(p_{jk} > p_{ctr} | D_s, M_{opt}) < c_f$. When needed, a similar safety stopping rule based on the posterior probability can be used to monitor toxicity at interims.

We adopt Bayesian model selection approach to select the best fitted model and use it to make interim decisions. Bayesian model averaging approach described in Section 12.3.4 can also be used to estimate p_{jk} and make interim decisions. In addition, here we consider equal randomization, which is easy to implement and yields good operating characteristics when combined with the futility and superiority rules described above. The adaptive randomization and curtailed rules in the MIDAS design can also be adopted here when appropriate.

2.5 Bayesian Adaptive Enrichment Design

The enrichment design is another effective CID to achieve precision medicine in the presence of patient heterogeneity. The enrichment design is motivated by the idea that heterogeneity of patient response to an experimental treatment, E, may be due to biological covariates that modify the effects of E at the cellular or molecular level. If differences in drug effects are due to biological covariates such as gene or protein expression, then only a subset of "E-sensitive" patients defined by those biological covariates may respond favorably to E. Precision medicine uses biological covariates to restrict administration of drug to an identified subset of E-sensitive patients, avoiding futile use of E in non-sensitive patients unlikely to benefit from E.

The enrichment design that focuses on E-sensitive patients provides an efficient approach in such settings. Most existing enrichment designs assume based on pre-clinical data that an E-sensitive subgroup is known, and moreover that E is substantively efficacious in that subpopulation. However, due to important differences between pre-clinical settings and human biology, data from clinical studies often show that one or both of these assumptions are false. Therefore, the key problems are how to use biological covariates to (1) identify the E-sensitive subgroup and (2) determine whether E provides an improvement over a standard control therapy, C, in the subgroup.

Park et al. (2021) propose a Bayesian randomized Group Sequential (GS) Adaptive Enrichment Design (AED) that compares an experimental treatment E to a control C based on survival time Y, and uses an early response indicator Z as an ancillary outcome to assist with adaptive variable selection and enrichment. Initially, the design enrolls patients under broad eligibility criteria. At each interim decision, models for regression of Y and Z on covariates are updated by performing covariate selection, re-fitting the models using newly selected covariates to define E-sensitive patients, and using this to update the Personalized Benefit Index (PBI) and eligibility criteria. Enrollment of each cohort is restricted to the most recent adaptively identified treatment-sensitive patients. Group sequential decision cutoffs are calibrated to control overall type I error and account for the adaptive enrollment restriction.

2.5.1 Design Structure

Consider a two-arm clinical trial with patients randomized to $E(G = 1)$ or $C(G = 0)$ in a fixed ratio. For each patient, we observe a covariate vector $x \in \mathbb{R}^p$ at enrollment, a short-term response indicator Z, and a time-to-event endpoint Y. In cancer trials, Z may be the indicator of $\geq 50\%$ tumor shrinkage at some point after treatment, and Y typically is the progression-free survival or the overall survival time. For right-censoring of Y at follow up time U when an interim decision is to be made, we define the observed event time $Y^o = \min(Y, U)$ and event indicator $\delta = I(Y \leq U)$.

In treatment arm $G = 0$ or 1, let $\pi(x, G, \theta_Z) = \Pr(Z = 1 | G, x, \theta_Z)$ denote the response rate of Z for a patient with covariates x, and let $h_G(y | x, Z, \theta_Y)$ denote the hazard function of Y at time y for a patient with covariates x and response indicator Z, where θ_Z and θ_Y are the model parameter vectors. At each decision, the AED design adaptively selects two subvectors of x to identify patients expected to benefit more from E than C in terms of Z or Y. The first subvector, x_Z, is identified by doing variable selection based on the difference in response probabilities $\Delta_Z(x, \theta_Z) = \pi(x, 1, \theta_Z) - \pi(x, 0, \theta_Z)$ in the regression model for $(Z | G, x)$. The second subvector, x_Y, is identified by doing variable selection based on the hazard ratio $\Delta_Y(x, \theta_Y) = h_1(y | x, Z, \theta_Y)/h_0(y | x, Z, \theta_Y)$ in the regression model for $(Y | Z, G, x)$. To accommodate the fact that a covariate predictive of a higher tumor response probability often is predictive of longer survival and so x_Z and x_Y may share common terms, selection of these two subvectors are based on correlated vectors of latent variable selection indicators to account for association. This will be described later.

The schema of the AED design is shown in Figure 2.2. The AED design enrolls a maximum of N patients sequentially in cohorts of sizes $c_1, \cdots, c_K$, with $\sum_{k=1}^{K} c_k = N$. The trial begins by enrolling patients under broad eligibility criteria for the first cohort of c_1 patients. When the first cohort of patients' outcomes have been evaluated, the subvectors x_Z and x_Y are determined and used to compute a PBI, given formally below. The PBI is used to define the subgroup of E-sensitive patients, and the comparative tests are defined in terms of the E-sensitive patients. If the trial is not terminated early due to either superiority or futility, then only E-sensitive patients are enrolled in the second cohort. This process is repeated group sequentially until the end of the trial. If the maximum sample size N is reached, a final analysis is done when all patients' follow-ups have completed.

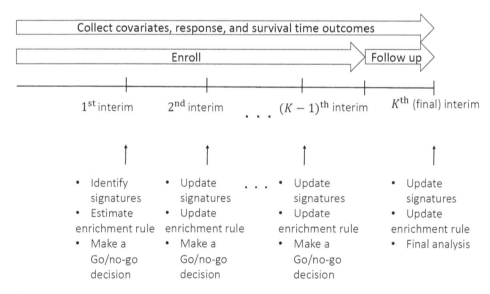

FIGURE 2.2
Schema of the enrichment design.

2.5.2 Probability Model

The joint distribution $(Y, Z \mid G, x)$ is modeled as a mixture of the conditional distribution of $(Y \mid Z, G, x)$ weighted by the marginal distribution of $(Z \mid G, x)$. Here we assume that Z always is observed before Y.

The marginal distribution of $(Z \mid G, x)$ is modeled using the probit regression $\pi(x_i, G_i, \theta_Z) = \Phi(\tilde{x}_i^T \beta_Z + G_i \tilde{x}_i^T Y_Z)$, where $i = 1, \cdots, n$, indexes patients, $\tilde{x} = (1, x^T)^T$, β_Z is the vector of covariate main effects, and $Y_Z = (\gamma_{Z,0}, \cdots, \gamma_{Z,p})^T$ is the vector of additional E-versus-C treatment-covariate interactions, with the main experimental versus control effect $\gamma_{Z,0}$.

The conditional distribution of $(Y \mid Z, G, x)$ is modeled using a proportional piecewise exponential (PE) hazard model (Ibrahim et al., 2005; Kim et al., 2007; McKeague and Tighiouart, 2000; Sinha et al., 1999). With a partition of the time axis into M intervals $I_m = (\tau_{m-1}, \tau_m)$ for $m = 1, \cdots, M$, with $0 = \tau_0 < \tau_1 < \cdots < \tau_M < \infty$, the proportional PE hazard function is

$$h\left(y \mid Z, G, x, \theta_Y\right) = \phi_m exp\left(x^T \beta_Y + G \tilde{x}^T Y_Y + \alpha_Y Z \right) I(y \in I_m), \ m = 1, \cdots, M,$$

where $\phi_m > 0$ is the hazard on the mth subinterval, α_Y is the main effect of response ($Z = 1$) on the hazard of Y, and $\theta_Y = (\phi_1, \cdots, \phi_M, \beta_Y^T, Y_Y^T, \alpha_Y)^T$ the parameter vector.

2.5.3 Sequentially Adaptive Variable Selection

To identify subvectors of x that identify patients more likely to benefit from E, joint variable selection is performed on x in the two submodels $(Y \mid Z, G, x)$ and $(Z \mid G, x)$, accounting for the possibility that a covariate predictive of one outcome may also be predictive of the other.

In the joint likelihood function of Z and Y, for each $t = Z$ or Y, let ψ_t denote the regression coefficient vector, excluding the intercept, so $\psi_Z = (\beta_{Z,1}, \cdots, \beta_{Z,p}, \gamma_{Z,0}, \cdots, \gamma_{Z,p})$, and $\psi_Y = (\beta_{Y,1}, \cdots, \beta_{Y,p}, \gamma_{Y,0}, \cdots, \gamma_{Y,p})$.

Park et al. (2021) perform Bayesian spike-and-slab variable selection (Mitchell and Beauchamp, 1988; George and McCulloch, 1993; Ishwaran and Rao, 2005) for each submodel $t = Z$ or Y. This approach uses sparse posterior coefficient estimates to determine variables to be included in the submodel. For each t, let $\lambda_t = (\lambda_{t,1}, \cdots, \lambda_{t,2p+1})^T$ be a vector of latent variable selection indicators corresponding to (x, G, Gx). The jth variable in (x, G, Gx) is included in the submodel for outcome t if $\lambda_{t,j} = 1$ and excluded if $\lambda_{t,j} = 0$. We restrict the variable selection algorithm to satisfy *the strong hierarchy interaction* constraint (Liu et al., 2015) in each submodel so that, if the interaction term Gx_j is included, then the main effect term x_j corresponding to Gx_j and G also must be included.

To accommodate the fact that some covariates may be predictive of treatment effects on both Z and Y, a "joint variable selection" strategy is adopted in Park et al. (2021) by endowing λ_Z and λ_Y with a joint distribution to borrow information about covariate effects on Z and Y. To account for correlation, a bivariate Bernoulli distribution is assumed for $(\lambda_{Z,j}, \lambda_{Y,j})$, for $j = 1, \cdots, 2p + 1$.

Denote $p_{Z,j} = \Pr(\lambda_{Z,j} = 1)$ and $p_{Y,j} = \Pr(\lambda_{Y,j} = 1)$ the marginal probabilities that the jth variable is included in the submodels $(Z \mid G, x)$ and $(Y \mid Z, G, x)$, respectively, and let

$$\rho_j = \frac{\Pr(\lambda_{Y,j} = 1, \lambda_{Z,j} = 1) / \Pr(\lambda_{Y,j} = 0, \lambda_{Z,j} = 1)}{\Pr(\lambda_{Y,j} = 1, \lambda_{Z,j} = 0) / \Pr(\lambda_{Y,j} = 0, \lambda_{Z,j} = 0)}$$

denote the odds ratio for the jth pair of latent variables. We denote by $\mathcal{B}(p_{Z,j}, p_{Y,j}, \rho_j)$ the joint Bernoulli distribution of $(\lambda_{Z,j}, \lambda_{Y,j})$.

The spike-and-slab prior model used for the joint variable selection is

$$\psi_{Z,j} \mid \lambda_{Z,j} \sim (1 - \lambda_{Z,j}) N(0, \tau^2_{Z,j}) + \lambda_{Z,j} N(0, u^2_{Z,j} \tau^2_{Z,j}), \ j = 1, \ldots, 2p+1, \tag{2.18}$$

$$\psi_{Y,j} \mid \lambda_{Y,j} \sim (1 - \lambda_{Y,j}) N(0, \tau^2_{Y,j}) + \lambda_{Y,j} N(0, u^2_{Y,j} \tau^2_{Y,j}), \ j = 1, \ldots, 2p+1, \tag{2.19}$$

where $u_{Z,j}, \tau^2_{Z,j}, u_{Y,j}, \tau^2_{Y,j}, j = 1, \ldots, 2p+1$ are prespecified hyperparameters. We choose large $u_{Z,j}$ and small $\tau_{Z,j}$ in (2.18) so that $\lambda_{Z,j} = 1$ implies a nonzero estimate of $\psi_{Z,j}$, whereas $\lambda_{Z,j} = 0$ implies that the covariate corresponding to $\psi_{Z,j}$ has a negligible effect on Z. Similar choices are applied to (2.19) to obtain sparse vectors of coefficient estimates for Y. The latent indicator variables are assumed to follow the prior distributions $(\lambda_{Z,j}, \lambda_{Y,j}) \mid p_{Z,j}, p_{Y,j}, \rho_j \sim \mathcal{B}(p_{Z,j}, p_{Y,j}, \rho_j)$ for $j = 1, \ldots, p+1$ and $\lambda_{Z,j} \sim \text{Bernoulli}(p_{Z,j})$ and $\lambda_{Y,j} \sim \text{Bernoulli}(p_{Y,j})$ for $j = p+2, \ldots, 2p+1$. To ensure the strong hierarchical property, the following constraints are imposed

$$p_{Z,j} = p_{Z,j-p-1} p_{Z,p+1} \min\{p_{Z,j-p-1}, p_{Z,p+1}\}, \ j = p+2, \ldots, 2p+1, \tag{2.20}$$

$$p_{Y,j} = p_{Y,j-p-1} p_{Y,p+1} \min\{p_{Y,j-p-1}, p_{Y,p+1}\}, \ j = p+2, \ldots, 2p+1, \tag{2.21}$$

During the trial, joint variable selection is performed at each interim stage to obtain the subvectors x_z and x_Y. While this procedure may miss informative covariates in x_Y early in the trial, due to an insufficient number of observed events for Y, as the trial progresses the probabilities of identifying truly important covariates with interactive effects increase.

2.5.4 Adaptive Enrichment

For each cohort $k = 1, \ldots, K$, let d_k be the accumulated number of events (i.e., $Y_i = Y_i^o$) at the time when the kth adaptive enrichment is performed, and let $n_k = \sum_{j=1}^{k} c_j$ be the total number of patients enrolled in the first k cohorts. Let $D_k = \{(Y_i^o, \delta_i, Z_i, G_i, x_i), i = 1, \ldots, n_k\}$ be the accumulated data, $x_Z^{(k)}$ and $x_Y^{(k)}$ the selected subvectors at the kth interim decision, and ϵ_1 and ϵ_2 be design parameters specified to quantify minimal clinically significant improvements in response probability and survival, respectively. We define the Personalized Benefit Index (PBI) for a patient with covariate vector x as

$$\Omega(x \mid D_k) = (1 - \omega_k) Pr\left\{\Delta_Z\left(x_Z^{(k)}, \theta_Z\right) > \epsilon_1 \mid D_k\right\} + \omega_k Pr\left\{\Delta_Y\left(x_Y^{(k)}, \theta_Y\right) < \epsilon_2 \mid D_k\right\}, \tag{2.22}$$

where the weight is $\omega_k = d_k / n_k$. The PBI depends on x only through the selected subvectors $x_Z^{(k)}$ and $x_Y^{(k)}$, that is, $\Omega(x \mid D_k) = \Omega(x_Z^{(k)}, x_Y^{(k)} \mid D_k)$. It is a weighted average of the posterior probabilities that a patient with covariates x will benefit from E more than C, defined in terms of the comparative treatment effect parameters $\Delta_Z(x_Z^{(k)}, \theta_Z)$ and $\Delta_Y(x_Y^{(k)}, \theta_Y)$. Early in the trial, when there are few observed event times, the PBI will depend on Z more than on Y. Later into the trial when more events occur, the weight $(1 - \omega_k)$ for the response probability difference becomes smaller and the weight ω_k for the survival hazard ratio component becomes larger, so the PBI depends more on the survival time data. A patient with biomarker profile x is considered eligible for enrollment into the $(k+1)$st cohort of the trial if their PBI is sufficiently large, formalized by the rule

$$\Omega(x \mid D_k) = \Omega\left(x_Z^{(k)}, x_Y^{(k)} \mid D_k\right) > v\left(\frac{n_k}{N}\right)^g, \tag{2.23}$$

for $k = 1, \ldots, K-1$.

2.5.5 Bayesian Sequential Monitoring Rules

The kth interim decisions are based on D_k, the accumulated data from k successive cohorts. Patients within each cohort are homogeneous, but patients may be heterogeneous between cohorts since different cohorts may have different eligibility criteria because the variable selection is repeated and the PBI is refined during the trial. Let

$$\mathcal{X}_k = \left\{ x: \Omega\left(x_Z^{(k)}, x_Y^{(k)} \mid D_k\right) > v\left(\frac{n_k}{N}\right)^g \right\}$$

denote the set of the covariates satisfying the eligibility criteria used for the $(k+1)$st cohort.

At this point in the trial, the covariate-averaged long-term outcome treatment effect is defined as

$$T_{Y,k}(\theta) = \int_{\mathcal{X}_k} \Delta_Y\left(x_Y^{(k)}, \theta_Y\right) \hat{p}_k\left(x_Y^{(k)}\right) dx_Y^{(k)},$$

where $\hat{p}_k(x_Y^{(k)})$ denotes the empirical distribution of $x_Y^{(k)}$ on the set $\mathcal{X}_k$. Since these expectations are computed over the selected enrichment set $\mathcal{X}_k$, i.e., the patients who are expected to benefit more from E than C in the kth cohort, $T_{Y,k}(\theta)$ is a treatment effect in the sense of precision medicine. Note that E is more effective than C for patients with $x \in \mathcal{X}_k$ if $T_{Y,k}(\theta)$ is sufficiently small.

Denoting the number of events in the jth cohort by e_j, we define the test statistic at the kth analysis as the weighted average of the treatment effects, $\bar{T}_{Y,k}(\theta) = \sum_{j=1}^k \omega_{Y,j} T_{Y,j}(\theta)$, where $\omega_{Y,j} = e_j / \sum_{l=1}^k e_l$ (Lehmacher and Wassmer, 1999). Note that $T_{Y,j}(\theta)$ is calculated based on the data observed at the interim time, so it must be updated at each later interim decision time as Y is a time-to-event endpoint. Let b_1 denote the hazard ratio (e.g., ≤ 1) under which E is deemed superior to C in the long-term endpoint Y, and let b_2 denote the hazard ratio (e.g., ≥ 1) under which E is deemed inferior to C. The values of (b_1, b_2) typically are prespecified by the clinicians. Let (B_1, B_2) be prespecified probability cutoffs that should be tuned through simulation studies. For the kth interim analysis, the decision rules are as follows:

1. **Superiority**: Stop the trial for superiority of E over C in $\mathcal{X}_k$ if $\Pr\{\bar{T}_{Y,k}(\theta) < b_1 \mid D_k\} > B_1$.

2. **Futility**: Stop the trial for futility of E over C in $\mathcal{X}_k$ if $\Pr\{\bar{T}_{Y,k}(\theta) > b_2 \mid D_k\} > B_2$.

3. **Final Decision**: If the trial is not stopped early, at the last analysis ($k = K$), conclude that E is superior to C in the final E-sensitive subset $\mathcal{X}_k$ if $\Pr\{\bar{T}_{Y,k}(\theta) < b_1 \mid D_k\} > B_1$ and otherwise conclude that E is not superior to C in $\mathcal{X}_k$. To account for the possibility that only a very small proportion of patients may benefit from E, the following additional futility stopping rule may be included at each interim. For a prespecified threshold $0 < q < 1$ based on practical considerations, the futility rule stops the trial if the estimated proportion of E-sensitive patients in the trial is $< q$. The authors recommend to use a value in the range .01- .10 in practice.

At the end of the trial, identification of the final E-sensitive subset $\mathcal{X}_k$ based on PBI involves all covariates, because the Bayesian spike-and-slab variable selection method does not necessarily drop covariates with little or no contribution to identify $\mathcal{X}_k$. To facilitate practical use, one can simplify the E-sensitive subset identification rule by dropping covariates that have low posterior probability (i.e., <.10) of being selected in the prediction model of (Y, Z).

In practice, logistical limitations will often limit the number of interim decisions to 1, 2, or 3. Based on these considerations, as a rule of thumb, a reasonable time to initiate the adaptive enrichment is after 1/3 to 1/2 of the maximum number of patients have been enrolled.

We refer the reader to the original article by Park et al. (2021) for more details of the design (e.g., prior distributions on the parameters, estimation procedure, a model elaboration for situations where Y is observed before Z can be evaluated, the generalization of the joint variable selection algorithm to the case where the predictors may be correlated, details of determining the design parameters $v > 0$ and $g > 0$, procedure to calibrate the values of (B_1, B_2), and simulation studies).

2.6 Summary

In this chapter, we have discussed several Bayesian adaptive design examples to illustrate complex innovative design. These designs have demonstrated a wide range of applications in practice and provided effective tools to improve the efficiency and success rate of drug development. Considering multiple endpoints and risk-benefit tradeoff better reflects the medical decisions in practice and thus provides a more efficient way to optimize treatment regimens. In a basket trial that evaluates the treatment effect of a targeted therapy in multiple cancer types simultaneously, the Bayesian hierarchical model and its variants can be used to borrow information across cancer types. In platform designs that simultaneously investigate multiple agents, the use of a master protocol provides an efficient approach to drop futile agents, graduate effective agents and add new agents during the course of the trial. In the presence of patient heterogeneity, the enrichment design is an effective way to use biomarkers to adaptively identify the sensitive subgroup and determine whether the experimental agent provides an improvement over the standard control therapy in the sensitive subgroup. The design strategies and methodologies described in this chapter can be combined and modified to better address challenges in specific clinical trials.

References

Barker, A., Sigman, C., Kelloff, G., Hylton, N., Berry, D., Esserman, L. (2009). I-SPY 2: an adaptive breast cancer trial design in the setting of neoadjuvant chemotherapy. *Clinical Pharmacology & Therapeutics*, 86(1), 97–100.

Berry, S., Carlin, B., Lee, J., Muller, P. (2010). *Bayesian Adaptive Methods for Clinical Trials*. Chapman & Hall/CRC Biostatistics series.

Berry, SM., Broglio, KR., Groshen, S., et al. (2013). Bayesian hierarchical modeling of patient subpopulations: efficient designs of phase II oncology clinical trials. *Clinical Trials*, 10(5), 720–734.

Brody, J., Kohrt, H., Marabelle, A. and Levy, R. (2011). Active and passive immunotherapy for lymphoma: proving principles and improving results. *Journal of Clinical Oncology*, 29(14), 1864–1875.

Bryan, LJ., Gordon, LI. (2015). Releasing the brake on the immune system: the PD-1 strategy for hematologic malignancies. *Oncology (Williston Park)*, 29(6), 431–439.

Cha, E. and Fong, L. (2011). Immunotherapy for prostate cancer: biology and therapeutic approaches. *Journal of Clinical Oncology*, 29(27), 3677–3685.

Chen TT. (1997). Optimal three-stage designs for phase II cancer clinical trials. *Statistics in Medicine*, 16(23), 2701–2711.

Chu, Y., and Yuan, Y. (2018a). A Bayesian basket trial design using a calibrated Bayesian hierarchical model. *Clinical Trials*, 15(2), 149–158.

Chu, Y., and Yuan, Y. (2018b). Blast: Bayesian latent subgroup design for basket trials. *Journal of the Royal Statistical Society: Series C (Applied Statistics)*, 67(3), 723–740.

Couzin-Frankel, J. (2013). Cancer immunotherapy. *Science*, 342(6165), 1432–1433.

Eilers, PH. and Marx, BD. (1996). Flexible smoothing with B-splines and penalties. *Statistical Science*, 11(2), 89–102.

Fan, J. and Gijbels, I. (1996). *Local Polynomial Modelling and Its Applications*. Boca Raton: CRC Press.

Flaherty, KT., Puzanov, I., Kim, KB., Ribas, A., McArthur, GA., Sosman, JA., O'Dwyer, PJ., Lee, RJ., Grippo, JF., Nolop, K. and Chapman, PB. (2010). Inhibition of mutated, activated BRAF in metastatic melanoma. *New England Journal of Medicine*, 363(9), 809–819.

Fleming, GF., Sill, MW., Darcy, KM., McMeekin, DS., Thigpen, JT., Adler, LM., Berek, JS., Chapman, JA., DiSilvestro, PA., Horowitz, IR. and Fiorica, JV. (2010). Phase II trial of trastuzumab in women with advanced or recurrent, HER2-positive endometrial carcinoma: a Gynecologic Oncology Group study. *Gynecologic Oncology*, 116(1), 15–20.

Freidlin, B., and Korn, EL. (2013). Borrowing information across subgroups in phase II trials: is it useful?. *Clinical Cancer Research*, 19(6), 1326–1334.

Gatzemeier, U., Groth, G., Butts, C., Van Zandwijk, N., Shepherd, F., Ardizzoni, A., Barton, C., Ghahramani, P. and Hirsh, V. (2004). Randomized phase II trial of gemcitabine-cisplatin with or without trastuzumab in HER2-positive non-small-cell lung cancer. *Annals of Oncology*, 15(1), 19–27.

George, EI., McCulloch, RE. (1993). Variable selection via gibbs sampling. *Journal of the American Statistical Association*, 88(423), 881–889.

Green, PJ. and Silverman, BW. (1993). *Nonparametric Regression and Generalized Linear Models: A Roughness Penalty Approach*. New York: Chapman and Hall.

Green, PJ. (1995). Reversible jump Markov chain Monte Carlo computation and Bayesian model determination. *Biometrika*, 82(4), 711–732.

Hobbs, B., Carlin, B., Mandrekar, S., Sargent, D. (2011). Hierarchical commensurate and power prior models for adaptive incorporation of historical information in clinical trials. *Biometrics*, 67(3), 1047–1056.

Hobbs, B., Landin, R. (2018). Bayesian basket trial design with exchangeability monitoring. *Statistics in Medicine*, 37(25), 3557–3572.

Humphrey RW, Brockway-Lunardi LM, Bonk DT, et al. (2011). Opportunities and challenges in the development of experimental drug combinations for cancer. *Journal of the National Cancer Institute*, 103(16), 1222–1226.

Ibrahim, JG., Chen, MH. (2000). Power prior distributions for regression models. *Statistical Science*, 15(1), 46–60.

Ibrahim, JG., Chen, MH., Sinha, D. (2005). *Bayesian Survival Analysis*. Wiley Online Library.

Ishwaran, H., Rao, JS. (2005). Spike and slab variable selection: frequentist and Bayesian strategies. *The Annals of Statistics*, 33(2), 730–773.

Jiang, L., Nie, L., Yuan, Y. (2020). Elastic priors to dynamically borrow information from historical data in clinical trials, arXiv, 2021(06083). DOI: 10.1111/biom.13551

Jiang, L., Li, R., Yan, F., Yap, T., Yuan, Y. (2021). Shotgun: a Bayesian seamless phase I-II design to accelerate the development of targeted therapies and immunotherapy. *Contemporary Clinical Trials*, 104, 106338.

Jung SH, Carey M, Kim KM. (2001). Graphical search for two-stage designs for phase II clinical trials. *Controlled Clinical Trials*, 22(4), 367–372.

Kaufman, HL. (2015). Precision immunology: the promise of immunotherapy for the treatment of cancer. *Journal of Clinical Oncology*, 33(12), 1315–1317.

Khamsi R. (2011). Combo antibody efforts up, despite regulatory uncertainties. *Nature Medicine*, 17(8), 907.

Kim, S., Chen, M., Dey, DK., Gamerman, D. (2007). Bayesian dynamic models for survival data with a cure fraction. *Lifetime Data Analysis*, 13(1), 17–35.

Lehmacher, W., Wassmer, G. (1999). Adaptive sample size calculations in group sequential trials. *Biometrics*, 55(4), 1286–1290.

Lin Y, Shih WJ. (2004). Adaptive two-stage designs for single-arm phase IIA cancer clinical trials. *Biometrics*, 60(2), 482–490.

Liu, C., Ma, J., and Amos, CI. (2015). Bayesian variable selection for hierarchical gene–environment and gene–gene interactions. *Human Genetics*, 134(1), 23–36.

Liu, S., Yuan, Y. (2015). Bayesian optimal interval designs for phase I clinical trials. *Journal of the Royal Statistical Society: Series C (Applied Statistics)*, 64, 507–523.

Liu, S., Guo, B., Yuan, Y. (2018). Bayesian phase I/II trial design for immunotherapy. *Journal of the American Statistical Association*, 113(523), 1016–1027.

Makkouk, A., and Weiner, GJ. (2015). Cancer immunotherapy and breaking immune tolerance: new approaches to an old challenge. *Cancer Research*, 75(1), 5–10.

McKeague, IW., Tighiouart, M. (2000). Bayesian estimators for conditional hazard functions. *Biometrics*, 56(4), 1007–1015.

Mitchell, TJ., Beauchamp, JJ. (1988). Bayesian variable selection in linear regression. *Journal of the American Statistical Association*, 83(404), 1023–1032.

Park, Y., Liu, S., Thall, P., Yuan, Y. (2021). Bayesian group sequential enrichment designs based on adaptive regression of response and survival time on baseline biomarkers. *Biometrics*, doi: 10.1111/biom.13421.

Pardoll, D. (2012). The blockade of immune checkpoints in cancer immunotherapy. *Nature Review Cancer*, 12(4), 252–264.

Prahallad, A., Sun, C., Huang, S., Di Nicolantonio, F., Salazar, R., Zecchin, D., Beijersbergen, RL., Bardelli, A. and Bernards, R. (2012). Unresponsiveness of colon cancer to BRAF (V600E) inhibition through feedback activation of EGFR. *Nature*, 483(7387), 100–103.

Ruppert, D., Wand, MP. and Carroll, RJ. (2003). *Semiparametric Regression*. Cambridge: Cambridge University Press.

Schmidli, H., Gsteiger, S., Roychoudhury, S., O'Hagan, A., Speigelhalter, D., Neuenschwander, B. (2014). Robust meta-analytic-predictie priors in clinical trials with historical control information. *Biometrics*, 70(4), 1023–1032.

Simon R. (1989). Optimal two-stage designs for phase II clinical trials. *Controlled Clinical Trials*, 10(1), 1–10.

Sinha, D., Chen, MH., Ghosh, SK. (1999). Bayesian analysis and model selection for interval-censored survival data. *Biometrics*, 55(2), 585–590.

Spiegelhalter, DJ., Best, NG., Carlin, BP. and van der Linde, A. (2002). Bayesian measures of model complexity and fit (with discussion). *Journal of the Royal Statistical Society: Series B (Statistical Methodology)*, 64(4), 583–639.

Tang, R., Shen, J., Yuan, Y. (2018). ComPAS: A Bayesian drug combination platform trial design with adaptive shrinkage. *Statistics in Medicine*, 38(7), 1120–1134.

Tiacci, E., Trifonov, V., Schiavoni, G., Holmes, A., Kern, W., Martelli, MP., Pucciarini, A., Bigerna, B., Pacini, R., Wells, VA. and Sportoletti, P. (2011). BRAF mutations in hairy-cell leukemia. *New England Journal of Medicine*, 364(24), 2305–2315.

Thall, PF., Wathen, JK., Bekele, BN., Champlin, RE., Baker, LH. and Benjamin, RS. (2003). Hierarchical Bayesian approaches to phase II trials in diseases with multiple subtypes. *Statistics in Medicine*, 22(5), 763–780.

Thall PF, Wooten LH, Tannir NM. (2005). Monitoring event times in early phase clinical trials: some practical issues. *Clinical Trials*, 2(6), 467–478.

Topalian, SL., Weiner, GJ. and Pardoll, DM. (2011). Cancer immunotherapy comes of age. *Journal of Clinical Oncology*, 29(36), 4828–4836.

Woodcock, J., LaVange, L. (2017). Master protocols to study multiple therapies, multiple diseases, or both. *The New England Journal of Medicine*, 377(1), 62–70.

Yan, Wang, and Yuan, Ying. (2021). *Bayesian Adaptive Designs for Oncology Clinical Trials (in Chinese)*, People's Medical Publishing House Co.

Yin, G. (2011). *Clinical Trial Design*. Wiley.

Yuan Y, Yin G. (2011). Bayesian phase I/II adaptively randomized oncology trials with combined drugs. *The Annals of Applied Statistics*, 5(2A), 924–942.

Yuan, Y., Nguyen, HQ., Thall, PF. (2016). *Bayesian designs for phase I-II clinical trials*. CRC Press.

Yuan Y, Guo B, Munsell M, Lu K, Jazaeri A. (2016). MIDAS: a practical Bayesian design for platform trials with molecularly targeted agents. *Statistics in Medicine*, 35(22), 3892–3906.

Woodcock, J. and LaVange, LM. (2017). Master protocols to study multiple therapies, multiple diseases, or both. *New England Journal of Medicine*, 377(1), 62–70. doi: 10.1056/NEJMra1510062.

3

Validation Strategy for Biomarker-Guided Precision/Personalized Medicine

Yan Hou[1], Meijuan Li[2], and Kang Li[3]

[1]*Peking University, Beijing, China*

[2]*Foundation Medicine, Inc., Cambridge, MA, USA*

[3]*Harbin Medical University, Harbin City, Heilongjiang Province, China*

CONTENTS

DOI: 10.1201/9781003107323-3

3.1 Introduction

3.1.1 Definitions and Types of Biomarkers

In early 2016, the Food and Drug Administration (FDA) and the National Institutes of Health (NIH) published the first version of the glossary included in the Biomarkers, Endpoints and Other Tools (BEST) resource. A biomarker is defined as a characteristic which is measured as an indicator of normal biological processes, pathogenic processes, or responses to an exposure or intervention, including therapeutic interventions. Biomarker modalities include molecular, histologic, radiographic, or physiologic characteristics.

The seven categories of biomarkers are defined in the BEST glossary, which covers susceptibility/risk, diagnostic, monitoring, prognostic, predictive, pharmacodynamic/response and safety. The susceptibility/risk biomarker indicates the potential for developing a disease or medical condition in an individual who does not currently have the clinically apparent disease or the medical condition. These biomarkers may be detected many years before the appearance of clinical signs and symptoms. The diagnostic biomarker is used to detect or confirm the presence of a disease condition of interest or to identify subpopulation with a specific disease. The clinical sensitivity and specificity of the biomarker and the analytical performance of the detection method influence the biomarker test. The monitoring biomarker measures repeatedly for assessing the status of a disease or medical condition or for evidence of exposure to (or effect of) a medical product or an environmental agent. These measurements focus on the change in the biomarker's value. The prognostic biomarker is used to identify the likelihood of a clinical event, disease recurrence, or progression in patients who have the disease or medical condition of interest. These biomarkers are always identified from observational data and used to identify patients more likely to have a particular outcome (Polley et al. 2019, Scirica et al. 2016). The predictive biomarker is used to identify individuals who are more likely to respond to exposure to a particular medical product or environmental agent. The response could be a symptomatic benefit, improved survival, or an adverse effect. Prognostic biomarkers and predictive biomarkers cannot generally be distinguished when only patients who have received a particular therapy are studied (Nalejska et al. 2014).

To identify a predictive biomarker, it is common to compare a new therapeutic with a control in patients with and without the biomarker. A representative example of developing a predictive biomarker in medical product is predictive enrichment of the study population for a randomized controlled clinical trial, in which the biomarker is used either to select overall population or to stratify patients into biomarker positive and biomarker negative groups, with the primary endpoint being the effect in the biomarker positive group (FDA 2019). For instance, serum Vascular endothelial Growth Factor (VEGF) and fibronectin can predict clinical response to interleukin-2 (IL-2) therapy of patients with metastatic melanoma and renal cell carcinoma, and high levels of these proteins correlate with lacking clinical response to IL-2 therapy and shortening overall survival of patients (Sabatino et al. 2009). The pharmacodynamic/response shows that a biological response has occurred in an individual who has been exposed to a medical product or an environmental agent. Since these biomarkers do not necessarily reflect the effect of an intervention on a future clinical event, they may not be accepted surrogate endpoints. The safety is measured before or after an exposure to a medical product or an environmental agent to indicate the likelihood, presence, or extent of toxicity as an adverse effect. Ideally, a safety biomarker would be a signal of developing toxicity prior to clinical signs and before any irreversible damage occurs. In summary, biomarkers are used to diagnose medical conditions or predict risks of condition of interest, detect signs of medical condition in the early stage, choose the optimal treatment for patients, speed up effective drugs with few adverse events into market, provide the comprehensive picture of events and alternation over time within a cell or body.

3.1.2 Precision Medicine and Companion Diagnostic Device

Due to biological variability, only a subset of patients may benefit from therapeutic products. Indeed, a number of therapeutic products have been approved only for particular patient subpopulations (de Weers et al. 2011, Roth and Diller 2014, Grilo and Mantalaris 2019). Precision medicine stratifies patients by biological information (e.g., genes, RNA/DNA, proteins) and targets those patients most likely to respond to a specific treatment. While a number of names have evolved in this field, such as targeted treatment, individualized care and stratified treatments, the current preferred term is "precision medicine". With the development of whole genomic data sequencing, new disease pathways relevant to this disease are being discovered and more and more new therapeutic targets, as well as adverse drug effects and effective subpopulations, are being identified. Precision medicine treatment targets only responders, which means there is an increase in tolerability and treatment adherence in the clinical trials (Hersom and Jorgensen 2018, Hwang et al. 2015, Lin et al. 2017). It in turn improves health outcomes and ultimately, makes more efficient use of limited health services. Despite these achievements, the promise of personalized medicine for the right treatment, for the right patient, at the right time will remain unfulfilled without strong support for a Companion Diagnostic (CDx) test. CDx tests detect specific genetic mutations and biomarkers in those patients who are most likely to respond to precision medicine treatment, thus reduce the number of patients treated.

A CDx is officially defined as an In Vitro Diagnostic (IVD) device that provides information that is essential for the safe and effective use of a corresponding therapeutic product (FDA 2014). The FDA emphasizes four subareas for a CDx, and they are (i) identify patients who are most likely to benefit from the therapeutic product, (ii) identify patients likely to be at increased risk for serious adverse reactions as a result of treatment with the therapeutic product, (iii) monitor response to treatment with the therapeutic product for the purpose of adjusting treatment to achieve improved safety or effectiveness, and (iv) identify patients in the population for whom the therapeutic product has been adequately studied, and found to be safe and effective (FDA 2014). In the past few years, an increasing number of predictive biomarker assays have been developed to guide anticancer treatment (Harigopal et al. 2020, Hersom and Jorgensen 2018, Rothschild 2014, Shaw et al. 2014, Twomey and Zhang 2021). Prior to the entry of individuals into a clinical trial, CDx might identify a population that has a higher likelihood of response and safety. Recently, the CDx is often developed in parallel to the drug using the drug-diagnostic co-development model (Jorgensen and Hersom 2016, Mansfield 2014, Watanabe 2015) (Figure 3.1).

According to the FDA requirements, a CDx must be included in the indications for use in the labeling instructions for both the co-developed therapeutic product as well as the specific diagnostic device (FDA 2014). A complementary diagnostic is a medical device or test (typically a 'predictive biomarker assay') that aids the therapeutic decision-making process and which provides information that is helpful for the safe and effective use of a particular biological product. A complementary diagnostic can inform on improving the benefit/risk ratio (improve disease management, early diagnosis, patient risk stratification and drug monitoring) without restricting drug access (Scheerens et al. 2017). Complementary diagnostic tests were referred to but no requirement from a regulatory perspective to link

Drug Development

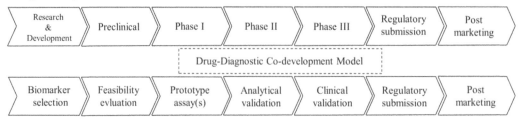

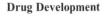

Diagnostic Development

FIGURE 3.1
Drug-diagnostic co-development model.

to a specific therapeutic, but complementary IVD information is included in the therapeutic product labeling(FDA 2014, Mansfield 2014). The Human Epidermal Growth Factor Receptor (HER) family of receptors plays a central role in the pathogenesis of several human cancers. They regulate cell growth, survival and differentiation via multiple signal transduction pathways and participate in cellular proliferation and differentiation. The family is made up of four main members: HER-1, HER-2, HER-3 and HER-4, also called ErbB1, ErbB2, ErbB3 and ErbB4, respectively (Riese and Stern 1998). The HER2 expression tests therapy is a CDx (Wolff et al. 2013). The subtype in breast cancer is not only used for patient stratification but also suitable for prognosis. The different biomarker purposes described are based on the clinical information obtained by the analysis. With the increasing use of biomarkers in daily routines, health authorities such as the European Medicines Agency (EMA) and the FDA have established guidance to regulate how to qualify and validate new biomarkers and the respective pre-analytical and analytical technology assays used to measure (EMA 2013, FDA 2014, Mansfield 2014). FDA approves for PD-L1immuno-histochemistry (IHC) 28-8 pharmDx complementary diagnostics in non-small cell lung cancer (NSCLC) for the cancer immunotherapy OPDIVO® (nivolumab) (Borghaei et al. 2015), and in recent years the FDA approves companion diagnostic for Nivolumab plus Ipilimumab in NSCLC(Hellmann et al. 2019, Hersom and Jorgensen 2018).

3.2 Validation Strategy of Biomarker Guided Therapy-Regulatory Perspectives

3.2.1 Clinical Validation of CDx Device and the Corresponding Therapeutic Product

Clinical validation is defined as the process that evaluates whether the biomarker can identify, measure, or predict a meaningful clinical, biological, physical, functional state, or experience in the specified context of use (FDA 2011, FDA 2018). The accuracy, precision and reliability of clinical validation determine the importance of a tool to be used in a specific clinical research setting and how to meaningfully interpret results. Clinical validation is conducted by planning to use, or promote the use of the biomarker in a specific patient population or for a special purpose. In clinical practice, sponsors of new therapeutic products are the primary entities conducting clinical validation. If new indication of an existing medical product would be developed, then the sponsor would be required to conduct clinical validation of biomarkers they use to make labeling claims. Evaluating the clinical utility of a novel biomarker requires a phased approach. Early-phase studies must prove that the biomarker is statistically associated with the clinical state of interest and provides sufficient information about the risk of disease status, the impacts of health and clinical decision above and beyond established biomarkers. Mid-phase studies describe how often this incremental change might alter decisions-making process.

3.2.2 Biomarker-Guided Trial Design

Biomarker-directed therapies from discovery to clinical practice are complex. The assay validation of biomarker assessment methods for reliability and reproducibility should be taken into consideration. For instance, when it comes to different assessment methods for multitudes of biomarkers, such as circulating tumor cells, Immunohistochemistry (IHC) and next generation sequencing and so on, how to validate them become so complex. Importantly, the choice of biomarker-guided trial design for biomarker validation is critical. This chapter focuses on trial designs for biomarker validation, including in the setting of the early-phase trials and confirmatory trials. The former mainly include those collecting data from previously well-conducted, Randomized Controlled Trials(RCTs) and the latter mainly consists of enrichment, all-comer and adaptive enrichment designs, (Mandrekar and Sargent 2011).

3.2.2.1 Retrospective Design

Limited to the time and expense required for prospective trials, it is an effective solution to test the performance of a biomarker using data from previously well-designed RCTs or a cohort or even a single-arm study that compare the performance of therapies performance stratified by a biomarker or a panel of biomarkers. The data from an RCT provides fundamentally essential for retrospective validation. In a single-arm or nonrandomized design, more complex statistical analysis methods are used to isolate the possible causal effect of the biomarker on therapeutic efficacy from the multitude of other factors that may influence the individualized decision (Mandrekar and Sargent 2009).

When the retrospective validation is appropriately conducted, it can help provide effective treatments to biomarker-defined patient subgroups in a timely manner that might otherwise be impossible due to ethical considerations. In particular, if a retrospective validation can be performed with data from two independent RCTs, this is considered to provide strong evidence for a robust predictive effect. One example that has been successfully validated using data collected from previous RCTs is KRAS, which is defined as a predictive biomarker of efficacy of panitumumab and cetuximab in metastatic colorectal cancer (Amado et al. 2008). In a prospectively specified analysis of data from a previously conducted randomized phase III trial of panitumumab versus best supportive care, KRAS status was assessed on 92% patients, and 43% having the KRAS mutation. The Hazard Ratio (HR) for treatment effect comparing panitumumab versus best supportive care on progression-free survival in the wild-type and mutant subgroups was 0.45 and 0.99, respectively, with a significant treatment by KRAS status interaction. This is representative of retrospective validation in the clinical trial with well-conducted RCTs.

As we know, the gold standard for predictive biomarker validation continues is a prospective RCT. Several designs have been developed and utilized in the field of clinical oncology for biomarker validation (Dong et al. 2016, Kubo et al. 2016, Lee et al. 2016, Perrone et al. 2016, Schultz et al. 2018, Sun et al. 2017, Zhang et al. 2017). Mandrekar and Sargent

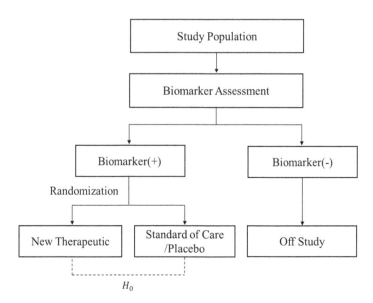

FIGURE 3.2
Enrichment design in which only biomarker-positive patients can benefit.

(2009) classify these designs into target/enrichment designs, unselected or all-comers designs and adaptive enrichment designs. The advantages and disadvantages along with real examples for these designs are presented.

3.2.2.2 Enrichment Design

Enrichment aims to utilize patient characteristics, such as demographic, pathophysiologic and genetic, to explore and identify the subpopulations that are more likely to respond to drug or other medical intervention. It can increase study power by decreasing heterogeneity and choosing an appropriate subpopulation. It also can identify a population with different outcome events, i.e., patients with severe disease or those in high-risk disease, which is called prognostic enrichment. In addition, it still can identify the subpopulation capable of responding to the treatment, which is called predictive enrichment.

Enrichment designs are always based on the paradigm that not all patients will benefit from the study treatment, but rather a subgroup of patients with a specific molecular feature (FDA 2019). This design, therefore, results in treatment benefit in the subgroup of the patient population defined by a specific marker status (Figure 3.2). This design is recommended to be used in the early stage to detect the unequivocal drug effect, and not the only study, at least not often. For example, HER2–positive patients demonstrate that trastuzumab (Herceptin; Genentech, South San Francisco, CA) combined with paclitaxel after doxorubicin and cyclophosphamide significantly improved Disease-Free Survival (DFS) among women with surgically removed HER2-positive breast cancer (Romond et al. 2005).

Two main issues should be considered in the enrichment design. Firstly, the reproducibility and accuracy of the assay must be well established before launching the trial, particularly the one with an enrichment design strategy. Second, it should sufficiently illustrate that patients with biomarker positive can benefit from this new therapy while the ones with negative biomarkers would not benefit from the same treatment (FDA 2019, Mandrekar and Sargent 2009). Generally speaking, three conditions are particularly appropriate for enrichment designs: (i) when therapies have modest absolute benefit in the unselected population, but might cause significant toxicity, (ii) therapeutic results are similar whereby a selection design would decrease damage to organs or not hurt, and (iii) an unselected design is ethically impossible based on previous studies.

3.2.2.3 Unselect or All-Comers Designs

In the unselected or all-comers designs, all patients who meet the eligibility criteria are enrolled into the trial. These designs can be further classified into sequential testing strategy designs, marker-based designs, or hybrid designs. These designs differentiate from each other by the protocol which specifies an approach to pre-specify or control overall type I and type II error rates, perform hypothesis testing (including a single hypothesis test, multiple tests, or sequential tests), and make a randomization schema. The critical considerations of these designs along with examples have been presented.

3.2.2.3.1 Sequential Testing Strategy Designs

Sequential testing designs are similar in principle to a standard RCT design with a single primary hypothesis, that is either tested in the marker-defined subgroup (denoted as $H_0^{(1)}$) first, and then tested in the entire population ($H_0^{(2)}$) if the subgroup analysis is significant, or in the overall population ($H_0^{(2)}$) first and then in a prospectively planned subset ($H_0^{(1)}$) (Figure 3.3). The first case is recommended where the treatment is assumed to be broadly effective, and the subset analysis is secondary. The latter (known as the closed testing procedure) is recommended when preliminary evidence strongly support that the treatment effect is the best in the biomarker-defined subgroup. Both these strategies are required to appropriately control for the type I error rates at the prespecified level in order to avoid inflating. Taking into account potential correlation arising from testing the overall treatment effect and the treatment effect within the biomarker-defined subgroup has also been proposed.

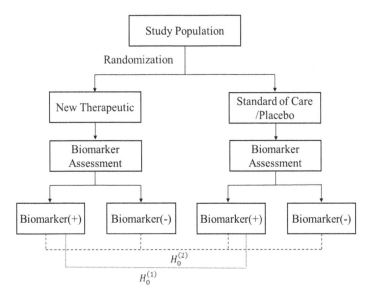

FIGURE 3.3
Sequential testing strategy design in which both biomarker-positive and biomarker-negative patients can benefit.

A typical example for this design comes from a US-based phase III trial testing cetuximab in addition to infusional fluorouracil, leucovorin and oxaliplatin as adjuvant therapy in metastatic colon cancer (Amado et al. 2008). While the trial has been amended to accrue patients only with KRAS–wild-type tumors, approximately 800 patients with KRAS mutant tumors have already been enrolled. The primary analysis in this study was performed at the prespecified 0.05 level in the patients with wild-type KRAS. A sample size of 1,035 patients with wild-type KRAS per arm would result in 515 total events, providing 90% power to detect an HR of 1.33 for this comparison using a two-sided log-rank test at a significance level of 0.05. If this subset analysis is statistically significant at significance level, then the efficacy of the regimen in the entire population will also be tested at 0.05 level, as this is a closed testing procedure. This comparison using all 2,910 patients will have 90% power to detect an HR of 1.27 comparing the two treatment arms, based on a total of 735 events.

3.2.2.3.2 Biomarker-Stratified Designs

The biomarker-stratified design aims to randomly assign patients into different intervention groups either based on the biomarker status. This design includes patients with both biomarker positive and biomarker negative who are treated with the same regimen, resulting in a significant overlap (driven by the prevalence of the marker) in the number of patients receiving the same treatment regimen in both arms (Figure 3.4). Three essential characteristics in biomarker-stratified designs were found as follows: (i) patients with a valid biomarker test result are randomized, (ii) prospectively specified sample size within each marker-based subgroup, (iii) biomarker-based randomization.

For settings where there is a candidate biomarker but not sufficient basis for using it to restrict eligibility, the biomarker stratified design is more appropriate. An example of the biomarker stratified design is known as MARVEL (Marker Validation of Erlotinib in Lung Cancer), of second-line therapy in patients with advanced non-small-cell lung cancer

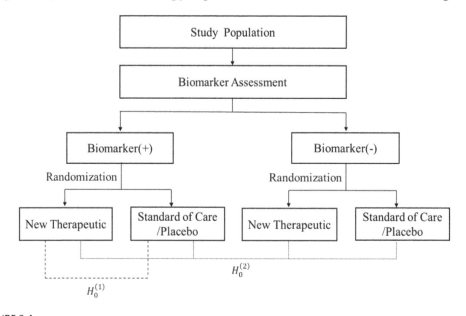

FIGURE 3.4
Biomarker-stratified designs in which both biomarker-positive and Biomarker-negative patients are randomly assigned to the new therapeutic under investigation.

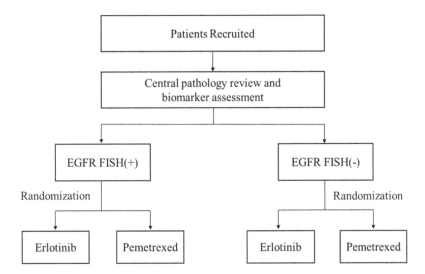

FIGURE 3.5
MARVEL (Marker Validation for Erlotinib in Lung Cancer) trial design. Stratified factors in this study: Eastern Cooperative Oncology Group (ECOG) performance status, gender, smoking status, histology, best response to prior chemotherapy. EGFR, epidermal growth factor receptor; FISH, fluorescent in situ hybridization.

(NSCLC) randomly assigned to pemetrexed or erlotinib (Figure 3.5). The detailed information can be seen in Twilt (2016). Stratifying the randomization is useful in particular because it ensures that all the patients enrolled in this study have received the treatment. However, the challenging issues in a prospective analysis plan include how to measure the test result which would be used in the primary analysis, how to control Family-Wise Error Rate (FWER), and how to determine the primary objective.

3.2.2.3.3 Hybrid Designs

Hybrid designs can be used when there is compelling prior evidence which shows detrimental effect of the experimental treatment for a specific biomarker-defined subgroup (i.e., biomarker-negative subgroup) or some indication of its possible excessive toxicity in that subgroup, thus making it unethical to randomize the patients within this population to the experimental treatment (Curran et al. 2012, Landes et al. 2019). This is shown in Figure 3.6.

This design is powered to detect differences in outcomes only in the biomarker-defined subgroup that is randomized to treatment choices based on the marker status, similar to an enrichment design strategy. However, unlike the enrichment design, the hybrid design provides additional information. Since all patients are screened for marker status to determine whether they are randomly assigned or assigned the Standard of Care (SOC), it seems prudent to include and collect specimens and follow-up these patients in the trial to allow for future testing for other potential prognostic markers in this population. This design is an appropriate choice when there is compelling prior evidence demonstrating the efficacy of a specific biomarker-defined treatment, thereby making it ethical to randomly assign patients with that particular marker status to this therapeutic.

3.2.2.4 Adaptive Enrichment Design

An adaptive enrichment design prospectively specifies a requirement on how the design elements can be modified to adapt to information accrued during the course of the trial,

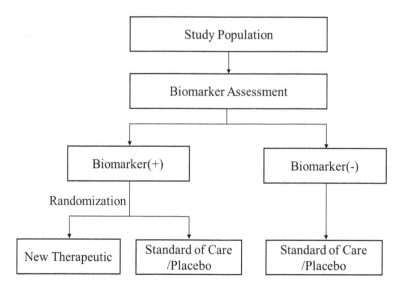

FIGURE 3.6
Hybrid design in which both biomarker-positive and biomarker-negative patients can benefit.

such as sample size adjustment, entry criteria revision and enrollment restriction to a sub-population based on interim analysis (Simon and Simon 2013). A typical example with adaptive enrichment design is displayed in Figure 3.7. Depending on the credentials of markers for patient enrichment, adaptive enrichment strategies can be classified as:

3.2.2.4.1 Adaptively Modifying Patient Enrollment

A randomized controlled trial can enroll both biomarker-positive and biomarker-negative patients. The trial can continue to enroll both subsets of patients if the interim analysis

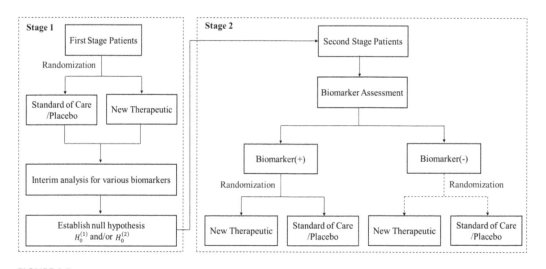

FIGURE 3.7
Adaptive enrichment design flowchart when the efficacy of biomarker-negative patients is much lower than that of biomarker-positive patients, enrollment of marker-negative patients could be reduced or stopped entirely.

results indicated the efficacy of biomarker-negative patients are not much worse than that of biomarker-positive patients within futility boundary; otherwise, accrual is limited to biomarker-positive patients until the originally planned total sample size is reached. A similar enrichment strategy involves enrolling only biomarker-positive patients during the initial stage, and continuously enrolling biomarker-positive patients and commencing accrual of biomarker-negative patients if interim results are not promising in biomarker-positive patients; otherwise, accrual stops.

3.2.2.4.2 Adaptive Threshold Strategy

It is assumed that a pre-specified biomarker score is given before launching the trial. However, the cut-off point for converting the score into a binary classifier that can maximize treatment effect in a subpopulation is unknown. Jiang (2007) describe an analysis plan in which the outcomes of all patients receiving the treatment were compared with control. If the difference is significant at pre-specified type I error rate, the new treatment is considered effective for the accrued patient population as a whole. Otherwise, a second stage test is performed using a pre-defined threshold of type I error rate, with the aim of finding the optimal cut-off point of the biomarker score for which the treatment effect is maximized in patients with biomarker scores above the threshold. The biomarker-adaptive threshold design is quite similar to the sequential testing strategy designs and can be implemented one of two ways: the new treatment is compared with the control in all patients at a prespecified significance level, and if not significant, a second stage analysis involving identifying an optimal threshold for the predictive marker is performed using the remaining alpha; or under the assumption that the treatment is effective only for a biomarker-driven subset, no overall treatment to control comparisons are made, instead, the analysis focuses on the identification of optimal threshold.

3.2.2.4.3 Adaptive Signature Design

Freidlin and Simon propose a design for the classifier development and the treatment effect evaluation in a single trial where the data were separated for developing classifier from the data used for evaluating treatment effect in subsets determined by the classifier (Freidlin and Simon 2005). The method involves dividing the data into a training set and a test set, using the training set to define a subset of patients who are most likely to benefit from the new treatment than from the control and then the test set to evaluate the treatment effects in patients who show the characteristics defined by that subset. In clinical practice, an external and independent dataset is preferred to evaluate the performance of this classifier.

In brief, three conditions are particularly appropriate for adaptive enrichment strategy: (i)treatment effect is uncertain in biomarker-positive and biomarker-negative patients before launching the trial, (ii)enrollment criteria revision may help increase accrual of a better responding subset, and (iii)the precise information on the performance of biomarker threshold values is unclear at the planning stage, in which defining an optimal cut-off value is needed to determine the enrichment subset.

3.2.3 Analytical Validation

The role of biomarkers in drug discovery and development has gained precedence over the years. As biomarkers become integrated into drug development and clinical trials, quality assurance and in particular assay validation becomes essential with the need to establish standardized guidelines for analytical methods used in biomarker measurements. The

FDA provides a precise depiction including quality aspects for the biomarker itself as well as for the assay according to measure it. Pursuant to the FDA definition, a valid biomarker assay is a biomarker measured in an analytical test system with well-established performance characteristics and for which an established scientific framework or body of evidence that elucidates the physiological, toxicologic, pharmacologic or clinical significance of the test results. Biomarker measurement can be assessed at different biological levels with different technologies; thus, the appropriate choice of the assay depends on both the application condition of the biomarker and the limitations of current technology. A number of assays can be used in the biomarker method validation process and range from the relatively low technology end such as IHC to immunoassays to the high technology end including platforms for genomics, proteomics and multiplex ligand-binding assays. For the clinical application beyond research, test systems for biomarker analysis need to be technically validated. The validation should cover the complete process including the use of the correct sample matrix, preanalytical procedures and the analytical measurement. The technical validation of biomarkers depends on all aspects of the analytical method including assay sensitivity, specificity, reliability and reproducibility (Findlay et al. 2000, Lee et al. 1995, Miller et al. 2001). Therefore, these factors should be taken into account. The validation process should consider additional factors, including regulatory requirements, potential risks for the patient associated with sampling procedures and operational risks for a drug program.

3.2.4 Biomarker Qualification

The FDA's Critical Path Initiative called for the establishment of a biomarker qualification process to enable progress in the drug development paradigm. In response to this, the Center for Drug Evaluation and Research (CDER) established a Biomarker Qualification Program (BQP) to qualify a biomarker for a specific Context of Use (COU). The BQP provides information to qualify biomarkers and make supporting information publicly available; to facilitate uptake of qualified biomarkers in the regulatory review process, and to encourage the identification of new biomarkers to be used in drug development and regulatory decision-making. Once a biomarker is qualified, sponsors can use it for the qualified COU in drug development programs without CDER review of the supporting information.

The FDA has issued guidance for industry on pharmacogenomic data submissions and in classifying the various types of genomic biomarkers and their degree of validity: exploratory biomarkers, probable valid biomarkers and known valid biomarkers (Park et al. 2004). Exploratory biomarkers lay the fundamental for probable or known valid biomarkers and can be used to fill in gaps of uncertainty about disease targets or variability in drug response, bridge the results of animal model studies to clinical expectation, or used for the selection of new compounds. The qualification process is introduced to bridge the gap from an exploratory biomarker to a probable or known valid biomarker and this validation process requires an efficient and reliable process map for biomarker validation. The exploratory biomarkers are helpful to fill in gaps of uncertainty about disease targets or variability in drug response, bridge the results of animal model studies to clinical expectation, or used for the selection of new compounds(Lesko and Atkinson 2001). A probable valid biomarker seems to have predictive performance for clinical outcomes but has not been widely accepted. The advancement from probable valid to known valid lies in the achievement of a broad consensus in cross-validation experiments which include the independent validation of the biomarker by replicating the outcome at different sites.

A known valid biomarker is defined as "a biomarker that is measured in an analytical test system with well-established performance characteristics and for which there is widespread agreement in the medical or scientific community about the physiologic, toxicologic, pharmacologic, or clinical significance of the test results." In the case of a process map that involves the biomarker validation in clinical trials, the regulatory agency will review the biomarker validation package in terms of the usefulness of the predictive biomarker in clinical benefit.

Biomarker qualification is also observed in the co-development of biomarkers (in the form of diagnostic tests) and drugs with the use of these biomarkers limited to the drug's application. Co-development imposes the necessity to generate specific guidelines describing analytical test validation, clinical test validation and clinical utility. To qualify a biomarker, the biomarker data should be reproducible and the studies should have adequate power to detect if the biomarker can be used as indicated in its COU. Thus, statistical design and analysis issues become important components of a biomarker qualification.

3.2.4.1 Design Considerations

As the biomarker or a panel of biomarkers moves from discovery phase to its confirmatory phase, key design elements, such as study statistical power, sample size, hypothesis-testing and analysis plan become increasingly important considerations. An early discussion with the Biomarker Qualification Review Team (BQRT) is highly recommended because each qualification is unique. Key design issues are the following:

3.2.4.1.1 Identification

Biomarker identification is a challenging issue, especially for composite biomarkers. Statistical methods for evaluating multiple predictors such as regression models with multiple covariates, ridge regression or Least Absolute Shrinkage and Selection Operator (LASSO) methods may be considered. Approaches such as tree-based, Support Vector Machine (SVM) or other machine learning methods may be able to identify nonlinear relationships and be more intuitive to clinicians.

3.2.4.1.2 Biomarker Levels

In some scenarios, the baseline measure of the biomarker is the desired measure, and a change in biomarker level is also needed. In the latter situation, biomarker levels are often measured relative to a baseline. When the intra-subject variability is greater than inter-subject variability, the linear change from baseline better characterizes the expression, while the relative change from baseline is preferred when the opposite holds.

3.2.4.1.3 Threshold

A good threshold is needed to distinguish patients with and without meaningfully different increases in the biomarker levels. Definition of the threshold can be complicated and may involve single or multiple time points, so care must be taken to establish relevance for each component of the COU, such as disease severity, intended population and sample size revision. Proper selection of thresholds is an important consideration for replicability and this concern can be mitigated if a large number of patients highly representative of the study population. The model selected to investigate the threshold should be as parsimonious as possible to avoid overfitting. Multiplicity may also be an issue when selecting thresholds.

3.2.4.1.4 *Reference Standards*

When a new biomarker is developed, no established gold standard biomarker can be used for comparing biomarker performance relative to the outcome of interest. In that situation, the use of all available information is a pragmatic approach. If a pseudo-gold standard is used as a reference, the new biomarker may have a lack of sensitivity, and its estimation may be biased. The extent of this bias depends on the correlation between the new and pseudo-gold standard biomarker. The use of adjudication committees to look at the event/nonevent data and how well the biomarker relates to the outcome may be considered to mitigate concern about bias.

3.2.4.2 **Analysis Considerations**

A prespecified, well-defined statistical analysis plan is critical in establishing the scientific credibility of a biomarker. A few key analysis considerations will be discussed:

3.2.4.2.1 *Cross-Validation (CV)*

CV plays an important role in learn and confirm paradigm. Traditionally, the data are split into a training and validation set or carried forward in a k-fold validation. However, the ideal validation should be performed in an externally independent set.

3.2.4.2.2 *Analysis Plan*

Important considerations when developing the analysis plan at the confirmatory stage include the following: (i) each hypothesis of interest relevant to the COU must be pre-specified, along with its relevant analysis plan; (ii) multiplicity adjustments, procedures to handle missing data and plans for any secondary comparison must be clearly described; (iii) if any confirmatory subgroup analysis is planned, it should be pre-specified with a cross validation or sequential testing strategy to prevent inflation of experiment-wise type I error.

3.2.4.2.3 *Interim Analysis*

Interim analyses are often pre-specified in the protocol and should be performed in both learning and confirming phases to ensure that the biomarkers are performing as expected. In earlier interim analysis the initial performance is judged by the learning phase criteria, modify biomarker thresholds or re-estimate sample size. Later interim may be to assess the performance improvements based on the modifications, including thresholds or to stop the trial based on futility. Each planned interim look needs to clearly identify its objective and any associated sample size re-estimation and the effect of the interim analysis on Type I error. If a limited COU is initially planned, the interim analysis may guide future development plans based on the learning phase information.

3.2.4.2.4 *Statistical Considerations in Biomarker Qualification*

An analytically validated method must be accepted to measure the biomarker. The relevant indices, such as Receiver Operation Characteristics (ROC), sensitivity and specificity of assay, normal ranges and variability of measurements. Patient characteristics or covariates that have an effect on biomarker expression should also be taken into account.

3.3 Complex Innovative Study Designs in Precision Medicine

3.3.1 Innovative Study Designs

3.3.1.1 Basket Trials Design for Integral Biomarkers

A basket trial studies a single targeted therapy among patients with multiple disease types or histology but characterized by a corresponding biomarker (Figure 3.8). Basket trial designs may be practically viewed as a collection of enrichment designs across different disease types or histology, it can be more efficient than multiple histology-specific enrichment trials conducted separately and are convenient to carry out. For example, after the approval of vemurafenib for BRAFV600 mutation-positive metastatic melanoma, a phase II basket trial of vemurafenib for multiple nonmelanoma cancers with BRAFV600 mutation was conducted with an objective response as the primary endpoint (Kaley et al. 2018).

In addition, they also inherit all of the advantages and disadvantages, with the same practical considerations as elaborated earlier. One unique challenge facing basket trials is the balance between feasibility and the exchangeability (e.g., histology agnostic) hypothesis, given the potential heterogeneity across different disease types. Meanwhile, all patients enrolled with the same biomarker can be questionable if not at all unrealistic, since this approach ignores the prognosis heterogeneity across different histology and assume disease subtype is not prognostic at all. In the case of vemurafenib for patients with BRAFV600 mutations, response to treatment was high when the primary site was melanoma but low when the primary site was colorectal cancer. One important consideration when designing discovery basket trials is whether randomization should be used or not. The nonrandomized basket trial may be clearly preferred because of its feasibility and close connection to the conventional single-arm phase II design traditionally used in

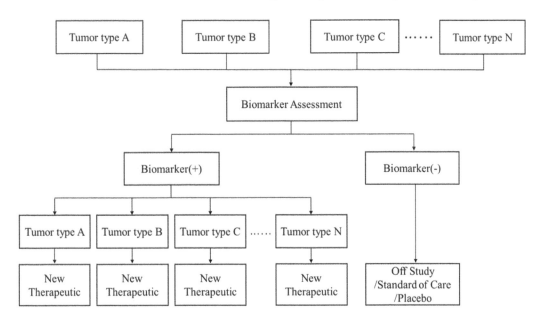

FIGURE 3.8
Basket trials for integral biomarkers.

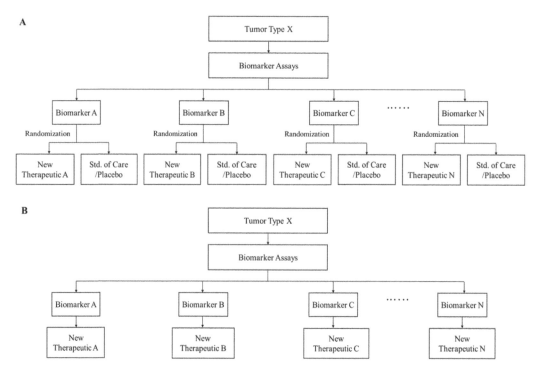

FIGURE 3.9
Umbrella trials for integral biomarkers with randomization (A) and nonrandomization (B).

early-stage development. However, nonrandomized basket design practically mandates objective response to be the only choice of the primary endpoint, because it is generally considered the only interpretable efficacy endpoint without a comparator.

3.3.1.2 Umbrella Trials for Multiple Integral Biomarkers

Multiple experimental therapeutics within a single disease histology are evaluated with umbrella design. A centralized molecular screening platform and a multiplex assay are used to simultaneously obtain the biomarkers that determine eligibility and treatment. Patients with biomarkers of interest are allocated into mutually exclusive biomarker-specific sub-trials, which use either nonrandomized or randomized enrichment designs (Figure 3.9). Statistical considerations, including sample size justification and interim analyses for efficacy and futility, are largely driven by needs within each of the sub-trials. Using sequential development features such as phase II/III designs and interim analyses that permit adaptation to findings, these trials adaptively provide the necessary flexibility for the umbrella trial objectives as a whole. When there are multiple candidate regimens that are of interest equally for some or all biomarker cohorts, umbrella trials also can be designed solely for discovery objectives. For example, in the BATTLE-1 trial, patients with chemotherapy-refractory NSCLC are assayed for four candidate biomarkers to be allocated to a total of five marker strata (including one nonmatched) and then randomly assigned to one of four drug regimens (Kim et al. 2011). One implication of conducting umbrella trials is that an explicit rule governing how to match biomarkers and candidate regimens needs to be pre-specified. Therefore, umbrella trials also provide a unique opportunity to evaluate whether a rule-based policy that matches biomarkers and drugs is effective.

3.3.1.3 Platform Trials

A common feature for both basket and umbrella trials is that within each biomarker-defined cohort a nonrandomized or randomized enrichment design is implemented. With the emergent use of molecular profiling, basket trials and umbrella trials, as well as extensions discussed here, can be collectively called platform trials. These trials consist of multiple enrichment sub-trials defined by molecular profiles and use a centralized screening platform and common data collection infrastructure. Such a protocol provides substantial flexibility in terms of discontinuing unpromising investigations, carrying forward favorable early results to definitive testing in a phase II/III framework, and introducing new sub trials as targets and agents are identified using the aforementioned adaptive design methods for single-biomarker settings. The NCI-MATCH (National Cancer Institute Molecular Analysis for Therapy Choice ClinicalTrials.gov identifier: NCT02465060) trial is a multiple targeted-therapy basket trial designed to evaluate whether biomarkers may exist in advanced solid tumors and lymphoma that are refractory to standard first-line therapy.

3.3.2 Statistical Consideration in Precision Medicine

As we know, the confirmatory subgroup is always clearly defined in the protocol, but it should be identified through exploratory analysis in early-stage clinical trials, as well as the throughout analysis from retrospective cohort. A number of statistical methods or machine learning methods have been developed to identify the subgroup based on biomarker(s), such as interactive tree, recursive splitting tree and regression model). The interactive tree can automatically identify the interaction and optimize the subgroup analysis in the best way, and most importantly, it can more effectively demonstrate the interaction between intervention and covariates. Since subgroup identification is essentially an exploratory study, it is mainly concerned with the interaction between the treatment and the co-participants and the consistency between the subgroups in terms of efficacy and futility analyses. Therefore, it is not necessary to control type I error.

Subgroup analysis for confirmatory clinical trials should be predefined in the protocol and analysis plan. In confirmatory clinical trials, FWER must be controlled in the strong sense. In other words, biomarker-based subgroup analyses in confirmatory clinical trials face the inflated type I error rate, i.e., the probability of erroneously concluding significant treatment effect when there is no effect in the study populations, due to multiple testing of treatment effects in subpopulations and overall population. These procedures ensure FWER control in a strong sense. The stepwise multiple testing procedure which asymptotically controls the familywise error rate at a desired level. Compared to related single-step methods, this procedure is more powerful since it often will reject more false hypotheses. Fallback procedure is another widely used technique in clinical trials to control the familywise error rate when multiple primary hypotheses are tested. Other procedures, such as Holm and Hochberg procedures, gatekeeping procedure and Hommel procedure.

3.3.2.1 Fixed Sequence Procedure

It is a stepwise multiple testing procedure that is constructed using a pre-specified sequence of hypotheses. When there are multiple hypotheses, these hypotheses can be ordered according to their importance. All tests will be performed at the 0.05 level following the pre-specified order. Once one hypothesis is tested not significantly, all subsequent

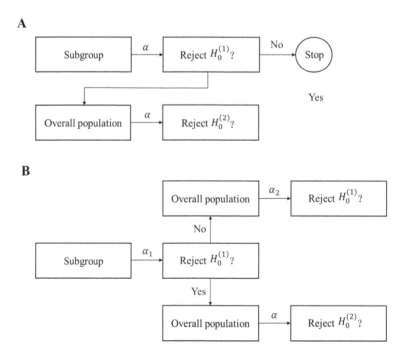

FIGURE 3.10
Multiple hypotheses with fixed sequential procedure (A) and fallback procedure (B) to control familywise error rate.

tests will not be performed (Figure 3.10 A). Power will be maximized as long as previous hypotheses are rejected, but minimized if a previous hypothesis is not rejected. Another disadvantage for this procedure is that the ordering of multiple hypotheses based on the clinical importance is subjective in nature.

3.3.2.2 Fallback Procedure

Unlike the standard Bonferroni adjustment, testing hypotheses with fallback procedure proceeds in an order determined a priori. As long as hypotheses are rejected, the type I error rate can be accumulated, later hypotheses are more powerful than under the Bonferroni procedure. Unlike the fixed sequence test, the fallback test allows that the full alpha of 0.05 is split for a series of hypotheses in a pre-specified order and the hypotheses in late order can still be tested if the previous hypothesis is not rejected (Figure 3.10 B) (Wiens 2003, Wiens and Dmitrienko 2005). However, Hommel and Bretz showed that in certain situations, the fallback procedure might violate the inherent hierarchical relationships among the hypotheses (Hommel and Bretz 2008). The details about fallback procedure can refer to (Dmitrienko et al. 2013, Wiens and Dmitrienko 2005, Wiens and Dmitrienko 2010), and for applications of fixed sequence multiple testing procedures in different fields, see Alosh and Huque (Alosh and Huque 2009, Alosh and Huque 2010). Qiu et al.(2015) also developed new multiple testing procedures to deal with the situation in which the hypotheses are pre-ordered based on prior knowledge and tested based on the p-values.

Notably, no procedure is universally optimal. The best procedure depends on the power to reject the various hypotheses, something that is never known with certainty, and the goals of the analyses. If the most important goal is to demonstrate a difference on the first hypothesis or all hypotheses, the fixed-sequence procedure performs best. However, the fixed sequence often has the highest chance of obtaining inconsistent results between the two independent studies, which makes it less appealing.

It is important to realize that predefined subpopulations are subsets of the overall population and the test statistics corresponding to the subpopulations and overall population are positively correlated. Therefore, using the joint distribution of the test statistics to determine the threshold values of test statistics can help improve the power of tests. However, it should be cautious of utilizing these methods in clinical practice and additional requirements from regulatory perspective should be taken into account. Because precision medicine research raises so many challenging issues that can only be solved by clinicians in multidisciplinary teams, basic scientists and statisticians who can collaborate on study design, analysis and interpretation.

3.4 Case Studies

3.4.1 Prognostic Enrichment—Oncology Studies

Trials intended to show reduced events or delayed recurrence of tumors are more likely to be approved in patients with high-risk for such events, such as genetic factors or other characteristics. For example,

a. Selection of high risk patients – Prostate cancer: D'Amico et al. (2004) report that in men with localized prostate cancer, the rate of rising in the Prostate-Specific Antigen (PSA) level, the PSA velocity (PSA increase > 2ng/ml during the prior year before diagnosis), predicts prostate cancer mortality after radical prostatectomy with almost 100% accuracy over a ten-year period. There were essentially few deaths from prostate cancer (many from other causes) and the recurrence rates were not that different. Therefore, to show a survival effect of a drug on patients with prostate cancer, a clinical trial must enroll patients with high risk of mortality.

b. Selection of high-risk patients – Breast cancer: Fan et al. (2006) applied five different gene-expression profiling methods, intended to identify a number of distinct prognostic profiles or gene sets to predict breast cancer recurrence rate, to 295 patient samples treated with local therapy: tamoxifen, tamoxifen plus chemotherapy, or chemotherapy alone. They found that four of the five gene profiling methods had high rates of concordance in their striking ability to predict the outcome, one of them is a 70-gene profile based on which the relapse-free survival and overall survival. The implications for patient selection are obvious, i.e., studies should select poorer prognosis patients to have a better chance of showing a drug effect, whether the endpoint is recurrence or survival.

3.4.2 Predictive Enrichment Design —Breast Cancer

Estrogen Receptors (ERs) and Progesterone Receptors (PRs) as biomarkers for response to endocrine therapy breast cancer: It has been shown that patients with breast cancer treated with tamoxifen, a selective estrogen receptor modulator, have a response rate of approximately 70% when their tumors express both ERs and PRs, have only 20% response rate when their tumors express either ERs or PRs, and have merely less than 5% response rate when their tumors are both ER and PR negative (Early Breast Cancer Trialists' Collaborative Group 2005). Therefore, testing breast cancer specimens for expression levels of ERs and PRs has been common practice for endocrine therapy decisions in early- and late-stage breast cancer treatment.

3.4.3 Predictive Enrichment – Melanoma

BRAF (B-Raf proto-oncogene) V600E as a biomarker to BRAF kinase inhibitor in melanoma: the BRAF encodes a cytoplasmic serine/threonine kinase regulates the mitogen-activated protein kinase signal transduction pathway, and controls several important cell functions including cell growth and proliferation. An activating mutation in codon 600 of exon 15 (V600E) of BRAF gene has been identified in multiple neoplasms, such as melanoma, colorectal carcinoma and Langerhans cell histiocytosis (Loo et al. 2018). A randomized phase III trial was performed to compare vemurafenib, a BRAF kinase inhibitor, with dacarbazine in patients who had metastatic or unresectable melanoma and BRAF V600E mutation. The results found that the response rate was 48% for patients who received vemurafenib versus 5% for those treated with dacarbazine, and that a relative reduction of 63% in the risk of death was associated with vemurafenib (Chapman et al. 2011).

3.4.4 Predictive Enrichment – MSI – High in PD-1/PD-L1

Microsatellite Instability (MSI) as a biomarker of response to immune checkpoint inhibitors: Programmed cell death protein 1/programmed cell death ligand one (PD-1/PD-L1) plays a crucial role in the progression of tumor by altering immune system. Therefore, PD-L1 protein expression detected by IHC can enrich for response to PD-1/PD-L1 inhibitors in a variety of tumor types. However, response rate of PD-1/PD-L1 inhibitors is only 10–20% in unselected patients, but 50% in Microsatellite Instability-high (MSI-high) tumors, which leads to FDA's approval of pembrolizumab in colorectal and endometrial carcinoma for MSI-high or deficient mismatch repair tumors (Havel et al. 2019, Kowanetz et al. 2018, Schrock et al. 2019).

3.4.5 Adaptive Enrichment Design – Breast Cancer

As another example that leads to regulatory approval, a clinical trial in women with newly diagnosed, locally advanced breast cancer is designed to evaluate the effect of investigational drugs added to standard of care compared with standard of care alone on pathological complete response rate. The treatment phase involves testing multiple investigational drugs that are thought to target identified tumor's biomarkers that are also used at baseline for selecting possibly responders. Interim responses are then used to inform treatment assignment strategies for patients who remain in the study (Barker et al. 2009).

3.5 Concluding Remarks

Speeding up new discoveries from bench to bedside is the ultimate goal of clinical and translational research. Analytical validity of a companion biomarker or diagnostic test whose development is just as critical as drug development. Analytical and clinical validation of biomarkers should be driven by a combination of scientific, clinical, statistical and ethical considerations and biological qualification is critical for the process. Biomarker-driven clinical trials allow us to investigate patient heterogeneity on the basis of molecular profiling, which consequently introduces new opportunities and challenges. Comparing with the conventional paradigm, biomarker-driven clinical trials have key design elements and practical challenges. These designs require more thorough planning and comprehensive evaluation on the study objectives, the credential of biomarker's clinical utility, different design and analysis plans, biological mechanism, evidence from preclinical and early clinical trials, prevalence of each subpopulation and so on. Precision medicine focuses on individual variations in genetics as well as differences in environments and lifestyles that will affect the efficacy and safety of a given treatment. When properly designed and implemented with adequate resources, especially appropriate validation methods, biomarker-driven clinical trials may efficiently and effectively generate evidence on biomarker-based personalized disease management, thereby enhanced opportunities for drug and companion diagnostics development.

References

Alosh, M. and M. F. Huque (2009). A flexible strategy for testing subgroups and overall population. *Stat Med*, **28**(1), 3–23.

Alosh, M. and M. F. Huque (2010). A consistency-adjusted alpha-adaptive strategy for sequential testing. *Stat Med*, **29**(15), 1559–1571.

Amado, R. G., M. Wolf, M. Peeters, et al. (2008). Wild-type KRAS is required for panitumumab efficacy in patients with metastatic colorectal cancer. *J Clin Oncol*, **26**(10), 1626–1634.

Barker, A. D., C. C. Sigman, G. J. Kelloff, et al. (2009). I-SPY 2: an adaptive breast cancer trial design in the setting of neoadjuvant chemotherapy. *Clin Pharmacol Ther*, **86**(1), 97–100.

Borghaei, H., L. Paz-Ares, L. Horn, et al. (2015). Nivolumab versus docetaxel in advanced nonsquamous non-small-cell lung cancer. *N Engl J Med*, **373**(17), 1627–1639.

Chapman, P. B., A. Hauschild, C. Robert, et al. (2011). Improved survival with vemurafenib in melanoma with BRAF V600E mutation. *N Engl J Med*, **364**(26), 2507–2516.

Curran, G. M., M. Bauer, B. Mittman, et al. (2012). Effectiveness-implementation hybrid designs: combining elements of clinical effectiveness and implementation research to enhance public health impact. *Med Care*, **50**(3), 217–226.

D'Amico, A. V., M. H. Chen, K. A. Roehl, et al. (2004). Preoperative PSA velocity and the risk of death from prostate cancer after radical prostatectomy. *N Engl J Med*, **351**(2), 125–135.

de Weers, M., Y. T. Tai, M. S. van der Veer, et al. (2011). Daratumumab, a novel therapeutic human CD38 monoclonal antibody, induces killing of multiple myeloma and other hematological tumors. *J Immunol*, **186**(3), 1840–1848.

Dmitrienko, A., R. B. D'Agostino, Sr. and M. F. Huque (2013). Key multiplicity issues in clinical drug development. *Stat Med*, **32**(7), 1079–1111.

Dong, S. J., X. J. Cai and S. J. Li (2016). The clinical significance of MiR-429 as a predictive biomarker in colorectal cancer patients receiving 5-Fluorouracil treatment. *Med Sci Monit*, **22**, 3352–3361.

Early Breast Cancer Trialists' Collaborative Group (2005). Effects of chemotherapy and hormonal therapy for early breast cancer on recurrence and 15-year survival: an overview of the randomised trials. *Lancet*, **365**(9472), 1687–1717.

EMA (2013). Guideline on clinical evaluation of diagnostic agents. *European Medicines Agency, Amsterdam, The Netherlands*.

Fan, C., D. S. Oh, L. Wessels, et al. (2006). Concordance among gene-expression-based predictors for breast cancer. *N Engl J Med*, **355**(6), 560–569.

FDA (2011). Guidance for industry – E16 biomarkers related to drug or biotechnology product development: context, structure, and format of qualification submissions. *The United States Food and Drug Administration, Silver Spring, Maryland.*

FDA (2014). Guidance for industry and food and drug administration staff – in vitro companion diagnostic devices. *The United States Food and Drug Administration, Silver Spring, Maryland.*

FDA (2018). Guidance for industry – bioanalytical method validation guidance for industry. *The United States Food and Drug Administration, Silver Spring, Maryland.*

FDA (2019). Guidance for industry – enrichment strategies for clinical trials to support determination of effectiveness of human drugs and biological products. *The United States Food and Drug Administration, Silver Spring, Maryland.*

Findlay, J. W., W. C. Smith, J. W. Lee, et al. (2000). Validation of immunoassays for bioanalysis: a pharmaceutical industry perspective. *J Pharm Biomed Anal*, **21**(6), 1249–1273.

Freidlin, B. and R. Simon (2005). Adaptive signature design: an adaptive clinical trial design for generating and prospectively testing a gene expression signature for sensitive patients. *Clin Cancer Res*, **11**(21), 7872–7878.

Grilo, A. L. and A. Mantalaris (2019). The increasingly human and profitable monoclonal antibody Market. *Trends Biotechnol*, **37**(1), 9–16.

Harigopal, M., D. Kowalski and A. Vosoughi (2020). Enumeration and molecular characterization of circulating tumor cells as an innovative tool for companion diagnostics in breast cancer. *Expert Rev Mol Diagn*, **20**(8), 815–828.

Havel, J. J., D. Chowell and T. A. Chan (2019). The evolving landscape of biomarkers for checkpoint inhibitor immunotherapy. *Nat Rev Cancer*, **19**(3), 133–150.

Hellmann, M. D., L. Paz-Ares, R. Bernabe Caro, et al. (2019). Nivolumab plus ipilimumab in advanced non-small-cell lung cancer. *N Engl J Med*, **381**(21), 2020–2031.

Hersom, M. and J. T. Jorgensen (2018). Companion and complementary diagnostics-focus on PD-L1 expression assays for PD-1/PD-L1 checkpoint inhibitors in non-small cell lung cancer. *Ther Drug Monit*, **40**(1), 9–16.

Hommel, G. and F. Bretz (2008). Aesthetics and power considerations in multiple testing–a contradiction? *Biom J*, **50**(5), 657–666.

Hwang, T. J., L. S. Lehmann and A. S. Kesselheim (2015). Precision medicine and the FDA's draft guidance on laboratory-developed tests. *Nat Biotechnol*, **33**(5), 449–451.

Jiang, W., B. Freidlin and R. Simon (2007). Biomarker-adaptive threshold design: a procedure for evaluating treatment with possible biomarker-defined subset effect. *J Natl Cancer Inst*, **99**(13), 1036–1043.

Jorgensen, J. T. and M. Hersom (2016). Companion diagnostics-a tool to improve pharmacotherapy. *Ann Transl Med*, **4**(24), 482.

Kaley, T., M. Touat, V. Subbiah, et al. (2018). BRAF Inhibition in BRAF(V600)-Mutant Gliomas: Results From the VE-BASKET Study. *J Clin Oncol*, **36**(35), 3477–3484.

Kim, E. S., R. S. Herbst, Wistuba, II, et al. (2011). The BATTLE trial: personalizing therapy for lung cancer. *Cancer Discov*, **1**(1), 44–53.

Kowanetz, M., W. Zou, S. N. Gettinger, et al. (2018). Differential regulation of PD-L1 expression by immune and tumor cells in NSCLC and the response to treatment with atezolizumab (anti-PD-L1). *Proc Nat Acad Sci USA*, **115**(43), E10119–E10126.

Kubo, T., Y. Kawano, N. Himuro, et al. (2016). BAK is a predictive and prognostic biomarker for the therapeutic effect of docetaxel treatment in patients with advanced gastric cancer. *Gastric Cancer*, **19**(3), 827–838.

Landes, S. J., S. A. McBain and G. M. Curran (2019). An introduction to effectiveness-implementation hybrid designs. *Psychiatry Res*, **280**, 112513.

Lee, C. K., L. Davies, V. J. Gebski, et al. (2016). Serum Human Epidermal Growth Factor 2 Extracellular Domain as a Predictive Biomarker for Lapatinib Treatment Efficacy in Patients With Advanced Breast Cancer. *J Clin Oncol*, **34**(9), 936–944.

Lee, J. W., J. D. Hulse and W. A. Colburn (1995). Surrogate biochemical markers: precise measurement for strategic drug and biologics development. *J Clin Pharmacol*, **35**(5), 464–470.

Lesko, L. J. and A. J. Atkinson, Jr. (2001). Use of biomarkers and surrogate endpoints in drug development and regulatory decision making: criteria, validation, strategies. *Annu Rev Pharmacol Toxicol*, **41**, 347–366.

Lin, J. Z., J. Y. Long, A. Q. Wang, et al. (2017). Precision medicine: In need of guidance and surveillance. *World J Gastroenterol*, **23**(28), 5045–5050.

Loo, E., P. Khalili, K. Beuhler, et al. (2018). BRAF V600E mutation across multiple tumor types: correlation between DNA-based sequencing and mutation-specific immunohistochemistry. *Appl Immunohistochem Mol Morphol*, **26**(10), 709–713.

Mandrekar, S. J. and D. J. Sargent (2009). Clinical trial designs for predictive biomarker validation: theoretical considerations and practical challenges. *J Clin Oncol*, **27**(24), 4027–4034.

Mandrekar, S. J. and D. J. Sargent (2011). Design of clinical trials for biomarker research in oncology. *Clin Investig (Lond)*, **1**(12), 1629–1636.

Mansfield, E. A. (2014). FDA perspective on companion diagnostics: an evolving paradigm. *Clin Cancer Res*, **20**(6), 1453–1457.

Miller, K. J., R. R. Bowsher, A. Celniker, et al. (2001). Workshop on bioanalytical methods validation for macromolecules: summary report. *Pharm Res*, **18**(9), 1373–1383.

Nalejska, E., E. Maczynska and M. A. Lewandowska (2014). Prognostic and predictive biomarkers: tools in personalized oncology. *Mol Diagn Ther*, **18**(3), 273–284.

Park, J. W., R. S. Kerbel, G. J. Kelloff, et al. (2004). Rationale for biomarkers and surrogate end points in mechanism-driven oncology drug development. *Clin Cancer Res*, **10**(11), 3885–3896.

Perrone, F., G. Baldassarre, S. Indraccolo, et al. (2016). Biomarker analysis of the MITO2 phase III trial of first-line treatment in ovarian cancer: predictive value of DNA-PK and phosphorylated ACC. *Oncotarget*, **7**(45), 72654–72661.

Polley, M. C., E. L. Korn and B. Freidlin (2019). Phase III precision medicine clinical trial designs that integrate treatment and biomarker evaluation. *JCO Precis Oncol*, **3**.

Qiu, Z.Y., W.G. Guo, and G. Lynch (2015). On generalized fixed sequence procedures for controlling the FWER. *Stat Med*, **34**(30), 3968–3983.

Riese, D. J., 2nd and D. F. Stern (1998). Specificity within the EGF family/ErbB receptor family signaling network. *Bioessays*, **20**(1), 41–48.

Romond, E. H., E. A. Perez, J. Bryant, et al. (2005). Trastuzumab plus adjuvant chemotherapy for operable HER2-positive breast cancer. *N Engl J Med*, **353**(16), 1673–1684.

Roth, E. M. and P. Diller (2014). Alirocumab for hyperlipidemia: physiology of PCSK9 inhibition, pharmacodynamics and Phase I and II clinical trial results of a PCSK9 monoclonal antibody. *Future Cardiol*, **10**(2), 183–199.

Rothschild, S. I. (2014). Ceritinib-a second-generation ALK inhibitor overcoming resistance in ALK-rearranged non-small cell lung cancer. *Transl Lung Cancer Res*, **3**(6), 379–381.

Sabatino, M., S. Kim-Schulze, M. C. Panelli, et al. (2009). Serum vascular endothelial growth factor and fibronectin predict clinical response to high-dose interleukin-2 therapy. *J Clin Oncol*, **27**(16), 2645–2652.

Scheerens, H., A. Malong, K. Bassett, et al. (2017). Current status of companion and complementary diagnostics: strategic considerations for development and launch. *Clin Transl Sci*, **10**(2), 84–92.

Schrock, A. B., C. Ouyang, J. Sandhu, et al. (2019). Tumor mutational burden is predictive of response to immune checkpoint inhibitors in MSI-high metastatic colorectal cancer. *Annals Of Oncology*, **30**(7), 1096–1103.

Schultz, M., L. J. H. Rasmussen, M. H. Andersen, et al. (2018). Use of the prognostic biomarker suPAR in the emergency department improves risk stratification but has no effect on mortality: a cluster-randomized clinical trial (TRIAGE III). *Scand J Trauma Resusc Emerg Med*, **26**(1), 69.

Scirica, B. M., D. L. Bhatt, E. Braunwald, et al. (2016). Prognostic implications of biomarker assessments in patients with Type 2 diabetes at high cardiovascular risk: A secondary analysis of a randomized clinical trial. *JAMA Cardiol*, **1**(9), 989–998.

Shaw, A. T., D. W. Kim, R. Mehra, et al. (2014). Ceritinib in ALK-rearranged non-small-cell lung cancer. *N Engl J Med*, **370**(13), 1189–1197.

Simon, N. and R. Simon (2013). Adaptive enrichment designs for clinical trials. *Biostatistics*, **14**(4), 613–625.

Sun, K., J. Park, M. Kim, et al. (2017). Endotrophin, a multifaceted player in metabolic dysregulation and cancer progression, is a predictive biomarker for the response to PPARgamma agonist treatment. *Diabetologia*, **60**(1), 24–29.

Twilt, M. (2016). Precision Medicine: The new era in medicine. *EBioMedicine*, **4**, 24–25.

Twomey, J. D. and B. Zhang (2021). Cancer immunotherapy update: FDA-approved checkpoint inhibitors and companion diagnostics. *AAPS J*, **23**(2), 39.

Watanabe, A. (2015). [companion diagnostics for solid tumors]. *Rinsho Byori*, **63**(11), 1310–1315.

Wiens, B. L. (2003). A fixed sequence Bonferroni procedure for testing multiple endpoints. *Pharm Stat*, **2**(3), 5.

Wiens, B. L. and A. Dmitrienko (2005). The fallback procedure for evaluating a single family of hypotheses. *J Biopharm Stat*, **15**(6), 929–942.

Wiens, B. L. and A. Dmitrienko (2010). On Selecting a Multiple Comparison Procedure for Analysis of a Clinical Trial: Fallback, Fixed Sequence, and Related Procedures. *Stat Biopharm Res* **2**(1), 11.

Wolff, A. C., M. E. Hammond, D. G. Hicks, et al. (2013). Recommendations for human epidermal growth factor receptor 2 testing in breast cancer: American Society of Clinical Oncology/College of American Pathologists clinical practice guideline update. *J Clin Oncol*, **31**(31), 3997–4013.

Zhang, X., Y. Zhang, H. Tang, et al. (2017). EGFR gene copy number as a predictive/biomarker for patients with non-small-cell lung cancer receiving tyrosine kinase inhibitor treatment: a systematic review and meta-analysis. *J Investig Med*, **65**(1), 72–81.

4

Model-Informed Drug Development

Haochen Liu and Fangrong Yan

China Pharmaceutical University, Nanjing, China

CONTENTS

DOI: 10.1201/9781003107323-4

4.1 Introduction

Quantitative models that leverage our understanding of physiology, disease processes and pharmacology are routinely applied to inform drug development [1]. Model-Informed Drug Development (MIDD) is the most recent term commonly used to describe the application of a wide range of quantitative models in drug development to facilitate the decision-making process [1].

At present, MIDD has garnered much attention as a potential enabler of efficient drug development [2]. The integration of model-based approaches into drug development and regulation has taken decades to conceptualize the MIDD [3]. The development of MIDD went through five phases. Firstly, early academic efforts employed quantitative physiological modeling to facilitate drug development (e.g. pioneered the use of non linear mixed effects modeling to describe pharmacokinetic variability and associate patient characteristics with variability) which laid the technical foundation for quantitative clinical pharmacology models to become tools to facilitate drug development [3]. Secondly, in the late 1990s, Sheiner introduced the "learn-and-confirm" concept, which is widely accepted as a necessary approach to addressing important clinical development and practice questions [3, 4]. In parallel, drug development and regulatory organizations, recognizing the emerging value of MIDD, began establishing dedicated groups focusing on modeling and simulation as part of multidisciplinary product development and review teams [3]. Thirdly, the value of MIDD has been recognized by global health organizations and regulatory bodies as publicly communicated by agencies such as the European Medical Agency (European Union) and the Pharmaceuticals and Medical Devices Agency (Japan) [3]. The regulatory agency starts developing guidance for the application and regulatory acceptance of MIDD approaches [3]. Fourthly, aggregating and disseminating impact cases of MIDD application in drug development and regulatory review further highlighted the value and return on investment [3]. Fifthly, MIDD has demonstrably augmented the clinical trial enterprise by creating a platform to integrate knowledge about the disease, patient factors and drugs with similar mechanisms of action with information generated throughout a development program. The result has been more efficient clinical trials and increased the probability of technical and regulatory success [5].

As MIDD plays important role in drug development and regulation, integrative approaches to advancing MIDD are conducted by Food and Drug Administration (FDA) [1]: (i) develop its regulatory science and review expertise and capacity to support evaluation of model-based strategies and development efforts; (ii) convene a series of workshops to identify best practices for MIDD; (iii) conduct a pilot meeting program for MIDD approaches; (iv) publish draft guidances, or revise relevant existing guidance, on MIDD; (v) develop or revise relevant manuals of policy/procedures, standard operating procedures and/or review templates and training, as needed. Overall, MIDD-related programmatic activities are expected to promote early interactions between drug developers and regulatory scientists on key issues during product development [1].

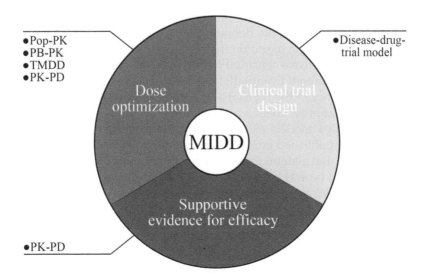

FIGURE 4.1
Application of model information drug development.

The regulatory application of MIDD can be broadly classified into four categories: supportive evidence for efficacy, clinical trial design, dose optimization and informing policy [1]. In this chapter, the models related to the above applications are introduced (Figure 4.1). For the application of supportive evidence for efficacy, the models for describing exposure-response (ER) relationships are introduced which contains classical Dose-response model, direct response Pharmacokinetic/Pharmacodynamic (PK/PD) model, mechanism based PK/PD model and quantitative systems biology model. For the application in clinical trial design, the quantitative disease-drug-trial models are introduced. For the application in dose optimization, population pharmacokinetic model, Physiologically Based Pharmacokinetic model (PB-PK), and Target-Mediated Drug Disposition Model (TMDD) are introduced. For regulatory application, two guidances published by FDA involving MIDD are introduced. In this chapter, some innovative thinking and modeling involving the above applications are introduced. (i) The application of quantitative systems biology models in drug development; (ii) The combined use of disease progression model and traditional trial design methods.

4.2 Exposure-Response Relationships

It has been a common practice for clinical pharmacologists at the FDA to identify supportive evidence of efficacy based on findings from clinical trials in a new drug application or a biological license application review [1]. The established exposure dose-response relationship generally provides critical evidence to support an efficacy claim of a product [1]. Several previous cases have illustrated that the ER relationships models play important role in addressing complex questions regarding efficacy. For example, when everolimus was developed to prevent graft loss after liver transplantation, a Unique Noninferiority (NI) trial was designed for ethical reasons [6]. Such a unique design, however, made the calculation of NI margin practically impossible based on the classic method recommended in the FDA's guidance [7]. Upon completion of the clinical trial, the efficacy results could not be interpreted with a reasonably defined NI margin. A novel ER-based method was applied to derive the NI margin based on the exposure and efficacy data from the control arm in the NI trial [8]. Extensive sensitivity analyses were conducted to address various concerns related to the method. Eventually, the derived NI margin served as the foundation to interpret the efficacy of the NI trial and became the essential part of the totality of evidence that led to the approval of everolimus for the new indication.

As the ER relationships models exhibit high value in addressing complex questions regarding efficacy, FDA published guidance for modeling ER relationships. In this section, based on this guidance, the general procedure for developing ER relationships models is introduced. Then several typical ER relationships models including PK/PD and quantitative systems biology model are also introduced.

4.2.1 Regulatory Guidance

The development of ER relationships models contains multiple steps including clinical trial design, biomarker selection and model development. In this section, the part of guidance involving model development is introduced.

4.2.1.1 General Considerations

Safety information and adequate and well-controlled clinical studies that establish a drug's effectiveness are the basis for approval of new drugs. ER data can be derived from these clinical studies, as well as from other preclinical and clinical studies, and provide a basis for integrated model-based analysis and simulation. Simulation is a way of predicting expected relationships between exposure and response in situations where real data are sparse or absent. There are many different types of models for the analysis of ER data (e.g. descriptive PD models or empirical models that link a PK model and a PD model). Descriptive or empirical model-based analysis does not necessarily establish causality or provide a mechanistic understanding of a drug's effect and would not ordinarily be a basis for approval of a new drug. Nevertheless, dose-response or PK/PD modeling can help in understanding the nature of ER relationships and can be used to analyze adequate and well-controlled trials to extract additional insights from treatment responses. This can suggest ways to optimize dosage regimens and to individualize treatment in specific patient subsets for which there are limited data. Creating a theory or rationale to explain ER relationships through modeling and simulation allows interpolation and extrapolation to better doses and responses in the general population and to subpopulations defined by certain intrinsic and extrinsic factors.

4.2.1.2 Essential Information for Modeling

In the process of PK/PD modeling, it is important to describe the following prospectively: (i) statement of the problem: the objectives of the modeling, the study design and the available PK and PD data; (ii) statement of assumptions. The assumptions of the model that can be related to dose-response, PK, PD and/or one or more of the following:

- The mechanism of the drug actions for efficacy and adverse effects
- Immediate or cumulative clinical effects
- Development of tolerance or absence of tolerance

- Drug-induced inhibition or induction of PK processes
- Disease state progression
- Response in a placebo group
- Circadian variations in basal conditions
- Influential covariates
- Absence or presence of an effect compartment
- Presence or absence of active metabolites and their contribution to clinical effects
- The PK model of absorption and disposition and the parameters to be estimated
- The PD model of effect and the parameters to be estimated
- Distribution of PK and PD measures and parameters
- Distributions of intra- and inter-individual variability in parameters
- Inclusion and/or exclusion of specific patient data.

4.2.1.3 Selection of the Model

In general, the model selection will be based on the mechanism of action of the drug, the assumptions made, and the intended use of the model in decision making. If the assumptions do not lead to a mechanistic model, an empirical model can be selected. In this case, the validation of the model predictability becomes especially important. The available data can also govern the types of models that can be used. The model selection process can be a series of trial and error steps. Different model structures or newly added or dropped components to an existing model can be assessed by visual inspection and tested using one of several objective criteria. New assumptions can be added when emerging data indicates that this is appropriate. The final selection of the model will usually be based on the simplest model possible that has reasonable goodness of fit, and that provides a level of predictability appropriate for its use in decision making.

4.2.1.4 Validation of the Model

Generally, we recommend that the predictive power of a model be dealt with during the study design as well as in the data analysis stages and that the study be designed to yield a predictive model. When plausible ER models are identified based on prior knowledge of the drug before conducting an ER study, the predictive power of the final models derived from the study results becomes a function of study design factors, such as number of subjects and sampling plan. The predictive power can be estimated through simulation, by considering distributions of PK, PD and study design variables. A robust study design will provide accurate and precise model parameter estimations that are insensitive to model assumptions. During the analysis stage of a study, models can be validated based on internal and/or external data. The ultimate test of a model is its predictive power and the data used to estimate predictability could come from ER studies designed for such a purpose. A common method for estimating predictability is to split the data set into two parts, build the model based on one set of data and test the predictability of the resulting model on the second set of data. The predictability is especially important when the model is intended to: (i) provide supportive evidence for primary efficacy studies, (ii) address safety issues, or (iii) support new doses and dosing regimens in new target populations or subpopulations defined by intrinsic and extrinsic factors or when there is a change in dosage form and/or route of administration.

4.2.2 Classical Dose–Response Model

The classical dose-response models contain various models, for instance, linear, logistic, E-max (simple, Sigmoid or standardized form), quadratic, exponential and linear in log-dose models [9–11]. However, these classical models are not used solely in MIDD studies. These models are usually embedded into other more complex models (e.g. PK/PD, quantitative systems biology model etc.). In this section, we list several standard classical dose-response models in Table 4.1.

The linear model is the simplest one. Its simplicity is an advantage. An example of a non-linear dose–response model is the E-max model: E_0 is the placebo effect, E_{max} is the asymptotic (associated to an" infinite dose") upper bound of effect, as compared to placebo, and $ED_{50}{}^h$ is the dose giving half of E_{max} as change from placebo. A more complex form of this model is its Sigmoid version, where an additional parameter is included, ensuring greater shape flexibility, the "Hill" exponent (the slope), h, reflecting the shape of the dose-effect curve. Other monotonic (as a function of dose) dose–response models can be considered: logistic, exponential, and linear in log-dose models. The quadratic model has the ability to describe a non-monotonic dose-response relationship, in a convex/U-shape (when $\beta_2 > 0$), or in a concave/umbrella-shape (when $\beta_2 < 0$).

4.2.3 Direct Response PK/PD Model

The direct response PK/PD model is based on the assumption that there is an effect compartment where drugs exhibit effects [12]. The concentration-effect relationships in the effect compartment are described by the classical dose-response models listed in the above section. For direct response PK/PD models, the measured concentration in plasma is directly linked to the effect-site concentration. Equilibrium between both concentrations is assumed to be rapidly achieved and thus their ratio is constant, under PK steady-state as well as non steady-state conditions [13]. Hence, the measured concentrations can directly serve as input function in the pharmacodynamic model component, thereby directly linking measured concentration to the observed effect. In that case, concentration and effect maxima would occur at the same time and affect vs. concentration plots would lack any hysteresis if the response is directly mediated [13].

Poon et al. provided an example for direct response PK/PD model. They developed a classical PK/PD model to link the serum concentration of the anti-human immunglobulin E (IgE) antibody CGP51901 for the treatment of seasonal allergic rhinitis to the

TABLE 4.1

Typical Classical Dose-Response Models. *d* Refers to the Dose and θ for the Vector of Parameters of the Dose-Response Function

Name	$f(d,\theta)$
Linear	$E_0 + \delta \times d$
E_{max}	$E_0 + E_{max} \cdot d/(ED_{50} + d)$
Sigmoid E_{max}	$E_0 + E_{max} \cdot d^h/(ED_{50}^h + d^h)$
Log linear	$E_0 + \delta \cdot \log(d + \textit{offset})$
Exponential	$E_0 e^{d/\delta}$
Quadratic	$E_0 + \beta_1 d + \beta_2 d^2$
Logistic	$E_0 + E_{max}/(1 + e^{(ED_{50} - d)/\delta})$

reduction of free IgE [14]. A two compartment model is employed to describe the pharma-cokinetics of CGP51901. The model is represented in Equation (4.1). In Equation (4.1) k_0, τ, and t are the infusion rate, duration of infusion, and the time elapsed after infusion, and α and β are the rate constants of distribution and elimination, respectively. The value k_{21} represents the rate constant of transfer between peripheral and serum compartment, and V_c is the central volume of distribution. The α (distribution) phase is the fast phase, and the β (elimination) phase is the slow phase of the concentration-time curve. The serum concentrations of free IgE and CGP 51901 can be described by means of an inhibition E_{max} model represented by Equation (4.2). The value IgE_0 is the free IgE level at 0 concentration of CGP 51901, and IC_{50} is the concentration of CGP 51901 at which 50% reduction of free IgE is achieved. The shape of response curve is determined with the IC_{50} and γ.

$$
\begin{cases}
c = Ae^{-\alpha t} + Be^{-\beta t} \\[2mm]
A = k_0 \dfrac{\alpha - k_{21}}{(\alpha - \beta)\,\alpha \cdot V_c}(1 - e^{-\alpha \tau}) \\[2mm]
B = k \dfrac{\beta - k}{(\beta - \alpha)\beta \cdot V_c}(1 - e^{-\beta \tau})
\end{cases}
\tag{4.1}
$$

$$
IgE = IgE_0 \left(1 - \frac{c^\gamma}{c^\gamma + IC_{50}^\gamma} \right)
\tag{4.2}
$$

4.2.4 Mechanism Based PK/PD Model

The direct response PK/PD models use empirical models to link the drug exposure and response directly which is only suitable for the condition that the response is directly mediated. However, the responses of many drugs are mediated by binding to targets which cannot be described by direct link. Therefore, to address the limitation of classical PK/PD model, the mechanism-based PK/PD model is developed.

The most significant difference between mechanism-based PK/PD models and classical PK/PD models is that mechanism-based PK/PD models contain specific expressions to quantitatively characterize processes on the causal path between plasma concentration and effect which is not considered in classical PK/PD models [15, 16]. These causal paths between plasma concentration and effect include: (i) drug target site distribution, (ii) drug target binding and activation, (iii) transduction mechanisms (including the homeostatic feedback mechanisms that might modulate the response), (iv) disease systems [15, 16]. To develop mechanism-based PK/PD models, the concepts of the above causal paths need to be introduced.

4.2.4.1 Drug Target Site Distribution

Most drugs have their target site outside the plasma. Hence, distribution to the site of action might represent a rate limiting step in the onset and the duration of the effect. This is often reflected in a delay, or 'hysteresis', of the pharmacological effect relative to the drug concentration in plasma. The so-called effect compartment model has been successfully applied to account for hysteresis caused by distribution to extracellular targets by passive diffusion.

4.2.4.2 Drug Target Binding and Activation

The modeling of drug target binding and activation can be regarded as a specific application of receptor theory in PK/PD modeling. According to receptor theory, the potency (i.e. EC_{50}), the intrinsic activity (i.e. E_{max}) and the slope factor are dependent on the properties of both the drug (i.e. the receptor affinity and the intrinsic efficacy) and the biological system (i.e. the receptor density and the transducer function relating receptor activation to pharmacological response) [16].

4.2.4.3 Transduction

In PK/PD modeling, the concept of 'transduction' refers to the processes that govern the transduction of target activation into the response in vivo [16]. Turnover or physiological indirect response models are widely used to account for delays in the time course of the pharmacological response relative to the time course of the drug concentration in plasma. Basically, drugs might stimulate or inhibit zero order input or first-order dissipation of drug response in a direct concentration-dependent manner.

4.2.4.4 Disease Systems

Ideally, drug treatment should slow down or even reverse the progression of the disease [16]. To estimate the actual treatment effect, it is essential to distinguish the time course of the drug effects from those caused by natural disease progression [16, 17]. Typically, disease systems analysis utilizes information on changes in a combination of biomarkers and clinical status as the basis for the modeling of the time course of disease progression in untreated and in treated patients [16].

The development of mechanism-based PK/PD model could be diversified dealing with different drugs and different diseases. Therefore, the procedures for development of mechanism-based PK/PD model are illustrated with an example. The research of Winter et al. provided an example for mechanism-based PK/PD model [18]. In this research, a mechanism-based PK/PD model was applied to estimate relative treatment effects of pioglitazone, metformin and glyclazide in type 2 diabetes mellitus. Firstly, the pharmacokinetic model is developed which follows the same procedures as the ordinary compartmental model.

Secondly, characterize the disease system. Usually, only the part of disease system related to drug targets is considered in the mechanism-based PK/PD model (This procedure may not be suitable to some complex disease systems. Under this condition, some other models will be developed which will be discussed in the next section.). In the research of Winter et al., a disease system based on the homeostatic feedback relationship between Fasting Plasma Glucose (FPG) and Fasting Serum Insulin (FSI). In the fasted or basal state, plasma glucose levels are primarily determined by endogenous glucose production in the liver. Most glucose uptake is to the brain, which is insulin-independent. If the FPG concentration rises, this stimulates the release and production of insulin by the β-cells in the pancreas, resulting in rising FSI concentrations. These elevated FSI concentrations, in turn, suppress the production of glucose by the liver, resulting in a reduction in FPG concentrations. Because brain function quickly deteriorates when plasma glucose concentrations become too low, FPG concentrations need to exceed a certain minimum threshold before they can stimulate the production of FSI. In healthy individuals, this homeostatic system of feedback relationships keeps FPG concentrations within their physiological range.

If the sensitivity to insulin in the liver is reduced, permanently elevated FSI concentrations are needed to suppress hepatic glucose production and maintain glycemic control. If, in addition to reduced insulin sensitivity, β-cell function is also impaired, insulin production becomes insufficient to maintain the high FSI levels required to suppress hepatic glucose production and fasting hyperglycemia. The above system is quantitatively characterized by Equation (4.3) to (4.5).

$$\frac{d\,\text{FSI}}{dt} = EF_B \cdot B \cdot (\text{FPG} - 3.5) \cdot k_{in}^{\text{FSI}} - \text{FSI} \cdot k_{out}^{\text{FSI}} \tag{4.3}$$

$$\frac{d\,\text{FPG}}{dt} = \frac{k_{in}^{\text{FPG}}}{EF_S \cdot S \cdot \text{FSI}} - \text{FPG} \cdot k_{out}^{\text{FPG}} \tag{4.4}$$

$$\frac{d\,\text{HbA}_{1c}}{dt} = \text{FPG} \cdot k_{in}^{\text{HbA1c}} - \text{HbA}_{1c} \cdot k_{out}^{\text{HbA1c}} \tag{4.5}$$

Here, the various k_{in} parameters are the influx rates and the k_{out} parameters are the efflux rate constants for FSI, FPG and glycosylated hemoglobin A1c (HbA_{1c}) turn-over, respectively. The coefficient B in Equation (4.3) represents the fraction of remaining β-cell function relative to normal functionality in healthy persons, and the coefficient S in Equation (4.4) represents the fraction of remaining hepatic insulin sensitivity relative to normal sensitivity in healthy persons. To describe the progression of disease, the coefficients B and S are considered to decline as asymptotic functions of time that go from 1 to zero as t goes from minus infinity to plus infinity shown in Equation (4.6) and (4.7).

$$B = 1 + e^{(b_0 + r_B t)} \tag{4.6}$$

$$S = 1 + e^{(s_0 + r_s t)} \tag{4.7}$$

Here, the parameters b_0 and s_0 represent a shift of the disease progression curves along the time axis: large values indicate that patients have a longer disease history and are further progressed at baseline. The parameters r_B and r_s determine the slope of the disease progression curves and hence the rate of change over time in B and S, respectively. Parameters EF_B and EF_s represent purely symptomatic effects that are switched on at start of treatment and switched off as treatment is discontinued.

Thirdly, the drug treatment effect needs to be linked to the above disease system. In the research of winter et al., the linear model and E_{max} model are employed to model drug target site distribution and drug target binding and activation respectively shown in Equation (4.8) and (4.9). FPG_0 is the baseline of FPG, E_{treat} is the drug treatment effect at time t, D_{exp} is the drug exposure level at time t and α presents the slope of the FPG status over time during drug treatment.

$$\text{FPG} = \text{FPG}_0 + E_{treat} + \alpha t \tag{4.8}$$

$$E_{treat} = \frac{E_{max} \cdot D_{exp}}{(EC_{50} + D_{exp})} \tag{4.9}$$

In summary, the development of mechanism-based PK/PD model contains three steps: PK model development, characterization of the disease system, and linking drug effect to disease system. The PK model development is similar to that in classical PK/PD model. The characterization of disease system should be based on the biological mechanism of the disease and the disease progression needs to be considered. Linking drug effect to disease system contains two parts of model selection: (i) modeling drug target site distribution, (ii) modeling drug target binding and activation. This step is similar to the direct link in the classical PK/PD. The effect compartment and classical dose-response models are usual candidate models respectively.

4.2.5 Quantitative Systems Biology Model

The direct response PK/PD model and mechanism based PK/PD model are described as empirical 'top-down' models which are usually employed in the clinical stage of drug development [19]. In recent years, a novel model, Quantitative Systems Biology model (QSB), is emerging. Unlike the previous top-down empirical PK/PD models, the QSB model is described as button up models [19]. The top-down models place greater reliance on obtaining experimental data on drug concentrations and associated biological responses collected over time and at various drug doses in specific systems of interest [20]. Inversely, the button up models usually apply quantitative methods to describe the dynamics of all intermediates of a particular pathophysiology network and then integrate the drug response model to the above network [19]. This significant difference from the top-down models makes that the QSB models can be widely used in almost all stages of new drug development including: (i) identify and evaluate targets, compounds, and biomarkers; (ii) understand preclinical models of disease, and; (iii) understand the mechanism of action of a compound [19]. The procedure for QSB development can be highly flexible. The QSB model is usually developed case by case. Therefore, in this section, a case study is used to illustrate the development of QSB.

In this section, the QSB model developed by Earp et al. is used to illustrate the development of QSB [21, 22]. Earp et al. developed a QSB model to optimize the corticosteroid therapy to treat Rheumatoid Arthritis (RA). Low-dose corticosteroid therapy has been recently implicated as a possible way of treating RA. But the inter-regulation processes between cytokines and endogenous corticosteroids could affect the effect of exogenous corticosteroids. Finding the optimal dosages and regimes of exogenous corticosteroids is a challenging problem. To address this issue, Earp et al. proposed to develop a QSB-PK/PD model. The QSB model is based on the mechanism of disease. Firstly, a mathematical model is developed to describe the system related to the disease. Ordinary Differential Equation (ODE) is the most common choice for this model. In the QSB model developed by Earp et al., a ODE system was established to describe the dynamic of cytokines and endogenous corticosteroids. TNF-α, IL-1β, and IL-6 increase immune cell trafficking and proliferation and cause up-regulation of GR and plasma CST [22]. In turn, Glucocorticoid Receptor (GR) and plasma corticosterone (CST) are thought to suppress cytokine expression by inhibiting the action of transcription factors nuclear factor - κB and activator protein 1. These inter-regulation processes between cytokines and endogenous corticosteroid account for limiting inflammation during progression and provide common factors for which dexamethasone (DEX) drug effects may be observed and used to explain treatment effects on disease endpoints. Overall disease progression is monitored by edema in the paw, and by femur and lumbar Bone Mineral Density (BMD). The production of edema is directly correlated with immune cell infiltration and pro-inflammatory cytokine concentrations. Bone production and loss have also been related to the presence of TNF-α, IL-1β, and IL-6. These cytokines not only reduce osteoblast activity, but are also thought to increase receptor activator of nuclear factor-κB (RANKL) expression and subsequent activation of osteoclasts. The above complex system was divided into several linked modules.

4.2.5.1 Corticosterone and GR Dynamics Module

The equation describing GR mRNA turnover is:

$$\frac{d\,GR_{mRNA}}{dt} = k_{in}^{GRm}(1 + T_{CYT})\left(1 - \frac{DR_N^{\gamma_{DR}}}{IC_{50\_DR}^{\gamma_{DR}} + DR_N^{\gamma_{DR}}}\right) - k_{out}^{GRm}GR_{mRNA} \tag{4.10}$$

$$k_{out}^{GR} = \frac{k_{in}^{GR}}{GR_0}\left(1 - \frac{DR_{N0}^{\gamma_{DR}}}{IC_{50\_DR}^{\gamma_{DR}} + DR_{N0}^{\gamma_{DR}}}\right) \tag{4.11}$$

$$\frac{d\,T_{cyt}}{dt} = k_{t\_cyt}(A_{cyt} - T_{cyt}) \tag{4.12}$$

$$A_{cyt} = \alpha_1(TNF\alpha_{mRNA} - TNF_0) + \alpha_2(IL1\beta_{mRNA} - IL1\beta_0) \tag{4.13}$$

k_{in}^{GRm} is the first-order production rate of GR mRNA. Drug bound to receptor is indicated by DR. After the DR complex translocates to the nucleus it is defined as DR_N. IC_{50_DR} is the concentration of DR_N required to inhibit GR mRNA production by 50%, and γ_{DR} is the Hill coefficient for inhibition by DR_N. The rate constant k_{out}^{GRm} describes the first-order loss for GR mRNA and is defined through the steady-state baseline condition. The variable T_{cyt} is representative of an overall cytokine protein expression and accounts for the slow onset of GR mRNA relative to the rapid rise in cytokine response. A_{cyt} is the contribution of pro-inflammatory cytokine mRNA on the production of T_{cyt}. The α_1 and α_2 are the intrinsic activities of each cytokine mRNA for producing cytokine protein, T_{cyt}.

4.2.5.2 Pro-Inflammatory Cytokine Dynamics Module

The impact of pro-inflammatory cytokines on each other was described by the transit compartment model which has been introduced in the above section.

$$\begin{cases} \dfrac{d\,T_{TNF\alpha}^n}{dt} = k_{t1}(T_{TNF\alpha}^{n-1} - T_{TNF\alpha}^n) \\[2mm] \dfrac{d\,T_{IL1\beta}^n}{dt} = k_{t2}(T_{IL1\beta}^{n-1} - T_{IL1\beta}^n) \\[2mm] \dfrac{d\,T_{IL6}^n}{dt} = k_{t3}(T_{IL6}^{n-1} - T_{IL6}^n) \end{cases} \tag{4.14}$$

T^n indicates the nth transit compartment relevant for the series of events that takes place prior to when disease onset is observed. The values of k_t indicate the turnover rate constant for each compartment in this series. The turnover of TNF-α mRNA is described by:

$$\frac{d\,\text{TNF}_{\text{mRNA}}}{dt} = k_{in}^{\text{TNF}\alpha} T_{\text{TNF}\alpha}^{n} \left(1 - \frac{\text{DR}_N^{\gamma_1}}{\text{IC}_{50\_\text{TNF}\alpha/\text{DR}_N} + \text{DR}_N^{\gamma_1}}\right)\left(1 - \frac{0.3\,\text{IL6}_{\text{mRNA}}}{\text{IC}_{50\_\text{TNF}\alpha/\text{IL6}} + \text{IL6}}\right) - k_{out}^{\text{TNF}\alpha}\text{TNF}_{\text{mRNA}} \quad (4.15)$$

$$k_{out}^{\text{TNF}\alpha} = k_{in}^{\text{TNF}\alpha}\left(1 - \frac{\text{DR}_{N0}^{\gamma_1}}{\text{IC}_{50\_\text{TNF}\alpha/\text{DR}_N}^{\gamma_1} + \text{DR}_{N0}^{\gamma_1}}\right)\left(1 - \frac{0.3\,\text{IL6}_0}{\text{IC}_{50\_\text{IL6}/\text{TNF}} + \text{IL6}_0}\right) \quad (4.16)$$

$k_{in}^{\text{TNF}\alpha}$ describes the first-order production rate dependent upon transit compartment $T_{\text{TNF}\alpha}^{n}$. DR_N is endogenous corticosterone bound with receptor in the nucleus, $\text{IC}_{50\_\text{TNF}\alpha/\text{DR}_N}$ is the concentration of DR_N required to inhibit TNF-α production 50%, and γ_1 is the Hill coefficient for the inhibition by DR_N. The term IL6_{mRNA} describes the amount of IL-6 mRNA and $\text{IC}_{50\_\text{TNF}\alpha/\text{IL6}}$ denotes the amount of IL6_{mRNA} necessary to inhibit TNF-α production 50% of maximal capacity (0.3). The rate constant $k_{out}^{\text{TNF}\alpha}$ describes the first-order loss for TNF-α mRNA and is defined through the steady-state baseline condition.

The turnover of IL-1β mRNA is described by

$$\frac{d\,\text{IL1}\beta}{dt} = k_{in}^{\text{IL1}\beta} T_{\text{IL1}\beta}^{n}\left(1 - \frac{\text{DR}_N}{\text{IC}_{50\_\text{IL1}\beta} + \text{DR}_N}\right)\left(1 - \frac{0.7\,\text{Rem}}{\text{IC}_{50\_\text{IL1}\beta/\text{Rem}} + \text{Rem}}\right) - k_{out}^{\text{IL1}\beta}\text{IL1}\beta_{\text{mRNA}} \quad (4.17)$$

$$k_{out}^{\text{IL1}\beta} = k_{out}^{\text{IL1}\beta}\left(1 - \frac{\text{DR}_{N0}}{\text{IC}_{50\_\text{IL1}\beta/\text{DR}_N} + \text{DR}_{N0}}\right) \quad (4.18)$$

$k_{in}^{\text{IL1}\beta}$ describes the first-order production rate dependent upon transit compartment $T_{\text{IL1}\beta}^{n}$. The $\text{IC}_{50\_\text{IL1}\beta}$ is the concentration of DR_N required to inhibit IL-1β mRNA production 50%. The term Rem describes an increase in other factors that control the decline in inflammation and is defined by $\text{Rem} = T_{\text{IL1}\beta}^{n} - R_{0\_\text{IL1}\beta}$. The parameter $\text{IC}_{50\_\text{IL1}\beta/\text{Rem}}$ denotes the amount of Rem necessary to inhibit IL-1β mRNA production to 50% of maximal capacity (0.7). The rate constant $k_{out}^{\text{IL1}\beta}$ describes the first-order loss rate-constant for IL-1β mRNA and is defined through the steady-state baseline condition Equation (4.18). The turnover of IL-6 mRNA is defined by

$$\frac{d\,\text{IL6}_{\text{mRNA}}}{dt} = k_{in}^{\text{IL6}} T_{\text{IL6}}^{n}\left(1 - \frac{\text{DR}_N^{\gamma_3}}{\text{IC}_{50\_\text{IL6}/\text{DR}_N}^{\gamma_{13}} + \text{DR}_N^{\gamma_3}}\right)\left(1 - \frac{0.8\,\text{Rem}}{\text{IC}_{50\_\text{IL6}/\text{Rem}} + \text{Rem}}\right) - k_{out}^{\text{IL6}}\text{IL6}_{\text{mRNA}} \quad (4.19)$$

k_{in}^{IL6} describes the first-order production rate dependent upon transit compartment T_{IL6}^{n}. The parameter $\text{IC}_{50\_\text{IL6}/\text{DR}_N}$ is the concentration of DR_N required to inhibit IL-6 mRNA production by 50%, and γ_3 is the Hill coefficient for inhibition by DR_N. The rate constant k_{out}^{IL6} describes the first-order loss for IL-6 mRNA and is defined through the steady state baseline condition:

$$k_{out}^{\text{IL6}} = k_{in}^{\text{IL6}}\left(1 - \frac{\text{DR}_{N0}^{\gamma_3}}{\text{IC}_{50\_\text{IL6}/\text{DR}_N}^{\gamma_3} + \text{DR}_{N0}^{\gamma_3}}\right) \quad (4.20)$$

4.2.5.3 Disease End Point Dynamics Module

Paw edema was modeled as production from natural growth (k_g), production from cytokines (k_{in_Paw}), and loss of the edema (k_{in_Paw}/R_{0_Paw}) that was produced by cytokines (i.e. when edema is not present only k_g affects paw size) as follows:

$$\frac{d\,\mathrm{PAW}}{dt} = k_g + k_{in\_paw}\mathrm{P_{CYT}} - \frac{k_{in\_PAW}}{\mathrm{PAW_0}}\mathrm{PAW} \tag{4.21}$$

$$\mathrm{P_{cyt}} = \pi_1(\mathrm{TNF}\alpha_{mRNA} - R_{0\_TNF\alpha}) + \pi_2(\mathrm{IL1}\beta_{mRNA} - R_{0\_mRNA}) + \pi_3(\mathrm{IL6}_{mRNA} - R_{0\_IL6}) \tag{4.22}$$

$\mathrm{P_{cyt}}$ describes the total contribution of cytokine mRNA to the overall edema. The values of π for each cytokine reflect intrinsic activities of each cytokine on the production of paw edema.

4.2.5.4 Drug Side Effect Dynamics Module

Bone mineral density was modeled from five different regions of interest (four femur, one lumbar). The major assumptions governing this model are 1) there are two types of bone, cancellous (Canc) and cortical (Cort), that contribute to BMD in each scan and 2) each region analyzed is composed of different fractions of cancellous and cortical bone. The parameters from the equations for the two types of bone turnover are the same for all regions; the only difference is the fraction of cancellous bone that is modeled for each specific region. Equations for cancellous and cortical bone mineral density are

$$\frac{d\,\mathrm{BMD_{cane}}}{dt} = k_{g\_canc}\mathrm{BMD_{cane}}\left(\mathrm{OB} - \mathrm{OC}\frac{\mathrm{BMD_{cane}}}{R_{max\_canc}}\right) \tag{4.23}$$

$$\frac{d\,\mathrm{BMD_{cort}}}{dt} = k_{g\_cort}\mathrm{BMD_{cort}}\left(1 + f_{cort}(\mathrm{OB} - 1) - [1 + f_{cort}(\mathrm{OC} - 1)]\frac{\mathrm{BMD_{cort}}}{R_{max\_cort}}\right) \tag{4.24}$$

The parameters k_g and $\mathrm{BMD_{max}}$ indicate the first-order growth constant and maximum value of bone density for each type. Hypothetical Osteoclast (OC) activity was described by the following compartment:

$$\frac{d\,\mathrm{OC}}{dt} = k_{OC}(1 + R_{cyt} - \mathrm{OC}) \tag{4.25}$$

$$\mathrm{R_{cyt}} = \rho_1(\mathrm{TNF}\alpha_{mRNA} - R_{0\_TNF\alpha}) + \rho_2(\mathrm{IL1}\beta_{mRNA} - R_{0\_IL1\beta}) + \rho_3(\mathrm{IL6}_{mRNA} - R_{0\_IL6}) \tag{4.26}$$

each ρ value indicates the individual contribution of that cytokine to the production of OC which stimulates bone loss. A hypothetical compartment for Osteoblasts (OB) was described by a transit compartment model:

$$\frac{d\,\mathrm{OB}}{dt} = k_{OB}(\mathrm{T_{OB}^n} - \mathrm{OB}) \tag{4.27}$$

4.2.5.5 Pharmacokinetics Module

After the disease network is characterized, the pharmacokinetics module is introduced to the network to describe the effect of the drug on the disease. In this case, the DEX exhibit effect by binding to the GR. Therefore, DEX affects the disease network through the variation of DR_N. The value of DR_N for the presence of the two CS is then calculated as the sum of concentrations of each drug bound to receptor in the nucleus:

$$DR_N = DR_{N\_C} + DR_{N\_D} \tag{4.28}$$

$$\frac{d\,DR_{N\_C}}{dt} = k_t DR_{CST} - k_{RE\_c} DR_{N\_C} \tag{4.29}$$

$$\frac{d\,DR_{N\_C}}{dt} = k_t DR_{DEX} - k_{RE\_D} DR_{N\_D} \tag{4.30}$$

k_T is the first-order rate constant for translocation of bound CST-GR complex to the nucleus. Bound CST-receptor complex (DR_{CST}) in the cytosol is

$$\frac{d\,DR_{CST}}{dt} = k'_{on\_C} \cdot CST \cdot GR - k_T DR_{CST} \tag{4.31}$$

bound DEX-GR complex (DR_{DEX}) in the cytosol is

$$\frac{d\,DR_{DEX}}{dt} = k_{on\_D} \cdot DEX \cdot GR - k_T DR_{DEX} \tag{4.32}$$

Concentrations of free GR in the presence of both CST and DEX is

$$\frac{d\,GR}{dt} = k_{syn\_GR} GR_{mRNA} - k_{dgr\_GR} GR - k'_{on\_c} CST \cdot GR - k_{on\_D} DEX \cdot GR + k_{RE\_c} RF \cdot DR_{N\_C} + k_{RE\_D} RF \cdot DR_{N\_D} \tag{4.33}$$

k_{syn_GR} is the first-order synthesis rate from GR mRNA and k_{dgr_GR} is the first-order loss rate constant. The parameters k_{RE_C} and k_{RE_D} describe the rates that corticosterone bound to receptor and dexamethasone bound to receptor return from the nucleus. Production of plasma CST concentrations is up-regulated by inflammation and is correlated with pro-inflammatory cytokines and inhibited by DEX-GR complex in the nucleus.

$$\frac{d\,CST}{dt} = k_{in\_cst}(1 + B_{cyt})\left(1 - \frac{DR_{N\_D}}{IC_{50\_CST} + DR_{N\_D}}\right) - \frac{k_{in\_CST}}{R_{0\_CST}} \tag{4.34}$$

k_{in_CST} is the first-order rate constant for the production of CST and IC_{50_CST} is the amount of DR_{N_D} required to inhibit production of CST 50%. The variable B_{CYT} is the influence of proinflammatory cytokines on CST up-regulation defined as

$$B_{cyt} = \beta_1(TNF\alpha_{mRNA} - R_{0\_TNF\alpha}) + \beta_2(IL1\beta_{mRNA} - R_{0\_IL1\beta}) \tag{4.35}$$

$\beta1$ and $\beta2$ are the intrinsic activities of each individual cytokine on CST up-regulation.

The most significant difference between the QSB model and other PK/PD is that the QSB model firstly characterizes the disease network and then links the pharmacokinetic model to the network which is inverse in the development of other PK/PD. This button up thinking makes QSB model getting more wide using drug development.

4.3 Study Design

A recent survey reported that pharmaceutical research and drug development is not efficient, for example, almost 50% of registration trials fail mainly because pharmaceutical companies employ one-size-fits-all development strategies [23]. To allow more efficient planning during the early phases of drug development there is a need for the accrual of disease and trial knowledge from across development programs [24]. Therefore, disease-drug-trial models are developed to representations of the time course of biomarker and clinical outcomes, placebo effects, a drug's pharmacologic effects, and trial execution characteristics for both the desired and undesired responses [24]. In this section, the general framework of disease-drug-trial models is introduced and then an example is employed to illustrate this model development.

4.3.1 Disease-Drug-Trial Models

The disease-drug-trial model contains three major submodels: disease model, drug model, and trial model (shown in Figure 4.2).

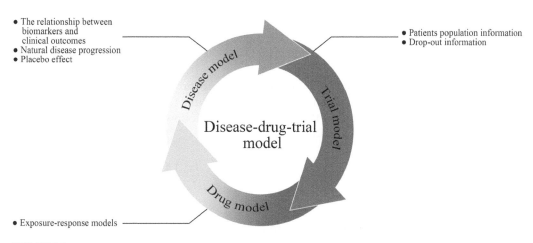

FIGURE 4.2
The conceptual depiction of quantitative drug-disease-trial models and their various submodels, including those for product features such as the biopharmaceutical characteristics.

4.3.1.1 Disease Model

The disease model represents three aspects of information: (i) the relationship between bio-markers and clinical outcomes, (ii) natural disease progression, and (iii) placebo effect. There are three general approaches to developing disease models: systems biology, semimechanistic and empirical models. The systems biology and semimechanistic/mechanistic models have been introduced in the above sections. Empirical disease model are merely mathematical models to interpolate between observed data. For instance, the relationship between the change in tumor size and survival is typically described using empirical parametric hazard models.

4.3.1.2 Drug Model

ER models are usually used for the drug model. The development of exposure-response models has been described in the above sections. The most challenging issue in drug model development is that how to bridge the ER across patients and healthy subjects. The report of Wang et al. provided a case which used a linear model to bridge the exposure response across patients and healthy subjects for a potential drug to treat insomnia [25].

4.3.1.3 Trial Model

Missing data due to dropouts could lead to biased interpretations of efficacy and safety [26]. The dropouts information is essential not only for designing better trials, but for optimizing therapeutic value and pharmacoeconomics. Therefore, modeling dropout pattern is the core task for trial models (some reports even termed trial model as dropout model). FDA recommended parametric hazard model for the development of trial model.

4.3.2 Case Study: Disease-Drug-Trial Model for Topiramate

Kalaria et al. developed a disease-drug-trial model for Topiramate [26]. They developed an empirical disease model to describe the disease progression. An exponential model was employed to describe the change in normalized BEF and BDF over time:

$$\mathrm{BF}(t) = BASL \cdot [1 - P_{\max}(1 - e^{-k_p t})] \tag{4.36}$$

BASL is the baseline BEF or BDF, $P_{\max}$ is the maximum proportional change in placebo response, and k_p is the rate constant associated with the time to achieve maximum placebo effect. The $E_{\max}$ model is selected as the drug model. The following equation described the bridging between disease model and drug model:

$$\mathrm{BF}(t) = BASL\,[1 - P_{\max}(1 - e^{-k_p t})]\left(1 - \frac{I_{\max}\mathrm{DOSE}}{ID_{50} + \mathrm{DOSE}}\right) \tag{4.37}$$

$I_{\max}$ is the maximum proportional change in drug response and ID_{50} is the dose required to achieve 50% of the maximal drug effect. A parametric hazard model was selected as the trial model:

$$h(t) = \lambda e^{\beta_1 \cdot \mathrm{BF}(t)} \tag{4.38}$$

Based on the simulation of above models, they find that for every unit increase in percent change from baseline in body weight (weight increase), the hazard for dropout increases by 18% and 125 and 150 mg should be considered to achieve a marked response.

4.4 Dose Optimization

In MIDD context, dosing regimen optimization can often be informed by modeling and simulation strategies. There are three major well-established quantitative methods for dosing regimen optimization: population pharmacokinetic model, physiologically based pharmacokinetic model (PB-PK) and Target-Mediated Drug Disposition model (TMDD). In this section, we introduce these three models.

4.4.1 Regulatory Guidance for Population Pharmacokinetic Model

Population PK analysis is a well-established, quantitative method that can quantify and explain the variability in drug concentrations among individuals. Population PK analysis integrates all relevant PK information across a range of doses to identify 60 factors that can affect a drug's exposure. In this section, several key points on Population PK modeling for regulatory review are listed [27].

4.4.1.1 Model Development

Some aspects of model development that are important for regulatory review are provided below: (i) model development issues can be addressed through several valid approaches, each with its own benefits and drawbacks. (ii) Covariate-parameter relationships can be established based on current knowledge of biology, physiology, or allometric principles. (iii) Issues regarding missing data, including missing covariates and data below the Limit of Quantification (LOQ), should be addressed with appropriate analysis methods. The sponsor should justify their methodological approach with regard to missing data and outliers and provide sensitivity analysis. (iv) Sponsors should specify how outliers are identified and handled in the analysis.

4.4.1.2 Model Validation

No single model validation method is generally sufficient to evaluate all components of a model. The following is a list of some of the GOF plots that are considered informative: (i) the Dependent Variable (DV) versus the Individual Predictions (IPRED), (ii) the DV versus Population Predictions (PRED), (iii) the absolute Individual Weighted Residuals (|IWRES|) versus IPRED or time, (iv) the Conditional Weighted Residuals (CWRES) versus PRED or time, (v) a representative sample of IPRED, PRED and observations versus time (one plot per subject), (vi) a histogram or Quantile-Quantile (Q-Q) plot of random effects, (vii) the correlations between random effects, (viii) the random effects versus covariates.

4.4.2 Population Pharmacokinetic Model

PopPK models aim at describing the average concentration-time profiles of drugs, while simultaneously quantifying the variability in the study population. The Nonlinear Mixed Effect Model (NMEM) contains fix effects and random effects. The concentration y_{ij}

measured in the individual i at time j of a population of N subjects taking the same drug is modeled by the structural PK model $f(x_{ij}, \theta_i)$. The NMEM assume that the structural PK model $f(x_{ij}, \theta_i)$ and average value of PK parameter vector θ have the same form in all subjects. Therefore, they are defined as the fixed effect. The individual PK parameter θ_i is considered as distributed around average value of PK parameter vector θ. The individual PK parameter θ_i associates the random effect (n_i). This distribution is assumed a priori to follow a given probability law, typically:

$$\begin{cases} \theta_i = \theta + \eta_i \text{ for normal distribution} \\ \ln \theta_i = \ln \theta + \eta_i \text{ for lognormal distribution} \end{cases} \tag{4.39}$$

There is a major limitation of NMEM that it only describes the variability of drugs concentration-time profiles and cannot summarize the factors which account for the variability. To address this issue, the covariates which characterize the factors responsible for heterogeneity in a population are usually introduced into NMEM. The covariates can be continuous (eg, bodyweight or age) or categorical (eg, sex or genetic polymorphisms). The influence of a covariate on a given PK parameter θ is described by:

$$\theta_i = g(\theta, z_i)e^{\eta_i} \tag{4.40}$$

$g(\theta, z_i)$ represents the function describing the relationship between the vector of relevant individual characteristics z_i and the individual PK parameter θ. n_i represents the individual random effect. As an example, drug clearance CL is often properly related to body weight according to the function:

$$CL = g(TVCL, \alpha; BW_i) = TVCL \left(\frac{BW_i}{BW_{std}} \right)^{\alpha} \tag{4.41}$$

TVCL indicating the typical population clearance, BW_{std} the standard value of body weight (typically 70 kg), BW_i the individual body weight, and α an allometric power coefficient.

Maximum Likelihood Estimations (MLEs), First Order Conditional Estimation (FOCE), and Expectation-Maximization Algorithms can be used to estimate the parameters of pop-PK models [28].

4.4.3 Physiologically Based Pharmacokinetic Model

The PB-PK model contains several blocks: Anatomy and physiology block, drug formulation block, drug absorption, drug distribution block and drug clearance block (shown in Figure 4.3).

4.4.3.1 Anatomy and Physiology Block

The physiology of the organism of interest is essential prior knowledge in PB-PK modeling and relevant organs are explicitly included in the model. Each organ is represented by its anatomical and physiological properties; for example, volume, tissue composition,

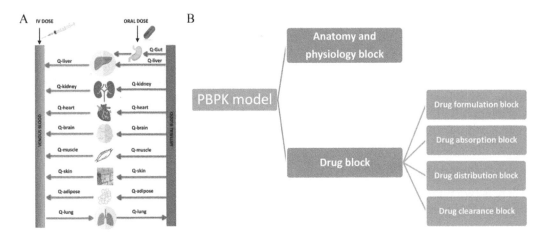

FIGURE 4.3
(A) The generic structure of a whole-body PB-PK model. (B) The composition of PB-PK model parameters.

and perfusion blood flow rates [29]. The anatomy and physiology block are represented by a set of ordinary differential equations. The parameters and ODEs are well established which are relatively fixed in different situations. These parameters and equations could be found in previous literatures [30–37]. However, the gastrointestinal physiology model is different from other organs. From a general perspective, the Gastrointestinal (GI) tract can be divided into several segments based on their anatomical and functional role: stomach, small intestine (duodenum, upper and lower jejunum, upper and lower ileum) and large intestine (cecum, colon ascendens, colon transversum, colon descendens, sigmoid and rectum) [29]. A well established model for gastrointestinal transit and absorption block termed as Advanced Compartmental Absorption and Transit (ACAT) which is relatively fixed in different situations could be found in previous literatures [38].

4.4.3.2 Drug Formulation Block

This block is oral dosage forms specific. This block describe the dissolution of oral dosage forms. There are three common dissolution models for modeling the dissolution of oral dosage forms: the Weibull model, Johnson model and z-factor model [39–41]:

$$\text{Weibull model: } x_d(t) = 1 - e^{-\frac{t^\beta}{\alpha}} \tag{4.42}$$

x_d is the amount dissolved at time t. The scale factor α and shape factor β are adjustable parameters which determine the shape of the dissolution curve.

$$\text{Johnson model: } \frac{dx_d}{dt} = \frac{3Dx_{s0}^{\frac{2}{3}}x_s^{\frac{1}{3}}}{\rho h r}\left(c_s - \frac{x_d}{V}\right) \tag{4.43}$$

$$\text{z-factor model: } \frac{dx_d}{dt} = \frac{3Dx_{s0}}{\rho h r}\left(\frac{x_s}{x_{s0}}\right)^{\frac{2}{3}}\left(c_s - \frac{x_d}{V}\right) \tag{4.44}$$

x_s is the amount of solid drug, D is the drug diffusion coefficient, x_{s0} is the initial amount of solid drug, ρ is the drug density, h is the diffusion layer thickness, r is the particle radius, c_s is the drug solubility, x_d is the total amount of dissolved drug at any time, and V is the estimated volume of dissolution medium. The above model can be bridged to the ACAT (Gastrointestinal transit and absorption block) by adjusting parameters c_s and V according to the physiology condition. This bridging can be used to establish an In Vitro – In Vivo Correlation (IVIVC) which providing a tool for optimizing the administered dosage form with a minimal number of in vivo animal experiments or clinical trials [29].

4.4.3.3 Drug Absorption Block

There is two types of drug absorption: passive and active processes. The passive process is described by permeability model:

$$\frac{dM_a}{dt} = \frac{2P_{eff}}{R} M_L \tag{4.45}$$

P_{eff} is the effective human permeability, R is the radius of the small intestine, M_a is the amount of drug absorbed, M_L is the amount of drug dissolved. The active process is mediated by transporter which is described by Michaelis–Menten equation:

$$v_a = \frac{V_{\max} c_d}{k_m + c_d} \tag{4.46}$$

v_a is the absorption rate, $V_{\max}$ is the maximum absorption rate, k_m is the Michaelis–Menten constant; c_d is the drug concentration.

4.4.3.4 Drug Distribution Block

A major advance in PB-PK modeling came with the use of calculation methods for organ/plasma partition coefficients, which describe steady-state ratios of the concentrations in the blood or plasma and the surrounding tissue [29]. There are multiple models for organ/plasma partition coefficients calculation. A popular model was proposed by Willmann et al. [42]:

$$k_{organ} = \frac{f_{water}^{organ} + f_{lipid}^{organ} \text{MA} + f_{protein}^{organ} k_{protein}^{organ}}{f_{water}^{plasma} + f_{lipid}^{plasma} \text{MA} + f_{protein}^{plasma} k_{HAS}^{plasma}} \tag{4.47}$$

The organ/plasma partition coefficients (k_{organ}) are calculated from the volume fractions of water (f_{water}), lipid (f_{lipid}) and proteins ($f_{protein}$) of the respective organ, and the lipid/water (MA) and protein/water partition coefficients ($k_{protein}$) of the compound.

4.4.3.5 Drug Clearance Block

Clearance is generally used to quantify elimination rates in liver, kidney, or other organs. At the body level, total plasma clearance (CL_{tot}) describes the sum of multiple clearance processes that occur simultaneously within multiple organs. Here, CL_{tot} is the apparent rate at which a compound is removed from the systemic circulation. In PB-PK modeling, the relative contribution of each organ to CL_{tot} can be further differentiated by quantifying the specific elimination rate in each organ.

There are two major drug clearance routes in the human body: liver clearance and renal clearance. At present, four models for describing the drug clearance in liver are developed including: well-stirred model, parallel tube model and dispersion model [43]. In the well-stirred model, the liver is conceived to be a single well-stirred compartment with intimate mixing between portal and hepatic arterial blood in the sinusoids which can be described by the following equation.

$$CL = \frac{Qf_B^u CL_{int}^u CL_{dif}}{CL_{int}^u (f_B^u CL_{dif} + Q) + QCL_{dif}} \tag{4.48}$$

Q is liver blood flow, CL_{int}^u is the free intrinsic clearance of unbound drug from liver water, CL_{dif} is the diffusional clearance of total drug between blood and liver tissue, and f_B^u is the fraction of unbound drug in the blood. In parallel tube model, the liver is conceptualized as a large number of identical cylindrical tubes, representing the sinusoids, that are arranged in parallel and with the hepatocytes, each having the same drug eliminating activity surrounding the cylinder which can be described by the following equation.

$$CL = Q\left(1 - e^{-f_B^u CL_{int}^u / Q}\right) \tag{4.49}$$

The dispersion model is the unifying form of well-stirred model and parallel tube model which can be described by the following equation.

$$\left\{ \begin{array}{l} CL = Q\left[1 - \dfrac{4a}{(1+a)^2 e^{(a-1)/2D_N} - (1-a^2)e^{-(a+1)/2D_N}}\right] \\[2mm] a = \sqrt{1 + 4R_N D_N} \end{array} \right. \tag{4.50}$$

The efficiency number (R_N) which describes the efficiency of drug removal by the liver and is equivalent under first-order conditions to $f_B^u CL_{int}^u / Q$. The axial dispersion number (D_N) is a measure of the dispersion or spread in residence times of drug molecules moving through the liver. When, $D_N \to \infty$, Equation (4.50) becomes the equation of well-stirred model. When $D_N \to 0$, Equation (4.50) becomes the equation of parallel tube model.

The renal clearance of drugs usually involves three processes: glomerular filtration, proximal tubular secretion, reabsorption from the distal tubule and collecting duct. Glomerular filtration is a passive process described by the following Equation [44]:

$$CL = P_1 + \frac{P_2}{P_1 \cdot BSA + 1} \tag{4.51}$$

BSA is the albumin concentration. P_1 and P_2 are regression factors with no physiology meaning. The proximal tubular secretion is an active process which is presumed to follow Michaelis-Menten kinetics based on total drug concentration in plasma. The reabsorption in kidney is can be described by parallel tube model.

4.4.4 Target-Mediated Drug Disposition

The term 'target-mediated drug disposition' was first introduced by Levy to describe drugs with PK properties markedly influenced by binding to their target [45, 46]. Mager et al. proposed a model for describing this process which is usually employed to characterize the pharmacokinetics of monoclonal antibodies. The proposed model is shown in Figure 4.4 [47]. The key feature of the model is that saturable, high-affinity binding of the drug to its pharmacologic target is responsible for observable nonlinear pharmacokinetic behavior. Drug in the central compartment (concentration, C_p; volume, V_c) binds (rate constant, k_{on}) to free receptors (or enzymatic sites) to form a drug-receptor complex (DR). The total binding capacity is R_{max} which imparts nonlinearity in distribution and sometimes in elimination. Once formed, DR may dissociate (rate constant, k_{off}) or in the case of receptor-mediated endocytosis, undergo internalization and degradation (rate constant, k_m). Unbound drug can also be directly eliminated (rate constant, k_{el}) or be subjected to non-specific tissue binding or distribution (amount, D_T; rate constants, k_{pt} and k_{tp}). The above system can be modeled by the following equations:

$$\frac{dc_p}{dt} = \ln(t) - (k_{el} + k_{pt})c_p + k_{tp}\frac{D_T}{V_c} - k_{on}(R_{max} - DR)c_p + k_{off} \cdot DR \qquad (4.52)$$

$$\frac{dD_T}{dt} = k_{pt}c_p V_c - k_{tp}D_T \qquad (4.53)$$

$$\frac{dDR}{dt} = k_{on}(R_{max} - DR)c_p - (k_{off} + k_m)DR \qquad (4.54)$$

In(t) describes the input divided by V_c for the system. R_{max} can be described by the following equation:

$$\frac{dR_{max}}{dt} = k_{syn} - k_m DR - k_{deg}(R_{max} - DR) \qquad (4.55)$$

k_{syn} is an apparent zero-order production rate constant, k_{deg} is a first-order degradation rate constant of free receptors.

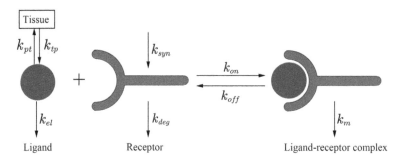

FIGURE 4.4
Pharmacokinetic model of target-mediated drug disposition.

4.5 Regulatory Application

The guidance for industry developed by FDA endorse the application of MIDD strategies in not only drug development but also regulatory evaluation. In this section, an example is introduced to illustrate the application of MIDD strategies in regulatory evaluation.

The guidance for industry pharmacokinetics in patients with impaired hepatic function: Study Design, Data Analysis, and Impact on Dosing and Labeling is an example for MIDD strategies application in regulatory evaluation. In this guidance, the population PK models are encouraged to help guide initial dosing in patients with impaired hepatic function. The principal task of population PK model is to correlate the hepatic functional (e.g. hepatic blood flow, serum albumin concentration, prothrombin time, or overall impairment scores such as Child-Pugh), and PK parameters (e.g. total body clearance, oral clearance, apparent volume of distribution, unbound clearance or dose-normalized area under the unbound concentration-time curve). A regression approach for continuous variables describing hepatic impairment and PK parameters is recommended by FDA.

References

1. Wang YN, Zhu H, Madabushi R, Liu Q, Huang SM and Zineh I. Model-Informed Drug Development: Current US Regulatory Practice and Future Considerations. Clinical Pharmacology & Therapeutics. 2019; 105(4):899–911.
2. Madabushi R, Wang Y and Zineh I. A Holistic and Integrative Approach for Advancing Model-Informed Drug Development. CPT: Pharmacometrics & Systems Pharmacology. 2019; 8(1):9–11.
3. Zhu H, Huang SM, Madabushi R, Strauss DG, Wang YN and Zineh I. Model-Informed Drug Development: A Regulatory Perspective on Progress. Clinical Pharmacology & Therapeutics. 2019; 106(1):91–93.
4. Sheiner LB. Learning Versus Confirming in Clinical Drug Development. Clinical Pharmacology & Therapeutics. 1997; 61(3):275–291.
5. Milligan PA, Brown MJ, Marchant B, Martin SW, van der Graaf PH, Benson N, Nucci G, Nichols DJ, Boyd RA, Mandema JW, Krishnaswami S, Zwillich S, Gruben D, et al. Model-Based Drug Development: A Rational Approach to Efficiently Accelerate Drug Development. Clinical Pharmacology & Therapeutics. 2013; 93(6):502–514.
6. De Simone P, Nevens F, De Carlis L, Metselaar HJ, Beckebaum S, Saliba F, Jonas S, Sudan D, Fung J, Fischer L, Duvoux C, Chavin KD, Koneru B, et al. Everolimus With Reduced Tacrolimus Improves Renal Function in De Novo Liver Transplant Recipients: A Randomized Controlled Trial. American Journal of Transplantation. 2012; 12(11):3008–3020.
7. Food and Drug Administration (FDA). Exposure-Response Relationships — Study Design, Data Analysis, and Regulatory Applications. Available at: https://www.fda.gov/regulatory-information/search-fda-guidance-documents/exposure-response-relationships-study-design-data-analysis-and-regulatory-applications. 2003.
8. Wang Y, Harigaya Y, Cavaille-Coll M, Colangelo P and Reynolds KS. Justification of Noninferiority Margin: Methodology Considerations in an Exposure-Response Analysis. Clinical Pharmacology & Therapeutics. 2015; 97(4):404–410.
9. Aouni J, Bacro JN, Toulemonde G, Colin P, Darchy L and Sebastien B. Design Optimization for Dose-Finding Trials: A Review. Journal of Biopharmaceutical Statistics. 2020; 30(4):662–673.
10. Pinheiro J, Bornkamp B, Glimm E and Bretz F. Model-Based Dose Finding Under Model Uncertainty Using General Parametric Models. Statistics in Medicine. 2014; 33(10):1646–1661.

11. Pinheiro JC, Bretz F and Branson M. Analysis of Dose–Response Studies—Modeling Approaches. In: Ting N, ed. Dose Finding in Drug Development. 2006; (New York, NY: Springer New York), pp. 146–171.

12. Megarbane B, Aslani AA, Deye N and Baud FJ. Pharmacokinetic/Pharmacodynamic Modeling of Cardiac Toxicity in Human Acute Overdoses: Utility and Limitations. Expert Opinion on Drug Metabolism & Toxicology. 2008; 4(5):569–579.

13. Derendorf H and Meibohm B. Modeling of Pharmacokinetic/Pharmacodynamic (PK/PD) Relationships: Concepts and Perspectives. Pharmaceutical Research. 1999; 16(2):176–185.

14. Racine-Poon A, Botta L, Chang TW, Davis FM, Gygax D, Liou RS, Rohane P, Staehelin T, van Steijn AMP and Frank W. Efficacy, Pharmacodynamics, and Pharmacokinetics of CGP 51901, an Anti-Immunoglobulin E Chimeric Monoclonal Antibody, in Patients with Seasonal Allergic Rhinitis. Clinical Pharmacology & Therapeutics. 1997; 62(6):675–690.

15. Danhof M, de Jongh J, De Lange ECM, Della Pasqua O, Ploeger BA and Voskuyl RA. Mechanism-Based Pharmacokinetic-Pharmacodynamic Modeling: Biophase Distribution, Receptor Theory, and Dynamical Systems Analysis. Annual Review of Pharmacology and Toxicology. 2007; 47:357–400.

16. Danhof M, de Lange ECM, Della Pasqua OE, Ploeger BA and Voskuyl RA. Mechanism-Based Pharmacokinetic-Pharmacodynamic (PK-PD) Modeling in Translational Drug Research. Trends in Pharmacological Sciences. 2008; 29(4):186–191.

17. Chan PLS and Holford NHG. Drug Treatment Effects on Disease Progression. Annual Review of Pharmacology and Toxicology. 2001; 41:625–659.

18. Winter WD, DeJongh J, Post T, Ploeger B, Urquhart R, Moules I, Eckland D and Danhof M. A Mechanism-Based Disease Progression Model for Comparison of Long-term Effects of Pioglitazone, Metformin and Gliclazide on Disease Processes Underlying Type 2 Diabetes Mellitus. Journal of Pharmacokinetics and Pharmacodynamics. 2006; 33(3):313–343.

19. Agoram BM and Demin O. Integration not Isolation: Arguing the Case for Quantitative and Systems Pharmacology in Drug Discovery and Development. Drug Discovery Today. 2011; 16(23):1031–1036.

20. Iyengar R, Zhao S, Chung S-W, Mager DE and Gallo JM. Merging Systems Biology with Pharmacodynamics. Science Translational Medicine. 2012; 4(126).

21. Earp JC, DuBois DC, Molano DS, Pyszczynski NA, Almon RR and Jusko WJ. Modeling Corticosteroid Effects in a Rat Model of Rheumatoid Arthritis II: Mechanistic Pharmacodynamic Model for Dexamethasone Effects in Lewis Rats with Collagen-Induced Arthritis. Journal of Pharmacology and Experimental Therapeutics. 2008; 326(2):546–554.

22. Earp JC, DuBois DC, Molano DS, Pyszczynski NA, Keller CE, Almon RR and Jusko WJ. Modeling Corticosteroid Effects in a Rat Model of Rheumatoid Arthritis I: Mechanistic Disease Progression Model for the Time Course of Collagen-Induced Arthritis in Lewis Rats. Journal of Pharmacology and Experimental Therapeutics. 2008; 326(2):532–545.

23. Lee JY and Gobburu JVS. Bayesian Quantitative Disease-Drug-Trial Models for Parkinson's Disease to Guide Early Drug Development. AAPS Journal. 2011; 13(4):508–518.

24. Gobburu JVS and Lesko LJ. Quantitative Disease, Drug, and Trial Models. Annual Review of Pharmacology and Toxicology. 2009; 49:291–301.

25. Wang Y, Bhattaram AV, Jadhav PR, Lesko LJ, Madabushi R, Powell JR, Qiu W, Sun H, Yim DS, Zheng JJ and Gobburu JVS. Leveraging Prior Quantitative Knowledge to Guide Drug Development Decisions and Regulatory Science Recommendations: Impact of FDA Pharmacometrics During 2004–2006. The Journal of Clinical Pharmacology. 2008; 48(2):146–156.

26. Kaaria SN, McElroy SL, Gobburu J and Gopalakrishnan M. An Innovative Disease-Drug-Trial Framework to Guide Binge Eating Disorder Drug Development: A Case Study for Topiramate. Cts-Clinical and Translational Science. 2020; 13(1):88–97.

27. Food and Drug Administration (FDA). Population Pharmacokinetics Guidance for Industry. 2019. Available at: https://www.fda.gov/regulatory-information/search-fda-guidance-documents/population-pharmacokinetics.

28. Guidi M, Csajka C and Buclin T. Parametric Approaches in Population Pharmacokinetics. Journal of Clinical Pharmacology. 2020; 00(0):1–17.

29. Kuepfer L, Niederalt C, Wendl T, Schlender JF, Willmann S, Lippert J, Block M, Eissing T and Teutonico D. Applied Concepts in PBPK Modeling: How to Build a PBPK/PD Model. CPT: Pharmacometrics & Systems Pharmacology. 2016; 5(10):516–531.

30. Agoram B, Woltosz WS and Bolger MB. Predicting the Impact of Physiological and Biochemical Processes on Oral Drug Bioavailability. Advanced Drug Delivery Reviews. 2001; 50:S41–S67.

31. Hoehme S, Brulport M, Bauer A, Bedawy E, Schormann W, Hermes M, Puppe V, Gebhardt R, Zellmer S, Schwarz M, Bockamp E, Timmel T, Hengstler JG, et al. Prediction and Validation of Cell Alignment along Microvessels as Order Principle to Restore Tissue Architecture in Liver Regeneration. Proceedings of the National Academy of Sciences of the United States of America. 2010; 107(23):10371–10376.

32. Liu XR, Smith BJ, Chen CP, Callegari E, Becker SL, Chen X, Cianfrogna J, Doran AC, Doran SD, Gibbs JP, Hosea N, Liu JH, Nelson FR, et al. Use of a Physiologically Based Pharmacokinetic Model to Study the Time to reach Brain Equilibrium: An Experimental Analysis of the Role of Blood-Brain Barrier Permeability, Plasma Protein Binding, and Brain Tissue Binding. Journal of Pharmacology and Experimental Therapeutics. 2005; 313(3):1254–1262.

33. Niederalt C, Wendl T, Kuepfer L, Claassen K, Loosen R, Willmann S, Lippert J, Schultze-Mosgau M, Winkler J, Burghaus R, Braeutigam M, Pietsch H and Lengsfeld P. Development of a Physiologically Based Computational Kidney Model to Describe the Renal Excretion of Hydrophilic Agents in Rats. Frontiers in Physiology. 2013; 3(494):1–16.

34. Tawhai MH and Bates JHT. Multi-Scale Lung Modeling. Journal of Applied Physiology. 2011; 110(5):1466–1472.

35. Thelen K, Coboeken K, Willmann S, Burghaus R, Dressman JB and Lippert J. Evolution of a Detailed Physiological Model to Simulate the Gastrointestinal Transit and Absorption Process in Humans, Part 1: Oral Solutions. Journal of Pharmaceutical Sciences. 2011; 100(12): 5324–5345.

36. Thelen K, Coboeken K, Willmann S, Dressman JB and Lippert J. Evolution of a Detailed Physiological Model to Simulate the Gastrointestinal Transit and Absorption Process in Humans, part II: Extension to Describe Performance of Solid Dosage Forms. Journal of Pharmaceutical Sciences. 2012; 101(3):1267–1280.

37. Thomas SR. Kidney Modeling and Systems Physiology. Wiley Interdisciplinary Reviews-Systems Biology and Medicine. 2009; 1(2):172–190.

38. Yu LX. An Integrated Model for Determining Causes of Poor Oral Drug Absorption. Pharmaceutical Research. 1999; 16(12):1883–1887.

39. Johnson KC and Swindell AC. Guidance in the Setting of Drug Particle Size Specifications to Minimize Variability in Absorption. Pharmaceutical Research. 1996; 13(12):1795–1798.

40. Takano R, Sugano K, Higashida A, Hayashi Y, Machida M, Aso Y and Yamashita S. Oral Absorption of Poorly Water-Soluble Drugs: Computer Simulation of Fraction Absorbed in Humans from a Miniscale Dissolution Test. Pharmaceutical Research. 2006; 23(6):1144–1156.

41. Tang YQ and Gan KS. Statistical Evaluation of in Vitro Dissolution of Different Brands of Ciprofloxacin Hydrochloride Tablets and Capsules. Drug Development and Industrial Pharmacy. 1998; 24(6):549–552.

42. Willmann S, Lippert J and Schmitt W. From Physicochemistry to Absorption and Distribution: Predictive Mechanistic Modelling and Computational Tools. Expert Opinion on Drug Metabolism & Toxicology. 2005; 1(1):159–168.

43. Wilkinson GR. Clearance Approaches in Pharmacology. Pharmacological Reviews. 1987; 39(1):1–47.

44. Hall S and Rowland M. Relationship Between Renal Clearance, Protein Binding and Urine Flow for Digitoxin, a Compound of Low Clearance in the Isolated Perfused Rat Kidney. Journal of Pharmacology and Experimental Therapeutics. 1984; 228(1):174.

45. Deng R, Jin F, Prabhu S and Iyer S. Monoclonal Antibodies: What are the Pharmacokinetic and Pharmacodynamic Considerations for Drug Development? Expert Opinion on Drug Metabolism & Toxicology. 2012; 8(2):141–160.
46. Levy G. Pharmacological Target-Mediated Drug Disposition. Clinical Pharmacology & Therapeutics. 1994; 56(3):248–252.
47. Mager DE and Jusko WJ. General Pharmacokinetic Model for Drugs Exhibiting Target-Mediated Drug Disposition. Journal of Pharmacokinetics and Pharmacodynamics. 2001; 28(6):507–532.

5

Real-World Data and Real-World Evidence

Xin Sun

Chinese Evidence-Based Medicine Center, West China Hospital, Sichuan University, Chengdu, China
NMPA Key Laboratory for Real World Data Research and Evaluation in Hainan, Chengdu, China
Sichuan Center of Technology Innovation for Real World Data, Chengdu, China

CONTENTS

DOI: 10.1201/9781003107323-5

5.1 What are Real-World Data and Real-World Evidence?

Real-World Data (RWD) is commonly defined as data collected in a non-randomized controlled trial setting, highlighting the representativeness of RWD for an actual diagnosis, treatment process, and patient health status in real medical or health care environment. In 2018, the US Food and Drug Administration (FDA) defined RWD as data relating to the health status of patients and/or delivery of health care, which are routinely collected from a variety of sources[1], including Electronic Health Records (EHRs), claims and billing activities, product and disease registries, patient-generated data, and data gathered from non-healthcare sources that can inform on health status, such as mobile devices. RWD can be collected for research purposes, such as from an observational study, or for non-research purposes, such as from monitoring, recording, and storage of various health-related data in routine practice.

Real-world evidence (RWE) is the clinical evidence derived from the analysis of RWD about the usage of a medical product and its potential benefits and harms. The use of RWE for regulatory purposes has attracted wide attention in the past few years, and it has been used for approval of new drugs and medical devices (often as a supplement to classical trials), approval of new indications or labelling changes, post-approval safety monitoring, coverage and payment decisions, and supporting healthcare practice decisions.

RWD has been widely used for a long time, even when they were not clearly defined. RWD research was originated from practical clinical trials, which was designed to determine the effectiveness of an intervention in a real-world setting. For instance, Kaplan *et.al.* conducted a multicenter, open-label, prospective study in 1993 to assess the efficacy and safety of ramipril in patients with essential hypertension[2]. In 1999, the Global Registry of Acute Coronary Events (GRACE), a large, prospective, multinational observational study of patients hospitalized with Acute Coronary Syndromes (ACE), was initiated to collect information through either active or passive surveillance approaches and provided a multicenter view of ACE management in real-world clinical practice[3]. Since the 1990s, more RWE has been developed around the world about various medical conditions and treatment strategies, using diverse research designs.

While RWD and RWE are playing an increasingly important role in health care decisions, challenges and special considerations in data sources, study designs, and analysis methods are worth discussing. In the following sections, we outlined the regulatory perspectives for RWE in different countries and regions (Section 2), discussed sources of RWD (Section 3), described methodological concerns on the design and analysis of RWE (Section 4), and presented six case studies of using RWD and RWE for regulatory decision making (Section 5).

5.2 Regulatory Perspectives

Increasing interest has emerged in the use of RWE to support regulatory decision making throughout the product life cycle – from primary approval to post-marketing surveillance. But using RWE for regulatory purposes is still challenged by the validity of causal inference, and methodological strategies are needed to ensure the quality of evidence. In face of these opportunities and challenges, national authorities in the US, Europe, China, and many other countries and regions have released policies and guidelines to instruct RWE generation and application in regulation, revealing an optimistic attitude towards RWD and RWE from the perspective of governments.

5.2.1 Current Use of RWE for Regulatory Purposes

The notion of using RWD to support regulatory decision-making is not new and RWD have been used for decades to monitor post-marketing safety and adverse events [4]. In December 2016, the 21st Century Cures Act opened the door to the potential use of RWD for formal drug approval in the FDA, which was a milestone progress of RWE use for regulatory purposes [5]. At the moment, RWE has been used to support regulatory decisions across the life cycle of drugs and medical products, from primary approval of a novel medical product, approval of supplemental indications, broadening the approved population to other disease stages or to pediatrics, to assessing the effectiveness and safety after accelerated approval [6].

Compared with Randomized Controlled Trial (RCT), the strengths of RWE include broader patient populations, representation of real clinical settings, lower costs and better feasibility in cases such as rare diseases [1]. However, the incorporation of RWE in regulatory decision-making still faces concerns on the validity of causal inference, and hence strategies are needed throughout evidence generation to ensure its quality [7].

5.2.1.1 Explicit Causal Question

A well-defined causal question should be able to be rephrased as an RCT that would answer it. For example, "Does obesity shorten life?" is not an explicit causal question because "obesity" cannot be randomized, while a similar question with randomizable interventions is explicit, such as "Does diet/exercise/gastric bypass surgery shorten life[8]?"

5.2.1.2 Data Appropriateness and Quality

Appropriate and high-quality data ensure that the derived RWE can serve its purpose in regulatory decision making, and hence should be evaluated before analysis. The appropriateness of data could be assessed from aspects such as representativeness of the population of interest, availability of critical data field, accurate data linkage, and adequate sample size and follow-up time [9]. The quality of data could be assessed from dimensions such as completeness, uniqueness, timeliness, validity, accuracy, and consistency [10]. More details are discussed in Section 3.

5.2.1.3 Selection of Study Design

The experimental design should be selected to match the causal question, because a flawed design could lead to invalid results even with statistical methods that appear to be appropriate[11,12]. More details are discussed in Section 4.

5.2.1.4 Complex Statistical Analysis

Various analytic techniques to minimize or eliminate confounding are needed, especially when dealing with observational data. For example, causal inference approaches, complex regression models, even artificial intelligence and machine learning approaches when necessary. More details are discussed in Section 4.

5.2.2 Regulatory Guidance and Policies

5.2.2.1 United States

In the US, the use of RWE/RWD for regulation was under discussion for a long time and hence the American government was more robust in the establishment of regulatory systems and guidelines.

As early as 2007, the Food and Drug Administration Amendments Act (FDAAA) required the Food and Drug Administration (FDA) to establish the risk identification of post-market and analysis database. In 2008, the FDA announced the Sentinel Initiative in response to the FDAAA to develop a national electronic safety monitoring system, and to achieve active monitoring of the safety of post-market medical products by using existing electronic health data, which lays a good foundation for the subsequent use of RWD[13]. In 2009, The American Recovery and Reinvestment Act (ARRA) gave a huge boost to Comparative Effectiveness Research (CER). RWD/RWE has become more widely used based on the real-world context of CER. The United States (US) Congress enacted into law the 21st Century Cures Act ("Cures Act") in December 2016, which encourages FDA to accelerate the development of drug regulatory decisions by the use of RWE for research[14]. As required by the 21st Century Cures Act, the FDA has been working to promote the use of RWE in drug development by "evaluating the potential use of RWD to generate RWE for product effectiveness to help support the approval of new drug indications." To guide future activities in this area, the FDA released "Use of Real-World Evidence to Support Regulatory Decision-Making for Medical Devices"[15] in August 2017 and "Framework for FDA's RWE Program"[16] in December 2018. The guidance describes sources of RWD and characterizes cases where RWE can be used to support regulatory decisions, including extended use indications, post-market surveillance, and conditional approvals. In addition, to better guide the use of RWD and RWE, the FDA has issued guidance "Use of Electronic Health Record Data in Clinical Investigations"[17] and "Submitting Documents Using RWD and RWE to FDA for Drugs and Biologics Guidance for Industry"[18].

5.2.2.2 Europe

The European Medicines Agency (EMA) system for RWE/RWD application is mainly established to focus on the collection and mining of medical information, emphasizing new collection methods and the possibility of in-depth data mining.

In 2013, the EMA issued the "Qualification opinion of a novel data-driven model of disease progression and trial evaluation in mild and moderate Alzheimer's disease", which discussed the technical details when using real-world observational data to construct disease prognostic models. In 2014, EMA also launched the pilot project on adaptive licensing to assess the feasibility of using observational study data to assist in decision making[19]. In 2016–2017, EMA issued successively the "Scientific Guidance on Post-authorisation Efficacy Studies"[20] and "Guideline on good pharmacovigilance practices: Module VIII-Post-authorisation safety studies"[21], to promote the use of RWD such as electronic medical data and registry data in post-market safety and efficacy assessments. In March 2017, EMA and the Heads of Medicines Agencies (HMA) jointly established the Big Data Working Group, which aims to use big data to improve regulatory decision-making and to raise the standard of evidence, with RWD being a subset of big data, including data from electronic health records, registry systems, hospital records, and health insurance[22]. Later on, EMA and HMA released a preliminary report in February 2019 to further explore the acceptability of RWE as a source of evidence[23], and a phase II report in January 2020 listing ten priorities to optimize these efforts[24]. Meanwhile, the Innovative Medicines Initiative, an EU public-private consortium, launched the GetReal Initiative in June 2018, to promote the adoption of quality RWE generation in the EU[25].

5.2.2.3 China

In China, the systematic use of RWE to support drug regulatory decisions is just in its early stage. However, the use of bevacizumab in combination with platinum-based chemotherapies was approved using evidence from three retrospective studies in 2018. The above shows that the national drug regulators have already begun to use RWE in their review practices.

In 2015, the State Council of the People's Republic of China released the "Action Plan for Promoting Big Data Development" that required to promote the development and sharing of public resource data, including big data of medical and health services, which coordinated and promoted the development and application of big data from a top-level design[26]. In 2017, the General Office of the CPC Central Committee and the General Office of the State Council issued the "Opinions on deepening the review and approval system reform to encourage innovation in drugs and medical devices"[27]. It is clearly pointed out that the early and mid-term indicators of clinical trials show efficacy and can predict its clinical value, they can be approved for marketing with conditions. Moreover, to better define real-world studies, outline the use and scope of RWE in drug development, explore the basic principles of RWE evaluation, and provide scientific and practical guidance for industry in using RWE to support drug development, China's Centre for Drug Evaluation (CDE) the Center for Medical Device Evaluation (CMDE), and the National Medical Products Administration (NMPA) issued a series of guidelines, namely "RWE to support drug development and approval guidelines (Trial Version)"[28], "The technical guidelines for real-world study to support the development and approval of pediatric drugs (Trial Version)"[29], "RWD for Medical Device Clinical Evaluation Technical Guidelines (Trial Version)"[30] and "Using RWD to generate RWE (Trial Version)"[31] This also marked the official opening of the national drug regulatory agencies from the regulatory level to build a framework system for the use of RWE.

5.2.2.4 Other Countries and Regions

In addition, other jurisdictions, including Canada, Japan and United Kingdom (UK), have made efforts to promote and support the use of RWE to varying degrees.

In Canada, RWE was brought into regulatory decision making in the 2016 Regulatory Review of Drugs and Devices initiative. In 2019, Health Canada issued a notice, "Optimizing the Use of Real-World Evidence to Inform Regulatory Decision Making"[32], and an article, Elements of Real-World Data/Evidence Quality throughout the Prescription Drug Product Life Cycle[33], designed to encourage industry to submit high-quality RWE and further promote its use and acceptability in regulatory decision-making.

In Japan, the use of RWD is currently limited to post-marketing studies[34]. In 2018, Japan's Pharmaceuticals and Medical Devices Agency (PMDA) updated the Good Post-marketing Study Practice to add considerations for using big data for post-marketing surveillance of drugs and collaborated with International Council for Harmonisation of Technical Requirements for Medicinal Products for Human Use (ICH) on the topic of using RWD for pharmacoepidemiological studies[35].

The British government highlighted the importance of using RWD to assess the quality and outcome of health services in the book "Equity and Excellence: liberating the National Health Service" published in 2010[36]. The Association of the British Pharmaceutical Industry (ABPI), in its publication "the vision for real world data-Harnessing the opportunities in the UK", has also made clear its desire to provide strategies to help the UK become a global RWD collection, analysis and use center[37].

5.3 Sources of RWD

To address regulatory issues, an ideal data source should cover a patient population with good stability and representativeness, and contain adequate information for evidence generation. Data might be needed on various information (e.g., demographics, symptoms, signs, laboratory and imaging results, medications, surgeries, and so forth) and throughout the entire or majority of disease course (e.g., from inpatient department, outpatient department, emergency department, over-the-counter, and so forth). When data from a single source could not provide all information needed, data linkage between different sources through a unique identifier might be necessary.

Based on how data are collected, RWD is divided into two categories: (i) data collected from routine patient care without research purposes, namely Routinely Collected Data (RCD); (ii) data collected using standardized forms for predefined research questions (i.e., primary data collection). RCD demand less human labor and time in data collection, but are prone to data unavailability and inaccuracies. Primary data collection contains data with high quality and validity for research, but substantial work is needed when setting it up. Increasing interest has emerges recently to set up registries on the basis of RCD, in order to reduce human labor while ensuring data quality.

In the current section, we discussed the availability of data, basic characteristics, scenarios, and strengths and limitations of these two sources of RWD.

5.3.1 Routinely Collected Health Data

RCD are data collected from routine clinical practices, which are generated to serve patient care without research purposes and can include clinical data, administrative and billing data. A distinct advantage of RCD is that it provides an adequate sample size with cost-effective and efficient data collection. Examples include Electronic Medical Records

(EMRs) or Electronic Health Records (EHRs), administrative claims data, safety or health surveillance data (e.g., infectious disease surveillance data, spontaneous reporting data), and birth or death registry[38,39].

EMRs may contain longitudinal patient records generated from primary or secondary patient care, and include information on hospital visits, symptoms and signs, medical histories, family histories, diagnoses, medications, procedures, laboratory tests, and imaging results. Although EMRs data reflect real-world clinical status of patients, the completeness of key research variables should be carefully assessed before further investigation, because EMRs data are prone to a high proportion of missing data. For example, primary care data may not capture information about in-hospital treatment, and prescription data may lack information about drug dispensing. In addition, the validity (e.g., sensitivity and specificity) of algorithms to identify variables of interest should be carefully validated. For example, patients with diabetes might be identified not only using the diagnosis for diabetes (either ICD codes or plain text), but also blood glucose from laboratory tests, prescription of antihyperglycemic drugs and insulin, and diagnosis for diabetic comorbidities. The process of EMR utilization often requires collaboration between various disciplines, such as epidemiology, statistics, clinical medicine, and information technology. EMRs have been used in a wide range of areas, including pharmacoepidemiologic safety studies, medication or medical devices monitoring, post-marketing safety surveillance, health economics, investigation of natural history of diseases and incidence, development of tools for real-time warning and assisting clinical decisions[1,22,23,40,41]. One of the best-known examples of EMR was the Clinical Practice Research Datalink (CPRD) in England, which has been proved to be of high quality and used in various healthcare research and pharmacovigilance[42-44].

Administrative claims data are data derived from payment interactions between defined patients and healthcare systems[45]. Examples include commercial insurance databases and government claims databases. They collect information about patient characteristics, disease diagnosis and billing and reimbursement for pharmacy dispensations or other medical services (e.g., hospitalization). Drug dispensing data in claims are one of the best data for drug exposure, because they are routinely audited to prevent fraud. However, diagnoses are considered less accuracy in claims than in EMR, because they are not directly tied to payment. Moreover, laboratory tests results and some confounding variables, such as smoking and drinking, are not available in administrative claims data. Administrative claims data have been used in comparative effectiveness or safety studies, drug utilization studies, health services research, and pharmacoeconomics[46]. A best-known example of administrative claims data is the Medicaid and Medicare database in the US[47].

Qualitative descriptions of the availability and completeness of variables is necessary before using RCD for research. The appropriateness of data for a particular research question should also be assessed, because different RCD databases contain different information and are consequently applicable to different research questions. It is crucial for generation of high-quality RWE that researchers choose data sources with consideration about its pros and cons, and when variables from a single data resource is inadequate, data linkage between multiple sources could be useful. We compared the scope of application, advantages, and disadvantages of EMR and administrative claims in Table 5.1.

Constructing a high-quality research database is crucial for conducting real world data research, because raw data from RCD are usually unlinked, unlabeled, contain unstructured texts, and hence uniform collection and cleaning rules are necessary[48,49]. An RCD-based research database should be established taking into consideration three key steps: data assessment, data extraction and data management (Figure 5.1).

TABLE 5.1

Comparison of EMRs vs. Administrative Claims

	EMR	Administrative Claims
Data Generation	Longitudinal patient records generated from routine patient care	Medical insurance reimbursement records of insured persons
Potentially available variables	Hospital visits, disease diagnoses codes, medication prescriptions or dispensing, procedures, laboratory tests, symptoms and signs, medical history, and family history.	Demographics, disease diagnosis, billing and reimbursement for pharmacy dispensations and other medical services (e.g., hospitalization)
Population coverage	Patients who visit medical institutions	Defined population with insurance
Strengths	Detailed information on hospital diagnosis and treatment; relatively high accuracy in diagnosis	Good representativeness; detailed information on medical cost; covering a long period of time
Limitations	Poor population representativeness; Lack of information on diagnosis and treatment outside of the hospital; part of data is unstructured; covering a short period of time	Lack of information on symptoms, signs, vaccination history, laboratory results and treatments; relatively low reliability of diagnosis
Applications	Pharmacoepidemiologic safety studies, pharmacovigilance, medication or medical devices monitoring, post-marketing safety surveillance, health economics, investigation on the natural history of disease and incidence, development of tools for real-time warning and clinical decisions	Comparative effectiveness or safety studies, drug utilization monitoring, health services research, and pharmacoeconomic studies

5.3.1.1 Data Assessment

Is a step to evaluate the appropriateness of data sources for defined research questions. As mentioned above, different data sources vary in variable availability and data quality, and hence the appropriateness of data should be assessed before any further exploration. The appropriateness is assessed from data quality and database accessibility. And data

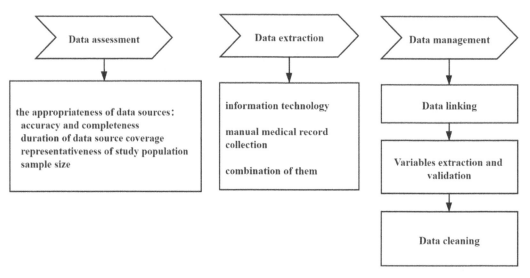

FIGURE 5.1
Three key steps for establishing an RCD-based research database.

quality is assessed from the accuracy and completeness of key variables, the period of time available, the representativeness of the study population, and the sample size of target population.

5.3.1.2 Data Extraction Method

Data Extraction Method is determined after access to the database is obtained. Three methods are commonly used for data extraction: data mining based on information technology, manual collection of medical records, and a combination of both. Different data extraction methods have their own advantages and disadvantages. Information technology-based data extraction is often accurate and efficient, but has limited feasibility and accuracy for unstructured text data and variables defined using complicated logical judgements and clinical experiences. Manual collection is useful for extracting unstructured information and complicated variables, but is time-consuming and labor-intensive, and is of limited use when dealing with a large sample size.

5.3.1.3 Data Management

Includes data linkage, variable extraction and data cleaning. (i) Data linkage: to determine unique patient identifiers; to link multiple data sources using the identifiers; to evaluate the ratio and accuracy of data linkage; (ii) variables extraction and validation: to extract variables using pre-defined variables extraction forms; to evaluate the accuracy of variable extraction; to describe the missing data, contradictory data, extreme values and abnormal values in each variable; (iii) data cleaning: to formulate variable dictionaries; to choose methods used to handle extreme values, abnormal values and missing values; to define the priority of contradictory data and the rules to structuralize text information. The formulation of data cleaning rules should be established considering the research questions, the clinical reality, and data distribution. Clear and explicit cleaning rules should be established for each variable. Both of the original data and cleaned variables should be retained.

5.3.2 Registry Database

A registry is often referred to as a patient registry because the primary population is patients with a certain medical feature. It is an organized system to collect longitudinal and consistent real-world data (clinical or other) through observational methods in a large defined patient cohort, in order to evaluate particular outcomes based on predefined objectives. The health information file(s) collected and formed through the patient registry is called the patient registry database[31,50-52].

Currently, three major types of patient registry databases, developed for different purposes and subjects, are used extensively for RWS. (i) **product registries**: collecting a series of data of patients exposed to a target health care product (e.g., drug or device) to evaluate the efficacy, safety, and cost-effectiveness of the intervention of the product in real-world clinical practice, and to support post-marketing regulation and decision-making; (ii) **disease or condition registries**: often established for major or rare diseases (e.g., Malignant tumors[53] or Albinism). The registry can be used to investigate the natural history of diseases, to assess the burden of diseases, to develop preventative and therapeutic interventions in the population, and to provide a scientific basis of enhanced accessibility of disease therapies. (iii) **Health service registries**: collecting information of patients exposed to target health services, in order to optimize the health service system,

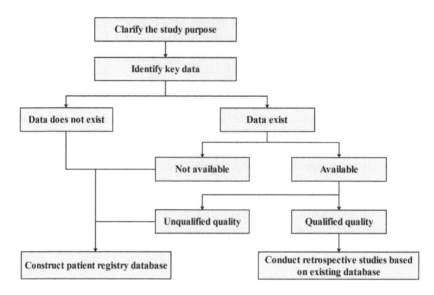

FIGURE 5.2
A flow diagram to determine the type of real-world data to use.

and to evaluate the health services effectiveness and health outcomes of the exposed population (e.g., liver transplant registry study[54]). Boundaries among these three registry databases are not clear-cut, with various degrees of crossover depending on the study aims and design.

In the actual research, we can determine whether to build a new patient registry database flowing the flow diagram in Figure 5.2. When constructing a new registry database is necessary, researchers can set up a registry with the following instructions[51].

5.3.2.1 Objectives and Feasibility

Should be fully considered before the commencement of database construction. A clear and specified objective is important for data collection. Feasibility should be considered from the following aspects: (i) funding and data sources are adequate, (ii) a multidisciplinary interdisciplinary team (e.g., clinical team, methodology team, data management team) can be organized to examine the feasibility; (iii) a research protocol identifying key types and sources of data can be helpful.

5.3.2.2 Patient Management (including Recruitment and Follow-Up) and Data Collection

Are two main steps of registry construction. Patient management process involves (i) identification of the target population, distribution of patients, and inclusion and exclusion criteria; (ii) recruitment of patients (e.g., telephone follow-up, online follow-up visits) and control of bias; (iii) follow-up plans and compliance maintenance. Data collection process should comprehensively consider: (i) design of the registry Case Report Form (CRF) and Data Management Plan (DMP); (ii) design of the Electronic Data Capture (EDC) system; (iii) selection of data sources; (iv) methods for data extraction and entry; (v) quality assessment and data standardization[55] (e.g., Clinical Data Interchange Standards Consortium); (vi) data storage and submission.

The processes of constructing a patient registry database are not fixed and can be reasonably adapted given different objectives and data sources. A well-developed patient registry database can comprehensively integrate multi-source data, obtain long-term outcomes, with high accuracy and integrity across a broad range of representative patients, and with more applications to answer questions regarding the efficacy, safety, and economic benefits and compliance of medication[31,56]. However, patient registry databases also have limitations: (i) not containing positive controls and untreated controls; (ii) introduces more difficulties in database operation and management; (iii) necessitating long follow-up and multidisciplinary team-working. Moreover, although the comprehensiveness of data can be improved when additional retrospective data or EMR data are used as complement, the feasibility of data standardization and linkage should be adequately examined.

5.3.3 Further Remarks

When using RWD, researchers should first examine comprehensively the reliability, validity, and specificity of variables, as well as the feasibility (affordability and completeness) of data collection, and then make an informed choice of the type of database. When routinely collected health data is incomplete and does not meet the need for the study, a special type of registry database, making use of existing RCD and prospectively collected data, can be constructed with proper data governance and management.

To help ensure the integrity of data, the ALCOA+CCEA[57,58] standards was promoted for researchers and audits, which identified data attributes of universal importance, including the attributable, legible, contemporaneous, original, accurate, complete, consistent, enduring, and available when needed. The detailed ALCOA+CCEA standards are shown in Table 5.2.

Construction and improvement of real-world databases are essential for development of pharmaceutical and medical technologies and for informing evidence-based healthcare decisions. RWD can be used not only as a complement of traditional RCT but also to represent patient populations encountered in real-world clinical practice. To make best use of RWD, scientific designs are needed for real-world databases, followed by complex data refinement and standardization to improve the rationality and reliability of RWE generation.

TABLE 5.2

ALCOA+CCEA Standards

Standards	Detailed Information
(A) attributable	The data can be traced back to the corresponding original records, data generator, generation time and modification record, etc.
(L) legible	The data should be clear and easy to read
(C) contemporaneous	The data should be recorded at the same time as when it occurred
(O) original	The data must be the first record made by the appropriate person and ensure the originality of the original records
(A) accurate	Ensure that all data required are captured and that data is captured in a consistent manner
(C) complete	Ensure the integrity of the data and original records and avoid missing data
(C) consistent	Ensure consistency between study data and source data
(E) enduring	The original records should be stored for a reasonable time for review and verification
(A) available	The original records should be stored in a reasonable way for review and verification

5.4 Study Designs and Analysis

5.4.1 Study Design

Designs about RWD for regulatory purposes include observational studies, pragmatic clinical trials, and trials with external RWD control. Distinguishing between these study designs helps researchers and policymakers take appropriate use of RWE to support regulatory decision-making.

5.4.1.1 Observational Study

Observational studies are studies without interventions, such as cohort studies, case-control studies, cross-sectional studies, case series, and so forth[16]. The type of design should be chosen according to research purpose and the availability and quality of data.

When designing a real-world observational study, the implementation process is as follows: (i) to clarify the research purpose; (ii) to construct the research question and hypothesis, with focus on five key elements: P (Population), I (Intervention), C (Control), O (Outcome), T (Timing); (iii) to evaluate the quality of database and key variables; (iv) to determine the appropriate type of study design; (v) to determine inclusion and exclusion criteria and to identify the study population; (vi) to determine the exposure and control group; (vii) to define the starting time of follow-up; (viii) to determine the endpoints; and (ix) to formulate the statistical analysis plan.

In the context of observational studies using RWD to generate RWE to support regulatory decisions, researchers should focus on the validity of results[14]. (i) **Quality of data**, such as the availability and quality of data on endpoints, the consistency in documentation, and the impact of missing data, which is the foundation to generate valid results. (ii) **Study design and analysis** is critical for ensuring confidence in results: Whether the study has an active comparator? Whether potentially unmeasured confounders and potential measurement variability are considered? Whether transparency about study design and analysis were examined before execution? (iii) **Sensitivity analyses and statistical analysis methods** should be prespecified.

The assignment of treatment in observational studies is based upon physicians' judgment, rather than randomization, which creates challenges for establishing causal inference. Hence, the identification and control of possible confounding factors and bias is an important consideration in the design and analysis of observational studies.

5.4.1.2 Pragmatic Clinical Trial

Pragmatic clinical trial (PCT) aims to estimate the effectiveness of an intervention in a setting close to routine clinical practice, which is a study design between RCT and observational study. Common design types for PCTs include[17]: (i) **individual PCTs**, which use individuals as observation units of trials; (ii) **cluster PCTs**, which use clusters as grouped units. Clusters in PCTs can be families, clinics, hospitals, or schools; (iii) **stepped wedge PCTs** is a special type of cluster PCTs, in which groups were randomly assigned to receive the intervention with different starting times. In stepped wedge PCTs, each group started the experimental intervention at different stage, and eventually all groups received the intervention. The type of design should be chosen on the basis of research purpose, research questions and research conditions. From the perspective of simpleness and efficiency, we give priority to individual PCTs.

The PRECIS-2 evaluation tool has been proposed to distinguish between RCT and PCT. Compared with RCTs, PCTs have the following characteristics[15]: (i) PCTs may have a broader inclusion/exclusion criteria; (ii) PCTs are usually applied in wider clinical practices; (iii) interventions for PCTs are more flexible; (iv) study procedures for PCTs may not actively promote adherence to treatment; (v) PCTs don't use placebo as control, and generally use conventional treatment, standard treatment, or recognized effective treatment as the control; (vi) follow-up and outcome measurements in PCTs are not fully standardized and optimized; (vii) PCTs are usually applied in an open-label condition, and hence may have more methodological concerns, such as measurement of bias.

Based on the characteristics of PCTs, some important considerations should be addressed when designing PCTs[14]: (i) whether the quality of data is applicable to support the generation of RWE? (ii) Whether the interventions and treatment strategies are well-suited to routine clinical practice? (iii) Whether the potential size sample is adequate, especially when outcomes are rare? (iv) Whether variations exist in endpoint evaluation and reporting among different study centers or different databases? (v) Whether the randomization method is used to control bias? (vi) When blinding of treatment is infeasible, outcomes that are less likely to be influenced by knowledge of treatment assignment should be used, such as objective outcomes (e.g., incidence of stroke, tumor size), in order to reduce bias due to lack of blinding.

PCTs involve complex interventions in a real practice setting and hence has more challenges in design and conduction. The methodological framework for PCTs is still under development at the moment, but since PCTs represent more realistic clinical situations and randomization could be applied, evidence obtained from PCTs is considered to be more reliable than that from purely observational studies.

5.4.1.3 Trial with External RWD as Control

The control arm of a study can be derived from external data, and in some cases, RWD can be used to generate external controls for trials. In some circumstances, standard RCT could be impractical or unethical and enough patients might not be recruited to achieve equal randomisation ratios, trials with external RWD controls are a possible type of evidence to support regulatory decisions, such as when standard treatment is lacking, in life-threatening diseases with limited treatment options, or rare diseases. As indicated by Gray et al in 2020, there are primarily two study designs making use of RWD as external controls: single-arm trials with external RWD controls (Supplemented SAT) and RCT with external RWD controls (Augmented RCT). In supplemented Single Arm Trial (SAT), control groups for SATs are solely provided by external RWD. In Augmented RCT, external RWD controls are used to add power to RCTs with small internal control groups (often N:1 randomisation ratio).

External RWD controls are classified into three categories according to the starting time[1] (Figure 5.3): (i) contemporaneous external controls, (ii) historical external controls, (iii) hybrid external controls. Contemporaneous external controls use prospective or contemporaneous retrospective RWD, which is collected on or after the enrollment of the first patient in the intervention group. Historical external controls use retrospective RWD collected before enrolling the first patient in the intervention group. Hybrid external controls include a mixture of both contemporaneous and historical external controls. Contemporaneous external controls using prospective data are preferable to other categories of external controls when temporal changes in the diagnostic criteria, medical procedures, or patient management exist potentially. For the same reason, using historical external controls is acceptable when there is no large temporal change.

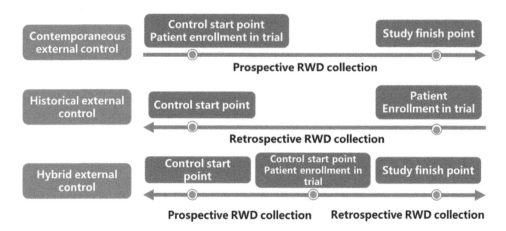

FIGURE 5.3
Three categories of external RWD controls, classified according to its starting time.

The comparability for external RWD controls to the treated group should be also examined on the basis of the underlying regulatory purpose. If the purpose is to provide supplemental historical data from diverse populations treated in real-world settings, the external controls can be defined more broadly than the treated group in trials. On the other hand, if the purpose is to establish a formal comparator group for primary drug approval, the external controls ought to be highly similar to the treated patients in trials.

There are some limitations to using external RWD controls. Firstly, selecting a comparable population could be difficult because of potential changes in medical procedures, variability in diagnostic criteria, classification criteria, outcome measures, patients baseline characteristics, and follow-up procedures. Secondly, ensuring the accuracy of research results could be challenging because the quality of external control data varies.

To mitigate potential bias and confounding in studies using RWD as external controls, a four-step approach was proposed to assist study design and analysis[59].

Step 1 - Key factors contributing to potential bias should be identified.

Step 2 - Baseline characteristics and potential confounders should be adjusted in analysis. Propensity score methods are frequently used for covariate balancing.

Step 3 - The potential bias should be assessed via quantitative bias analysis, which may be performed at multiple points during the design and analysis of an externally controlled study.

Step 4 - Outcomes from the external controls and the internal control group of an RCT should be combined using Bayesian dynamic borrowing analysis. In this method, power from the external controls is borrowed depending upon the internal control group.

Steps 1–3 is applicable for supplemented SATs without an internal control group. Step 4 is applicable in augmented RCTs with an internal control.

5.4.2 Statistical Analysis

Statistical analysis of RWD is much more complicated than that of RCTs. In this section, we provided a high-level overview of statistical analysis considerations for each design, and discussed the considerations of missing data and sensitivity analysis.

5.4.2.1 Statistical Analysis for Observational Studies

For observational studies, the statistical methods are primarily causal inference methods, where special attention needs to be paid to controlling or adjusting for confounding effects, in order to avoid deriving biased effect estimates. We discussed the main methods used in observational studies, including the methods for variable selection and variable adjustment.

(a) Variable Selection

Choosing all potentially relevant variables for modeling (including variables for confounders and risk factors) from a set of covariates plays an important role in the analysis of RWD. The approaches used to identify variables could be classified into two categories.

Researchers could first construct a causal network diagram, such as Directed Acyclic Graphs (DAGs) and the Single World Intervention Graph (SWIG), on the basis of expert opinion, to show the relationship among exposures, outcomes, and confounders. From the causal network, researchers identified risk factors, confounders, intermediate variables, time-varying confounders, collider variables, and instrumental variables. Risk factors and confounders need to be adjusted, while intermediate variables, collider variables, and instrumental variables cannot be included in the model. For time-varying confounders, special methods need to be considered, such as the G-methods, in order to get an unbiased result.

Alternatively, when constructing a causal network diagram is infeasible, for example for high-dimensional confounding factors in RWD, data-driven automatic variable selection methods can be considered. These selection methods empirically learn correlations among variables from the data and filter out variables related to treatment factors and/ or outcome variables as covariates. The simplest data-driven automatic approach is descriptive statistical analysis. For example, comparing variables between exposed and non-exposed groups allows identification of variables that are associated with exposure and outcome, and allows detection of unevenly distributed covariates between groups as potential confounders for adjustment. Some traditional variable selection procedures (forward selection, backward elimination, stepwise selection) and recently develop approaches (least absolute shrinkage and selection operator (Lasso) and machine learning) are more sophisticated.

The above two categories can be used in combination: professional knowledge is used to determine a set of potential variables, and then data-driven methods are used to select the covariates for final analysis. The advantage of the combination variable selection method is that it limits the dependence on expertise and reduces both the risk of over adjustment and the bias caused by confounders. However, some special issues should be highlighted: (i) many well-known variable selection procedures are designed for outcome prediction, instead of causal inference, and hence these procedures may work well for prediction, but not for causal inference. For example, propensity models only include the variables that guarantee exchangeability, and consequently covariates strongly associated with treatment but not exchangeability might not be included and this leads to estimates with large variances. (ii) No one approach is generally better than another, and each approach has different prerequisite assumptions, which may not be verified. (iii) The implementation of these variable selection procedures may be difficult, especially when dealing with high-dimensional variables with time-varying exposures. (iv) Machine learning estimators have been put forward in recent years, but it may get a variance that is too big to be useful and result in a meaningless causal inference; (v) the selection process of covariates must be transparent to the public.

(b) Variable adjustment

There is no randomization in most RWS (except for PCTs), leading to the existence of numerous confounding factors. Hence, controlling measured and unmeasured confounders is critical for RWS to achieve a reliable conclusion, and special statistic methods are needed. Two categories of approaches are used to adjust variables: traditional multivariate regression models and causal inference methods.

Multivariate Regression Models

Multivariate regression models are the most commonly used statistical analysis methods to adjust confounding factors in estimating the effects of treatment or exposure (table 5.1)[60]. The regression model is selected considering the forms of outcomes, exposure of interest, and study covariates. However, several important factors should be considered when applying these models: (i) the underlying assumptions of the model should be checked for the study data, for example, the proportional hazards assumption should be assessed for the Cox proportional hazards model. (ii) Whether important covariables are adjusted? (iii) The number of study subjects (and cases) is sufficient for model, typically the number of study subjects is at least 20 to 30 times the number of covariates, and the number of patients with an outcome event is recommended to be at least ten times the number of covariates. (iv) Whether aggregated covariates, such as propensity scores, are included when dealing with high-dimensional confounders? (v) Whether the non-linear form, such as polynomial, are taken into account for important covariates? (vi) Whether the interactions between different covariates are considered?

Causal Inference Methods

Counterfactual causal inference was one of the most important statistical ideas of the past 50 years, which has been commonly used in multiple areas such as econometrics and epidemiology. Based on the theoretical framework of counterfactual causal inference,

TABLE 5.3

Commonly Used Multivariate Regression Models

Outcome Measure	Single measure		Repeated Measure, Fixed Intervals	Repeated Measure, Variable Intervals
	No Clustering	Clustering (e.g., Multi-site Study)		
Dichotomous	Logistic regression	Multilevel (mixed) logistic regression, GLMM, GEE, Conditional logistic regression	Repeated measures ANOVA (MANOVA), GLMM, GEE	GLMM, GEE
Continuous	Linear regression	Multilevel (mixed) linear regression, GLMM, GEE	Repeated measures ANOVA (MANOVA), GLMM, GEE	GLMM, GEE
Aggregate or count data	Poisson regression, negative binomial regression model	Multilevel (mixed) Poisson regression, Multilevel (mixed) negative binomial regression		
Time-to-event	Cox proportional hazards model	Variance-adjusted Cox model or shared frailty model		

Note: ANOVA, analysis of variance; GEE, generalized estimating equation; GLMM, generalized linear mixed models; MANOVA, multivariate analysis of variance.

many methods are used for causal inference in observational studies. In this section, we discussed several of these casual inference methods: propensity score, disease risk score, and instrumental variables.

Propensity Scores　The propensity score was proposed by Rosenbaum and Rubin in 1983[61]. The propensity score is a function of the covariates, which is defined as the probability of receiving treatment (or exposure) conditional on observed covariates. In conventional analysis, the propensity score was typically estimated from regression models, such as a logistic regression or a probit regression of the treatment conditional on the covariates. In practice analysis, treatment variables are often multiple categorical or continuous, and hence generalized propensity scores should be used instead, the methods for which have been proposed by Imbens [62] and Hirano&Imbens [63], respectively. Generalized propensity scores can be estimated by regression model (such as logistic and probit regression model), machine learning (such as gradient boosting machine), the covariate balancing generalized propensity score based on generalized method of moments, and so forth.

The methods for causal inference through propensity scores included subclassification or stratification[64], matching[65], weighting[66], and regression adjustment[67]. Some cautions need to be addressed: (i) propensity scores cannot be used in an analysis with time-dependent confounders. (ii) Regression adjustment, subclassification or stratification, weighting, and greedy matching are not appropriate when there is a poor overlap in the propensity score distributions. (iii) Propensity scores may not work well if interventions change over time. (iv) The estimated propensity scores may not be stable when the treatment (or exposure) is rare, which could lead to the analysis being failed. (v) The covariates used to estimate propensity scores should be either true confounders or at least related to the outcome. (vi) Propensity scores matching can only ensure that measured covariates are being balanced, while unknown or unobserved confounders need to be assessed using sensitivity analysis. (vii) For subclassification or stratification, the distribution of the propensity score may differ between groups within some strata, and control of confounding is less effective than matching and weighting. (viii) The subjects who failed matching were excluded from the analysis, which reduces the precision of effect estimates and the validation for external replication; (ix) for weighting, when the propensity scores are extremely large or small, a robust estimator is needed; (x) for regression adjustment, balance in study covariates between groups should be carefully assessed.

Disease Risk Score　A basic assumption is needed for the propensity score method that the probability of receiving every value of treatment (or exposure) conditional on the covariates is greater than zero and less than one. Hence, the propensity scores are not appropriate if a particular combination of covariates makes a subject to be treated or exposed to have a definite probability of "one" or "zero"; at the same time, the propensity scores model becomes more complex if the treatment (or exposure) is rare or multiple.

The disease risk score is an alternative to the propensity score. It estimates the probability of an outcome occurring under specific covariates and a presumed no-exposure condition. Thus, disease risk score balance the covariates affecting the outcome between the groups, which is different from the propensity scores that balances the covariates affecting the treatment (or exposure). The disease risk score may be estimated by two ways. First, a regression model was constructed to estimate the propensity score relating the study outcome to the treatment (or exposure) and the covariates for the entire study population; then the disease risk score was computed as the fitted value from that regression model for each study subject, by setting the treatment (or exposure) status to non-treatment (or non-exposure).

The regression model also can be constructed only for the unexposed data, with the fitted values, and then computed for the entire data.

Similarly, to propensity scores, the disease risk score is often used for subclassification or stratification, matching, or to be directly included in model for adjustment as a continuous covariate along with treatment (or exposure). However, direct inclusion of the disease risk score as a continuous covariate for adjustment in the model performs poorly for controlling for confounders and bias[68]. The disease risk score is particularly useful in studies with a common outcome and a rare or complicated treatment (or exposure). In studies with a multilevel treatment (or exposure), in which some of the levels are infrequent, the disease risk score may be a good alternative to propensity scores.

Instrumental Variables   The multivariate regression models, propensity score, and disease risk score described above only adjust for measured covariates, but not unknown or unmeasured covariates. Instrumental variables, other than confounding/covariate control, is an alternative approach to validly estimate causal effects[69]. A variable can be defined as an instrumental variable if it meets three assumptions: (i) it is causally related to treatment (or exposure); (ii) it does not affect the outcome except through its potential effect on the treatment (or exposure); (iii) it is unrelated to the confounders of treatment (or exposure) and outcome. Two-stage least squares procedures and structural mean models are often employed when using instrumental variables.

Every method has relative advantages and disadvantages compared to other methods, and for the instrumental variable, the biggest advantage is that it does not need to adjust the unknown or unmeasured covariates. The most difficult step of this approach is to identify a high-quality instrument variable that meets the three assumptions, because assumptions (ii) and (iii) cannot be empirically verified. Moreover, relatively minor violations of these three assumptions may result in large biases in unpredictable or counterintuitive direction. Furthermore, to ensure the instrumental variable estimates are causally interpretable, homogeneity or monotonicity conditions are often needed. Homogeneity is often an implausible condition and monotonicity appeared credible in many settings. In non-homogeneous population, the causal effect estimate can only identify the average causal effect in a subpopulation of compliers and not in the entire population[70]. The requirement for monotonicity also brings up some concerns[71]: (i) the proportion of subpopulation of compliers is not identified; (ii) monotonicity is not a reasonable assumption in some observational studies; (iii) the partitioning of the population into subpopulations may not be justifiable.

5.4.2.2 *Statistical Analysis for Pragmatic Clinical Trials*

For the pragmatic non-randomized controlled trials, the methods discussed above could be employed. For the pRCTs, the statistical analysis was consistent with the basic principles of an interpretive randomized controlled trial, namely the Intention-To-Treat (ITT) analysis principle, using the Full Analysis Set (FAS) as the primary analysis data set. However, compared to RCTs, pRCTs are conducted in real-world settings where individual patient differences may be greater, standardization of the interventions received may be lower, patient compliance may be poorer, medical skills of clinical professionals may vary, and missing data may be greater. Hence, some issues should be addressed (i) there is a large heterogeneity in the study population and clinical setting of pRCT, and hence the statistical efficacy of the study results may be low, and a non-inferiority design should be used with caution; (ii) although the principle of randomization insulates the study from confounding factors, post-randomization confounding bias still need to be considered due to adherence issues.

Traditional ITT analysis in this context can gradually deviate from the original focus of the trial on efficacy. New methods such as instrumental variables could be employed; (iii) ITT analysis is not appropriate when the censor proportion is high, and in such cases, a more advanced method, for example the inverse probability weights method, could be used; (iv) as with multicenter RCTs, if the pRCT study population is from multiple centers, control for center effects is required. When the primary outcome variable is a continuous indicator, covariance analysis can be used; when the primary outcome variable is a categorical indicator, the Cochran-Mantel-Haenszel method can be considered. When there are other confounders or factors to be considered in addition to the central effect, a random effect model can be used; (v) Additional sensitivity analysis also is needed.

5.4.2.3 Statistical Analysis for Trials with RWD as the External Control

For trials using RWD as the external control, the main issue is how to combine the external control. For Bayesian dynamic borrowing analysis, the "power prior" approach and the Meta-Analytic Predictive prior (MAP) approach (including robust MAP and semiparametric MAP) can be applied.

5.4.2.4 Missing Data Considerations

Missing data are inevitable in RWS, and data for both outcomes and covariates can be missing. As such, the extent of missingness and its potential impact on analysis needs to be considered. Before proceeding with the primary analyses, it is important to use exploratory data analysis to characterize the missing patterns, in order to inform subsequent processing of missing data. Usually, missing data can be divided into three categories according to the missing mechanism: Missing Completely at Random (MCAR), Missing at Random (MAR), and Missing Not at Random (MNAR).

Choosing the right method for imputing and analyzing missing data is an effective means to reduce bias and increase efficiency. Including only the study subjects without missing data in the analysis is not recommended. The imputation method should be selected on the basis of the missing mechanism and the study question. For MCAR data, some researchers suggested analysis performed only with complete data, but it should be noted that this procedure reduced sample size and might affect efficiency. For MAR data, many statistical models can be used for data imputation, such as multiple imputation, traditional regression modeling methods, Markov Chain Monte Carlo methods, fully conditional specification, and so forth. For MNAR data, pattern mixture models can be used to construct different statistical models using missing and non-missing data for analysis, respectively. It should be noted that none of the three missing data mechanism assumptions is directly detectable and the mechanism for a specific database can only be justified by knowledge about the data collection process. In addition, it is difficult to identify the best missing data analysis method, and there is no method to obtain the same robust and unbiased estimates as the original complete data. The key to the best strategy for dealing with missing data lies in a sound design and implementation of the study.

5.4.2.5 Sensitivity Analysis

Sensitivity analysis is needed because each method has its own assumption, some assumptions cannot be verified in practice analysis. Therefore, sensitivity analysis is needed to address these assumptions with a view to evaluating the robustness of the causal inference results. We suggested the following steps: (i) to identify possible sources of bias on the basis of the causal structural model and the observed data; (ii) to use quantitative bias analysis methods, including both deterministic and probabilistic methods, to determine the extent of impact of bias on the results. In a formal quantitative bias analysis, one should construct the model using a minimal set of parameters governing this model, and then assign to the model all feasible values for each parameter, based on the literatures or expert knowledge[72]. Most commonly, the impact of each potential bias is modelled separately.

5.5 Case Studies

We presented several case examples to illustrate how RWD and RWE are used in drug development in fields like drugs for rare diseases (5.1–5.2) and post-marketing drug evaluation (5.3–5.6).

5.5.1 Using Registries to Support Cerliponase Alfa Approval

Cerliponase alfa (Brineura), an enzyme-replacement therapy, was approved in 2017 by FDA as the first treatment for neuronal ceroid lipofuscinosis type 2 (CLN2) disease. CLN2 disease, also known as late infantile neuronal ceroid lipofuscinosis (NCL) is a rare, autosomal recessive, pediatric neurodegenerative disease caused by gene mutation and is featured by difficulty in coordinating movements (ataxia). Patients often progressed to use of a wheelchair by late childhood. There were no other approved pharmacological treatments for CLN2 other than drugs for symptom management.

The approval of cerliponase alfa was supported by evidences ferived from the comparison of an intervention group from a single-arm trial, with an external control group from a natural history study[73,74]. A total of 24 symptomatic pediatric patients with CLN2 disease treated by cerliponase alfa were compared with 42 untreated CLN2 disease patients with similar but non-identical baseline characteristics[73]. The natural history study was conducted using the DEM-CHILD NCL database, which was a registry containing extensive retrospective and prospective natural history data collected from more than 500 patients with different forms of NCL throughout Europe[74].

The key question in this study was how to ensure that the external control group was as similar as possible to the treated group. To ensure the comparability, CLN2 disease patients in the registry were evaluated using similar eligibility criteria to those in the trial when selecting the historical controls, and efficacy conclusions were based on multiple analyses of the best matched patients and accounted for various confounding factors including age, genotype, and screening motor score[73,74].

Moreover, complex statistical analyses, including patient-level matching (1:1 ratio) and covariate adjustments were conducted to control for possible confounders and to support the conclusion on efficacy[74]. In addition, a sensitivity analysis with many-to-one matching between natural history patients and treated patients was done to confirm the robustness of the results[74]. Eventually, results from this study supported the indication of cerliponase alfa to slow the loss of ambulation in symptomatic pediatric patients with CLN2.

5.5.2 Using Electronic Medical Records to Support Asfotase Alfa Approval

Asfotase alfa (Strensiq), was approved in 2015 by FDA, for the treatment of patients with perinatal/infantile- and juvenile-onset Hypophosphatasia (HPP). HPP is a genetic, chronic, progressive, and life-threatening rare metabolic bone disease, characterized by low Alkaline Phosphatase (ALP) activity and defective bone mineralization that could lead to destruction and deformity of bones and other skeletal abnormalities. Asfotase alfa is an enzyme-replacement therapy used to reverse the skeletal mineralization defects in HPP.

The approval of Asfotase alfa for patients with the perinatal and infantile forms of HPP, was based on comparison of 68 treated patients from two multicenter, multinational, single-arm, interventional studies, with 48 patients with similar characteristics from a retrospective natural history study, who served as another type of external control[74,75]. These controls were patients diagnosed with or treated for severe pediatric hypophosphatasia at academic medical centers, whose data were obtained using a retrospective chart review of medical records[75].

Data of these medical records were abstracted according to pre-designed Case Report Forms (CRFs) by trained personnel. Extracted data included demographics, diagnostic history, clinical laboratory results obtained closest to the date of diagnosis, ALP gene mutation analysis results, and clinical course including comorbidities, complaint of developmental delays, hospitalizations, medications, therapies, and procedures[74]. In this study, data reliability, data quality and standardization of data collection are essential to generate valid RWEs.

Overall survival, skeletal health quantified radiographically on treatment, and ventilatory status was selected as the main outcome measures. Results showed that Asfotase alfa mineralized HPP skeleton, including the ribs, and improved respiratory function and survival in life-threatening perinatal and infantile HPP. The overall survival rate for treated patients at last observed point was 91.2% in the treated group versus 27.1% in the historical control group, and the median time to death was also longer in the treated group (1353 days vs 271 days)[75].

5.5.3 Using Post-Marking Surveillance Data to Evaluate Long-Term Safety and Effectiveness of Ipragliflozin

Ipragliflozin, an orally active, next-generation sodium-glucose transporter 2 (SGLT2) inhibitor, was approved in Japan for treating type 2 diabetes mellitus (T2DM) among adults in 2014, either alone or in combination with one of six other types of antihyperglycemic agents (metformin, pioglitazone, a sulfonylurea, an a-glucosidase inhibitor, a dipeptidyl-peptidase-4 inhibitor or nateglinide)[76]. SGLT2 inhibitors suppress glucose reabsorption at renal proximal tubules, thus stimulating glycosuria and leading to reductions in both fasting and postprandial blood glucose (and consequently a decrease in glycated hemoglobin [HbA1c] level), body weight and blood pressure in patients with T2DM. In addition, SGLT2 inhibitors also decrease cardiovascular risk, and improve hepatic function, and thus are recommended as the first-line oral medication for specific T2DM patients by the European Society of Cardiology and the European Association.

Ipragliflozin was approved with a series of pivotal phase III trials, demonstrating the safety and efficacy of Ipragliflozin in T2DM patients in Japan[76]. Post-marking evaluations of long-term safety and effectiveness of Ipragliflozin is warranted because T2DM is a progressive disease requiring life-long therapy and concerns remain about the potential Adverse Events (AEs) of SGLT2 inhibitor therapy.

Therefore, a long-term, multicenter post-marketing surveillance study (STELLA-LONG TERM [Specified drug use resulTs survEy of ipragLifLozin treAtment in type 2 diabetic patients: LONG-TERM use]), was conducted over an observation period of three years in routine clinical practice and registered more than 11,000 patients[77]. The study included Japanese patients newly initiated on ipragliflozin between 17 July 2014 and 16 October 2015 (data lock: 30 September 2019). Survey items included demographics, treatments, Adverse Drug Reactions (ADRs), vital signs, and laboratory variables.

Interim analyses covering periods of up to three months, twelve months, and two years after treatment initiation demonstrated that ipragliflozin was well tolerated, including in the elderly and other age subgroups, and maintained glycemic control and body weight reduction for up to 24 months after treatment initiation [78]. Results based on final safety and efficacy analysis sets (11,051 and 8,763 patients, respectively) showed a similar safety profile of ipragliflozin treatment in long-term, and constantly improved efficacy parameters for over three years [77].

5.5.4 Using Observational Data to Compare Real-World Safety of Bevacizumab with Ranibizumab

Comparative effectiveness research showed that Intravitreal Bevacizumab (IVB) and Intravitreal Ranibizumab (IVR) had equal efficacy for treatments of neovascular Age-Related Macular Degeneration (nAMD) and Diabetic Macular Edema (DME), but there was limited evidence comparing the incidence of Serious Systemic Adverse Events (SSAEs) and post-injection endophthalmitis between IVB and IVR treatments to support regulatory decision making. Moreover, findings from trials and small-sample retrospective studies were of limited generalizability to certain populations and rare SSAEs. Therefore, a prospective, multicenter, observational study, based on real-world medical records and patient interviews, was conducted to assess the safety profile of IVB and IVR in patients with retinal diseases[79].

This study included patients with retinal diseases from outpatient ophthalmology clinics of eight tertiary and teaching hospitals located in Central, Northern, and North-eastern Thailand between January 2013 and August 2014. These medical centers were chosen for their capacity to diagnose and treat retinal disorders with both IVB and IVR, which was determined by their diagnostic equipment, operating theatres, experienced retinal specialists, and other physicians who could deal with any complications arising from retinal diseases or anti-VEGF therapy.

Data of patients from included clinics were collected by patient interviews and medical record reviews, which were conducted at least once a month for a period of six months. Safety checks were performed via telephone calls when patients missed scheduled clinic visit for longer than a month. Hospital admission data from the National Health Security Office (NHSO)'s in-patient database and mortality data from the Ministry of Interior's civil registration database, were used to identify hospitalization due to SAEs and deaths occurring outside of study sites and during the follow-up period for all patients, including those who were lost to follow-up[79].

Finally, 6354 eligible patients treated with IVB or IVR were recruited from eight hospitals. For SSAEs, incidence rates were calculated with event free probabilities and were illustrated as Kaplan–Meier curves[79]. Data about individuals were censored at the time of loss to follow-up, consented withdrawal, drug switching from initial treatment to another, being event-free at the end of follow-up period, or death, whichever came first. SAEs with expectedly low incidence were combined as composite outcomes. Covariates were combined with the aim of achieving at least 5–10 Events Per Variable (EPV) to minimize bias and variability of estimates[79]. Missing data were not imputed, because it was assumed that patients went missing at random and treatment allocation between IVB and IVR was independent of the outcome of interest.

Univariable and multivariable time-to-event analyses were used to identify risk factors associated with systemic safety outcomes as well as to compare the risk of SSAEs between IVB and IVR groups[79]. Possible interactions between covariates were also considered in the model. Besides, the Propensity Score (PS) method was applied to minimize selection bias due to the imbalance of measured baseline covariates between these two groups, which was included as a continuous covariate in the multivariable time-to-event models, and it did not alter the results[79]. Results suggested that the rates of SAEs in both groups were low, and that the IVB and IVR treatments were not associated with significant risks of SAEs[79].

5.5.5 Using Pragmatic Trials to Compare the Effectiveness of Paliperidone Palmitate with Antipsychotic Treatment for Schizophrenia

Explanatory trials among relatively homogenous study populations under well-defined and highly controlled conditions demonstrated that treatments for schizophrenia with once-monthly paliperidone palmitate (PP) significantly delayed treatment failure, compared with daily oral antipsychotic (OA)[80]. However, explanatory trials typically exclude complicated patients, such as those with comorbid substance abuse and suboptimal disease management, who may be of particular interest to population health decision-makers as well as clinicians because these patients are more likely to be high resource utilizers. Another question of interest is whether the effectiveness of long-acting injectable (LAI) antipsychotic therapies is better than daily oral antipsychotic (OA) for treating schizophrenia in actual practice.

With these considerations in mind, a prospective, randomized, open-label, active-controlled, multicenter, pragmatic trial was conducted. The study consisted of a screening phase of up to two weeks, followed by a 15-month randomized treatment phase[81]. The study included adults with a current diagnosis of schizophrenia including patients typically excluded from antipsychotic treatment trials (e.g., those with a history of recent incarceration and comorbid substance abuse), allowed flexible treatment management decisions, and selected endpoint measures representing clinically important outcomes (e.g., hospitalization, treatment discontinuation). The study design also encouraged study participation after an initial treatment failure event, permitting evaluation of cumulative treatment failures during the entire trial period. The pragmatic analysis included all data related to treatment failures from randomization until the end of the 15-month period, regardless of whether subjects were maintained on their initial randomized treatment, which allowed for comparison of long-term treatment consequences.

Of the 693 subjects screened, 450 were randomly assigned (1:1) to either flexibly dosed, monthly PP (n = 230) or flexibly dosed, daily OA (n = 220)[81]. The OA medication used included aripiprazole, haloperidol, olanzapine, paliperidone, perphenazine, quetiapine, and risperidone, and subjects were allowed to switch between all types of oral medications during the 15-month follow-up when necessary. Finally, the intent-to-treat (ITT) population included 226 patients on PP and 218 patients on OA, of whom 41.2% and 40.4% completed 15 months of follow-up, respectively. The Mean Cumulative Function (MCF) of treatment failures and institutionalizations significantly favored PP compared with OA, suggesting that compared with OA, PP is not only more effective in delaying median time to treatment failure, but also reduces more treatment failures and institutionalizations[81]. This study resulted in an expansion of the FDA label in January 2018, which was the first example using RWE from a pragmatic trial in schizophrenia to support a regulatory decision[82].

5.5.6 Using Insurance Claims Data to Support Confirming Supplemental Indications for an Approved Drug (Telmisartan)

Telmisartan (Micardis), Angiotensin Receptor Blocker (ARB), was approved as an antihypertensive in 1998, and it was approved supplementarily in 2009 for cardiovascular risk reduction among patients aged 55 years or older who were unable to take angiotensin-converting enzyme inhibitors (ACE-Is) such as ramipril, based on evidence from the Ongoing Telmisartan Alone and in Combination with Ramipril Global Endpoint Trial (ONTARGET)[83]. To confirm these supplemental indications for telmisartan, a cohort study of patients newly prescribed with telmisartan or ramipril were conducted using insurance claims data, to compare health outcomes in real practice.

This study was conducted in commercially insured patients using the MarketScan health care database, which was a nationwide database capturing anonymized longitudinal health care data for more than 60 million commercially insured people in the United States[83]. Variables captured included inpatient and outpatient diagnostic codes, procedural codes, demographics and pharmacy dispensing of prescription drugs[83]. This study applied the same eligibility criteria and outcome measurements as that used in the ONTARGET, and used a composite of myocardial infarction, stroke, or hospitalization for congestive heart failure as the outcome[83].

Finally, 48053 eligible patients newly prescribed with telmisartan and 4665 patients with ramipril were included. To control for confounders, propensity score (PS) was calculated based on 74 patient characteristics including demographics, comorbid conditions, concurrent medications, and health care use measures, and then PS matching (1:1) with a caliper of 0.05 was used to balance patient characteristics[83]. Standardized differences were compared to evaluate the balance level after PS matching. An unstratified Cox proportional hazards regression was applied to compute hazard ratios (HRs) and 95% CIs, whose robustness was assessed by replicating it in a larger cohort derived with less stringent exclusion criteria[83].

This study based on real-world data from routine care provided findings similar to those found in the randomized clinical trial that used to approve telmisartan's supplemental indication[83]. It is one of the largest studies which analyzed real-world data to mirror a large randomized clinical trial that had established the clinical basis for a supplemental indication for a medication.

References

1. Burcu M, Dreyer NA, Franklin JM, et al. Real-world evidence to support regulatory decision-making for medicines: Considerations for external control arms. *Pharmacoepidemiol Drug Saf.* 2020;29(10):1228–1235.
2. Kaplan NM. The CARE study: a postmarketing evaluation of ramipril in 11,100 patients. The clinical altace real-world efficacy (CARE) investigators. *Clin Ther.* 1996;18(4):658–670.

3. Rationale and design of the GRACE (Global Registry of Acute Coronary Events) Project: a multinational registry of patients hospitalized with acute coronary syndromes. *Am Heart J.* 2001;141(2):190–199.

4. Li W, Ruan W, Lu Z, Wang D. Parity and risk of maternal cardiovascular disease: A dose-response meta-analysis of cohort studies. *Eur J Prevent Cardiol.* 2019;26(6):592–602.

5. Kesselheim AS, Avorn J. New "21st century cures" legislation: speed and ease vs science. *Jama.* 2017;317(6):581–582.

6. Franklin JM, Glynn RJ, Martin D, Schneeweiss S. Evaluating the use of nonrandomized real-world data analyses for regulatory decision making. *Clin Pharmacol Therap.* 2019;105(4):867–877.

7. Goodman SN, Schneeweiss S, Baiocchi M. Using design thinking to differentiate useful from misleading evidence in observational research. *Jama.* 2017;317(7):705–707.

8. Hernán MA, Taubman SL. Does obesity shorten life? The importance of well-defined interventions to answer causal questions. *Int J Obes (2005).* 2008;32 Suppl 3:S8–14.

9. Girman CJ, Ritchey ME, Zhou W, Dreyer NA. Considerations in characterizing real-world data relevance and quality for regulatory purposes: a commentary. *Pharmacoepidemiol Drug Saf.* 2019;28(4):439–442.

10. Gan Y, Jiang H, Li L, et al. A national survey of turnover intention among general practitioners in China. *Int J Health Plan Manag.* 2019; 35(2):482–493.

11. Petersen ML, van der Laan MJ. Causal models and learning from data: integrating causal modeling and statistical estimation. *Epidemiol (Cambridge, Mass).* 2014;25(3):418–426.

12. Rubin DB. For objective causal inference, design trumps analysis. *J The Ann Appl Stat.* 2008;2(3):808–840, 833.

13. Behrman RE, Benner JS, Brown JS, McClellan M, Woodcock J, Platt R. Developing the sentinel system–a national resource for evidence development. *N Engl J Med.* 2011;364(6):498–499.

14. U.S. Food and Drug Administration. Framework for FDA's Real-World Evidence Program. Accessed from: https://www.fda.gov/media/120060/download.

15. Gedeborg R, Cline C, Zethelius B, Salmonson T. Pragmatic clinical trials in the context of regulation of medicines. *Ups J Med Sci.* 2019;124(1):37–41.

16. Peng X SX, Tan J, Wang L, Nie X, Wang W, Wen Z, Sun Xin, On behalf of China real world data and studies alliance (China REAL). Technical guidance for designing observational studies to assess therapeutic outcomes using real-world data. *Chin J Evidence-Based Med.* 2019;19(7):1–8.

17. Wen Z LL, Liu Y, Guo X, Li H, Guo X, Chen J, Chen X, Fei Y, Sun X, On behalf of China REAL world data and studies alliance (ChinaREAL). Technical guidance for pragmatic randomized controlled trials. *Chin J Evidence-Based Med.* 2019;19(7):1–9.

18. U.S. Food & Drug Administration. Submitting Documents Using Real-World Data and Real-World Evidence to FDA for Drugs and Biologics Guidance for Industry. Available at: https://www.fda.gov/media/124795/download. Accessed December 2019.

19. European Medicines Agency. Pilot project on adaptive licensing. Available at:https://www.ema.europa.eu/en/documents/other/pilot-project-adaptive-licensing_en.pdf. Accessed 19 March 2014.

20. European Medicines Agency. Scientific guidance on post-authorisation efficacy studies. Available at: https://www.ema.europa.eu/en/documents/scientific-guideline/scientific-guidance-post-authorisation-efficacy-studies-first-version_en.pdf. Accessed 12 October 2016.

21. European Medicines Agency.Guideline on good pharmacovigilance practices (GVP) Module VIII – Post-authorisation safety studies (Rev 3). Available at:https://www.ema.europa.eu/en/documents/scientific-guideline/guideline-good-pharmacovigilance-practices-gvp-module-viii-post-authorisation-safety-studies-rev-3_en.pdf. Accessed 9 October 2017.

22. European Medicines Agency. Big data. Available at: https://www.ema.europa.eu/en/about-us/how-wework/big-data. Accessed 9 December 2019.

23. European Medicines Agency. HMAEMA joint big data Task Force: summary report. Available at: https://www.ema.europa.eu/en/documents/minutes/hma/ema-jointtask-force-big-data-summary-report_en.pdf. Accessed 9 December 2019.

24. European Medicines Agency. HMAEMA joint big data Task Force phase II report: 'evolving data-driven regulation. Available at: https://www.ema.europa.eu/en/documents/other/hma-ema-joint-big-data-taskforcephase-ii-report-evolving-data-drivenregulation_en.pdf. Accessed 22 January 2020.
25. EU/EFPIA. Innovative medicines initiative. GetReal initiative; 2019. Available at: https://www.imigetreal.eu/GetReal-Initiative. Accessed 9 December 2019.
26. The State Council of the People's Republic of China. Action Plan for Promoting Big Data Development. Available at: http://www.gov.cn/zhengce/content/2015-09/05/content_10137.htm. Accessed 31 August 2015.
27. The State Council of the People's Republic of China. Opinions on deepening the review and approval system reform to encourage innovation in drugs and medical devices. Available at: http://www.gov.cn/zhengce/2017-10/08/content_5230105.htm. Accessed 8 October 2015.
28. Center for Drug Evaluation, National Medical Product Administration, China. Real-world evidence to support drug development and approval guidelines (Trial Version). Available at: http://www.cde.org.cn/zdyz.do?method=largePage&id=303ca56a4ce06eb0.
29. Center for Drug Evaluation, National Medical Product Administration, China. The technical guidelines for real-world study to support the development and approval of pediatric drugs (Trial Version). Available at: http://www.cde.org.cn/zdyz.do?method=largePage&id=6d4b993 2c598599e.
30. Center for Medical Device Evaluation, National Medical Product Administration, China. Real World Data for Medical Device Clinical Evaluation Technical Guidelines (Trial Version). Available at: https://www.nmpa.gov.cn/xxgk/ggtg/qtggtg/20201126090030150.html.
31. Center for Drug Evaluation, National Medical Product Administration, China. Using real-world data to generate real-world evidence (Trial Version). Available at: http://www.cde.org.cn/news.do?method=largeInfo&id=eaed86b800e8d9d9.
32. Government of Canada. Optimizing the use of real world evidence to Inform regulatory decision-making. Health products and Food branch notice. Available at: https://www.canada.ca/en/health-canada/services/drugs-health-products/drug-products/announcements/optimizing-real-world-evidence-regulatory-decisions.html.
33. Government of Canada. Elements of real world data/evidence quality throughout the prescription drug product Life Cycle. Available at: https://www.canada.ca/en/services/health/publications/drugs-health-products/real-world-data-evidence-drug-lifecycle-report.html.
34. Ando T. Recent trend on utilization of real world data: challenges in Japan. Available at: https://www.pmda.go.jp/files/000226214.pdf.
35. Yoshiaki Uyama. PMDA's initiative on real world data utilization for regulatory purposes. https://www.pmda.go.jp/files/000232083.pdf.
36. Department of Health. Equity and Excellence: liberating the NHS. Available at: https://assets.publishing.service.gov.uk/government/uploads/system/uploads/attachment_data/file/213823/dh_117794.pdf.
37. Association of the British Pharmaceutical Industry. The vision for real world data-Harnessing the opportunities in the UK. Available at: https://www.abpi.org.uk/media/1378/vision-for-real-world-data.pdf.
38. Benchimol EI, Smeeth L, Guttmann A, et al. The reporting of studies conducted using observational routinely-collected health Data (RECORD) statement. *PLoS Med*. 2015;12(10):e1001885.
39. Langan SM, Schmidt SA, Wing K, et al. The reporting of studies conducted using observational routinely collected health data statement for pharmacoepidemiology (RECORD-PE). *BMJ (Clin Res Ed)*. 2018;363:k3532.
40. Frankovich J, Longhurst CA, Sutherland SM. Evidence-based medicine in the EMR era. *N Eng J Med*. 2011;365(19):1758–1759.
41. Ourth H, Nelson J, Spoutz P, Morreale AP. Development of a pharmacoeconomic model to demonstrate the effect of clinical pharmacist involvement in diabetes management. *J Manag Care Special Pharm*. 2018;24(5):449–457.

42. Bhaskaran K, Dos-Santos-Silva I, Leon DA, Douglas IJ, Smeeth L. Association of BMI with overall and cause-specific mortality: A population-based cohort study of 3·6 million adults in the UK. *Lancet Diabetes Endocrinol.* 2018;6(12):944–953.

43. Leite A, Thomas SL, Andrews NJ. Implementing near real-time vaccine safety surveillance using the clinical practice research datalink (CPRD). *Vaccine.* 2017;35(49 Pt B):6885–6892.

44. Ghosh RE, Crellin E, Beatty S, Donegan K, Myles P, Williams R. How clinical practice research datalink data are used to support pharmacovigilance. *Therap Adv Drug Saf.* 2019; 10:2042098619854010.

45. Strom BL, Kimmel SE, Hennessy S. *Pharmacoepidemiology 6th edition.* 2019.

46. Hennessy BLSSEKS. Pharmacoepidemiology 5th edition. 2012.

47. Bauchner H. Medicare and medicaid, the affordable care act, and US health policy. *Jama.* 2015;314(4):353–354.

48. Wen W, Jing T, Yan R, et al. Real-world data studies: update and future development. *Chin J Evidence-Based Med.* 2020;20(11):1241–1246.

49. Wen W, Pei G, Jing W, et al. Technical guidance for developing research databases using existing health and medical data. *Chin J Evidence-Based Med.* 2019;19(07):763–770.

50. Richard EG, Nancy AD, Michelle BL, editors.. Registries for evaluating patient outcomes: a user's guide. *US* Dep Health Hum Serv: Agency Healthcare Res Quality *(AHRQ).* 2014 Report No.: 13(14)-EHC111.

51. Jing T, Liangliang C, Wen W, Yanmei L, Guiting Z, Xin S. Real world study using observational designs: Plan for patient registry study and development of registry database. *Chin J Evidence-Based Med.* 2017;17(12):1365–1372.

52. Jing T, Xiaoxia P, Xiaochen S, et al. Technical guidance for developing patient registry databases. *Chin J Evidence-Based Med.* 2019;19(07):771–778.

53. Steliarova-Foucher E, Colombet M, Ries LAG, et al. International incidence of childhood cancer, 2001–10: A population-based registry study. *Lancet Oncol.* 2017;18(6):719–731.

54. Haldar D, Kern B, Hodson J, et al. Outcomes of liver transplantation for non-alcoholic steatohepatitis: A European liver transplant registry study. *J Hepatol.* 2019;71(2):313–322.

55. National Medical Product Administration, China. Technical Guidance for Clinical Trial Data Management. 2016; Available at: https://www.nmpa.gov.cn/directory/web/nmpa/xxgk/ggtg/qtggtg/20160729183801891.html.

56. Dhruva SS, Ross JS, Desai NR. Real-world evidence: Promise and peril for medical product evaluation. *P T.* 2018;43(8):464–472.

57. Group GIW. Reflection paper on expectations for electronic source data and data transcribed to electronic data collection tools in clinical trials. 2010; https://www.ema.europa.eu/en/documents/regulatory-procedural-guideline/reflection-paper-expectations-electronic-source-data-data-transcribed-electronic-data-collection_en.pdf.

58. Xueying L, Ruoqi S, Chen Y, et al. The selection of data governance model of clinical study based on real-world data. *Chin J Evidence-Based Med.* 2020;20(10):1150–1156.

59. Gray CM, Grimson F, Layton D, Pocock S, Kim J. A framework for methodological choice and evidence assessment for studies using external comparators from real-world data. *Drug Saf.* 2020;43(7):623–633.

60. AHRQ Methods for Effective Health Care. In: Velentgas P, Dreyer NA, Nourjah P, Smith SR, Torchia MM, eds. *Developing a protocol for observational comparative effectiveness research: a user's guide.* Rockville (MD): Agency for Healthcare Research and Quality (US) Copyright © 2013, Agency for Healthcare Research and Quality. 2013; Publication No.: 12(13)-EHC099.

61. Rosenbaum PR, Rubin DB. The central role of the propensity score in observational studies for causal effects. *Biometrika.* 1983;70(1):41–55.

62. Imbens G. The role of the propensity score in estimating dose-response functions. *Biometrika.* 2000;87(3):706–710.

63. Hirano K, Imbens GW. *The Propensity Score with Continuous Treatments.* Applied Bayesian Modeling and Causal Inference from Incomplete-Data Perspectives; 2004.

64. Rosenbaum PR, Rubin DB. Reducing bias in observational studies using subclassification on the propensity score. *J Am Stat Assoc.* 1984;79:516–524.

65. Rosenbaum PR, Rubin DB. Constructing a control group using multivariate matched sampling methods that incorporate the propensity score. *Am Stat.* 1985;39:33–8.

66. Hernán MA, Robins JM. Estimating causal effects from epidemiological data. *J Epidemiol Community Health.* 2006;60:578–86.

67. Reinisch J, Sanders S, Mortensen E, et al. In-utero exposure to phenobarbital and intelligence deficits in adult men. *JAMA.* 1995;274:1518–25.

68. Tadrous M, Mamdani MM, Juurlink DN, et al. Performance of the disease risk score in a cohort study with policy-induced selection bias[J]. *J Comp Eff Res,* 2015, 4(6): 607–614. DOI:10.2217/cer.15.40.

69. Angrist JD, Imbens GW, Rubin DB. Identification of causal effects using instrumental variables (with discussion). *J Am Stat Assoc.* 1996;91:444–72.

70. Angrist JD, Imbens GW, Rubin DB. Identification of causal effects using instrumental variables (with discussion). *J Am Stat Assoc.* 1996;91:444–72.

71. Hernán MA, Robins JM (2020). *Causal inference: What if.* Boca Raton: Chapman & Hall/CRC.

72. Lash TL, Fox MP, Fink AK. *Applying quantitative bias analysis to epidemiologic data.* New York: Springer; 2009.

73. Schulz A, Ajayi T, Specchio N, et al. Study of intraventricular cerliponase alfa for CLN2 disease. *N Engl J Med.* 2018;378(20):1898–1907.

74. Wu J, Wang C, Toh S, Pisa FE, Bauer L. Use of real-world evidence in regulatory decisions for rare diseases in the United States-current status and future directions. *Pharmacoepidemiol Drug Saf.* 2020;29(10):1213–1218.

75. Whyte MP, Rockman–Greenberg C, Ozono K, et al. Asfotase alfa treatment improves survival for perinatal and infantile hypophosphatasia. *J Clin Endocrinol Metab.* 2016;101(1):334–342.

76. Poole RM, Dungo RT. Ipragliflozin: first global approval. *Drugs.* 2014;74(5):611–617.

77. Nakamura I, Maegawa H, Tobe K, Uno S. Real-world evidence for long-term safety and effectiveness of ipragliflozin in Japanese patients with Type 2 diabetes mellitus: Final results of a 3-year post-marketing surveillance study (STELLA-LONG TERM). *Expert Opin Pharmacother.* 2021;22(3):373–387.

78. Maegawa H, Tobe K, Tabuchi H, Nakamura I. Baseline characteristics and interim (3-month) efficacy and safety data from STELLA-LONG TERM, a long-term post-marketing surveillance study of ipragliflozin in Japanese patients with type 2 diabetes in real-world clinical practice. *Expert Opin Pharmacother.* 2016;17(15):1985–1994.

79. Sangroongruangsri S, Chaikledkaew U, Kumluang S, et al. Real-world safety of intravitreal bevacizumab and ranibizumab treatments for retinal diseases in Thailand: A prospective observational study. *Clin Drug Investig.* 2018;38(9):853–865.

80. Alphs L, Benson C, Cheshire-Kinney K, et al. Real-world outcomes of paliperidone palmitate compared to daily oral antipsychotic therapy in schizophrenia: a randomized, open-label, review board-blinded 15-month study. *The Journal of clinical psychiatry.* 2015;76(5):554–561.

81. Alphs L, Mao L, Lynn Starr H, Benson C. A pragmatic analysis comparing once-monthly paliperidone palmitate versus daily oral antipsychotic treatment in patients with schizophrenia. *Schizophr Res.* 2016;170(2–3):259–264.

82. Baumfeld Andre E, Reynolds R, Caubel P, Azoulay L, Dreyer NA. Trial designs using real-world data: The changing landscape of the regulatory approval process. *Pharmacoepidemiol Drug Saf.* 2020;29(10):1201–1212.

83. Fralick M, Kesselheim AS, Avorn J, Schneeweiss S. Use of health care databases to support supplemental indications of approved medications. *JAMA Intern Med.* 2018;178(1):55–63.

6

AI/ML in Medical Research and Drug Development

Amir Nikooienejad and Haoda Fu

Advanced Analytics and Data Sciences, Eli Lilly and Company,
Lilly Corporate Center, Indianapolis, IN, USA

CONTENTS

6.1 Introduction

In this chapter we review some key contributions of artificial intelligence (AI) and machine learning (ML) methods in medical research and drug development. With the advent of novel methods and advancements in computational power in recent years, such approaches have been employed extensively in different applications more than ever before. Medical field and pharmaceutical industry have not been an exception. To review what has been done and provide an insight for future direction, it is not possible to list every contribution of AI/ML in this field all in one chapter. The intent, however, is to review fundamental or leading publications that has utilized or proposed a novel AI/ML based approach in different stages of drug development process or clinical research as a solution to the existing challenges. The reader is hence advised to consider those references as a potential lead to dig deeper into the subject for further research according to their goal. Before going into details, we first provide a brief definition of AI and ML and how to distinguish between them by pointing out their relationship with respect to each other and their differences. We then review different aspects of machine learning and discuss common methodologies related to deep learning and reinforcement learning. Those methods are vastly applied in different applications in academia and industry. There have been various survey and review articles published on this regard [Réda et al., 2020; Topol, 2019; Yu et al., 2019] to name a few, but here we try to explore AI/ML contribution from a new angle and by breaking the process down into different stages and provide more details.

The structure of this chapter is as follows. In Section 6.2, we review frequently used deep learning methods and introduce the foundation of reinforcement learning. Section 6.3 through 6.7 investigate applications of AI/ML methods in different stages of the drug development from drug discovery up to manufacturing and fault detection. In particular, the sections are structured as they sequentially occur in this industry. First, we start from target identification and molecular design in Section 6.3, and then transition into pharmacokinetics and pharmacodynamics topic in Section 4. After that, Section 6.5 zooms into some specific application of AI/ML in clinical trials, clinical practice, and healthcare system in general. Some recent interesting algorithms regarding personalized medicine are discussed in Section 6.6. An important piece of drug development process after FDA's approval is manufacturing of the drug in mass production with high quality standards. This is discussed in Section 6.7. The main point of all these sections is to provide the role of AI/ML and discuss how it has impacted and will shape the process in near future. Finally, Section 6.8 wraps up the chapter and provides a discussion around the current role of AI/ML in this field and its limitations.

6.2 AI, ML and Deep Learning Methods

It would be better to start from the question of what machine learning is, how it is related to artificial intelligence and where deep learning methods stand with respect to the other two. The concept of artificial intelligence has been around for a long time when in 1950s scientists wondered the tasks that are performed by humans can be automated and done by machines. The concept of symbolic AI was a common theme back then when it was believed that programmers can come up with large explicit rules for machines to reach human-level intelligence. However, it has only been in recent years that we have seen breakthroughs in the application ML mainly due to enhanced computational power with the advent of new processing units such as GPU or TPU, as well as state-of-the art means of data collection that has led to existence of massive high-quality data. One example of such valuable datasets is ImageNet [Deng et al., 2009], a dataset consisting of 1.4 million annotated images in 1,000 categories that has been used in training of countless of neural networks purposed for image analysis in various fields.

Not all methods in artificial intelligence pertain to learning though. We can consider machine learning as a subset of the artificial intelligence concept. The term learning here refers to something that sits in stark contrast with traditional hard coding of rules in classical programming, symbolic AI. In the latter the programmer provides rules and some data, and specific outcomes are produced with respect to the inputs, whereas in the former the data as well as expected outcome are the inputs, and the module is trained to come up with set of rules to match the given outcome to the given data. In other words, in classical programming rules are the input to the process but in modern machine learning the rules are the output of the process.

The idea of deep learning, where multiple layers of artificial neurons stacked together, is originally based on biological neurons in human brain and how we, as humans, perceive the world. It can be thought of as a flexible set of functions that are built upon many basic computational blocks called neurons [Roberts et al., 2021]. Deep learning is part of machine learning and with the emergence of brilliant algorithms in the last decade its impact has been manifested specially in the supervised learning paradigm. Today, almost all the fields of industry are benefiting from deep learning methods.

6.2.1 Supervised Learning

ML methods can be categorized into three major groups: supervised learning, unsupervised learning, and reinforcement learning. Supervised learning is perhaps the most common type of machine learning approaches in which the system is trained on a very large sample of previously collected labeled data to classify and predict the label of new data. Applications of supervised learning can include classifying images (MRI scans, biopsy images, pictures of packages on production line, etc.), signals from activity watches to determine specific behavior, video signals to detect certain objects and many other examples. There has been a remarkable advance in techniques and methods of utilizing Deep Neural Networks (DNN) in different aspects of supervised learning. The backbone of all these methods is Stochastic Gradient Descent (SGD) to minimize the loss function between the predicted and true outcome using input data at the training stage. Backward propagation, aka back prop, is the key step in calculating gradients to minimize the loss function. This concept has been very well illustrated in [LeCun et al., 2015] in the context of training multilayer network architectures used in DNNs. In the following, we briefly review some of the key breakthroughs in DNN that has facilitated its use in various applications in academia and industry more reliably than ever.

6.2.1.1 Convolutional Neural Networks

Convolutional neural networks also known as ConvNets or CNN, have shown to be a powerful tool in various problems mainly those that involve images, e.g., image segmentation, object detection and face recognition [Taigman et al., 2014]. Also, in natural language processing [Collobert et al., 2011] and speech recognition [Sainath et al., 2013]. According to [LeCun et al., 2015] the four key aspects of CNN that capture the properties of the input signal are local connections, shared weights, pooling and using many layers. Local neighboring pixels are usually highly correlated, which form a specific feature that can be repeated in other parts of the image. On the other hand, pooling combines similar features into one, for instance by using the maximum value of a grid of pixels of a specific size as the representative of the grid. This not only to reduce dimensionality but also makes the data invariant to small shifts and distortions in the image [LeCun et al., 2015]. Some examples of CNN in medical research are [Li et al., 2014; Yang and Yu 2021] for classification and object detection in medical imaging analysis or [Tsehay et al., 2017] for detecting prostate cancer on MRI images. More examples of CNN in medical research and clinical trials are discussed in Section 6.5.

6.2.1.2 Recurrent Neural Networks

Recurrent neural networks (RNN) are utilized for tasks that involves sequential data, such as language models or speech signals. In general, it is a perfect fit for any sequence generating tasks in medical research including drug discovery as we review in the next section. Training of such models is challenging due to their sequential nature, where the gradient either diminishes or explodes as the length of the sequence increases. However, thanks to [Hochreiter and Schmidhuber, 1997; El Hihi and Bengio, 1996] and [Sutskever, 2013], RNNs do not suffer from that issue anymore and can efficiently be trained. The introduction of concepts such as Long Short Term Memory (LSTM) [Hochreiter and Schmidhuber, 1997] and later Gated Recurrent Unit (GRU) [Cho et al., 2014; Chung et al., 2014] overcome issues of training RNNs and paved the way for their exploitation in real world problems. Major breakthroughs in the field of machine translation have occurred by exploiting LSTM [Sutskever et al., 2014]. RNNs also are the backbone of Natural Language Processing (NLP). The advent of Attention mechanisms mainly for recurrent networks [Bahdanau et al., 2014; Kim et al., 2017] advanced the field even further by allowing to model dependencies regardless of their distance in the sequence. Although, later through Transformer model, [Vaswani et al., 2017] generalized Attention mechanism out of RNN and added the capability to draw global dependencies between input and output of a DNN. Similar to CNN, we will review more applications of RNN in the pharmaceutical industry and clinical research in the following sections.

6.2.2 Unsupervised Learning

Unlike supervised learning, there are no labeled data in unsupervised learning. The goal is to detect patterns or structures within data that are hidden or has not been identified previously. Clustering is a great example for this type of ML and all clustering methods fall into this category. Anomaly detection or change point detection in time series data are other examples of unsupervised learning.

6.2.3 Reinforcement Learning

Reinforcement learning (RL) is a totally different paradigm than supervised or unsupervised learning, although some similarities may exist. In reinforcement learning an agent is interacting with the environment and learns how to make decision by trial and error. The system is reward-based and in this way the agent learns how to reach to the final goal by exploring the environment and finding new ways. This is like unsupervised learning in a sense that no labeled data is involved and there is no supervision either. The fundamental feature of RL that distinguishes it from other learning methods is that RL uses training data that evaluates actions rather than giving instructions by taking correct actions [Sutton and Barto, 2020].

Four main elements of RL are *policy, reward signal, value function* and optionally a *model* that governs the environment [Sutton and Barto, 2020]. Policy is a function that maps each state of the environment to an action, which can be deterministic or stochastic in nature. Reward specifies the immediate value of the action while value functions for each state represent the reward in the long run. The model of the environment, if known, are usually Markov transition matrices and the environments in RL can usually be modeled as Markov Decision Process or MDP in short. The ultimate goal of RL is to find the optimal solution to the underlying task by identifying the optimal action for any given situation or state (this is the optimal policy) that maximizes the expected cumulative reward also known as *total return*. This goal is a way to control the system, but unlike other control-based methods, RL does not require a correct or reliable mathematical model of the environment. Learning optimal policy can be done through experiencing the environment with trial and error. This makes RL methods quite attractive and puts it in a unique position in healthcare and medical field, where sequence of decisions needs to be made. For instance, with the goal of a patient's long-term benefit, what decisions should be made from the treatment to lifestyle modifications that are unique to the patient. This opens a new chapter in personalized engagement and smart coaching that, with the use of RL methods, can be done better than any time before. This is a space that not everything can be summarized in covariates, or it is not possible to find a right model to explain the problem, hence the traditional statistical methods would come short of delivering the optimum solution.

Another topic in RL that is highly relevant to the field of drug development, clinical trials, or medical research through personalization of treatments, investigating multiple treatments in clinical trials and/or managing a certain disease is multi-armed bandits. In this problem and at each time step the agent is faced with multiple actions (analogous to the arm of a slot machine in a casino, except that we have multiple arms here) and taking each action has a consequence (reward). The reward is random for each action and the goal is to maximize the expected total reward over time. The main challenge here is the trade-off between exploration and exploitation. Should the agent always try new arms to expand its knowledge about arms and explore (exploration), or as soon as it finds an arm with a relatively high reward it should stick with that to gain more rewards (exploitation). There are different ways to address this issue. Algorithms like E-greedy, Upper Confidence Bounds (UCB) and Thompson sampling [Chapelle and Li, 2011; Agrawal and Goyal, 2012] are the some of the most common ways to balance this trade-off.

A perhaps more practical version of multi-armed bandits is contextual bandit algorithm [Woodroofe, 1979; Chu et al., 2011; Agarwal et al., 2014] where the agent takes into account the context at each time step to adapt better to the environment in the real world. As context changes over time, the agent adapts itself and selection of actions changes accordingly. In fact, the motivating example in the first contextual bandit paper [Woodroofe, 1979] was related to clinical trials. Although, the scope of contextual bandit algorithm is now much broader.

Deep neural networks also play a seminal role in recent advances in RL approaches such as Deep Q-Networks [Mnih et al., 2015] or asynchronous methods for deep reinforcement learning [Mnih et al., 2016]. DNNs are used for value function approximation in situations where state space is continuous and a more complex non-linear features are required to describe the state spaces. Benefiting from all these advancements, reinforcement learning has gained a lot of attention in the past few years, and it spans a wide range of applications including but not limited to gaming, robotics, NLP, healthcare, finance and many more [Li, 2017]. Reaching superhuman level in the game of Go, Chess and Shogi by AlphaZero [Silver et al., 2018] and human-level control in Atari games through deep reinforcement learning [Mnih et al., 2015] are some examples of breakthroughs of RL in recent years. RL-based algorithms have proven to be advantageous in various parts of medical field such as managing Type 1 diabetes, personalized coaching, and clinical trials in general. We will review some instances of such algorithms in the following sections.

6.3 Target Identification and Molecular Design

In the current highly competitive landscape of drug development, big pharmaceutical companies are utilizing AI-related methods more than any time before in different stages of drug development. Drug discovery and target identification, as one of the crucial stages of drug development and pharmaceutical research, is certainly not an exception. High failure rate of clinical trials [Mullard, 2018] as well as enormous costs of running them are the main contributors. As a result, exploiting ML based approaches can help making the process more efficient and cost effective. As suggested by the title of this section, the application of AI/ML methods in this stage of drug development can be divided into two parts: target identification and molecular design.

6.3.1 Target Identification

Investigating an association between the outcome and some features such as gene expression, genomic pathways related to an underlying disease, key laboratory measurements, etc., is a first step towards identifying some targets. In such analysis, usually the sample size is much smaller than the number of features and therefore traditional feature selection approaches would fail to deliver results. Some modern statistical learning algorithms based on penalized likelihood method [Fan and Lv, 2008; Zou, 2006; Zou and Hastie, 2005] or high dimensional Bayesian variable selection algorithms such as [Nikooienejad et al., 2016, 2020; Shin et al., 2018; Narisetty and He, 2014] are parametric approaches to address this problem. On the other hand, XGBoost, a scalable tree boosting method described in [Chen and Guestrin, 2016] is a widely used machine learning approach that can be employed for this problem as a potential non-parametric solution. Deep neural networks have been recently used for target identification and drug re-purposing problem as described in [Zeng et al., 2020]. The deep learning methods can be useful in predicting drug-target interaction [Wen et al., 2017; You et al., 2019] as one of the crucial steps in drug discovery that can help in challenging the status quo of traditional methods in this field.

6.3.2 Molecular Design

High-throughput Screening (HTS) is an experimentation method that is especially used in drug discovery. Active compounds, antibodies or genes that modulate certain pathways can be rapidly identified by this method. It has been employed in small-molecule drug discovery for the past two decades [Schneider et al., 2020]. With big amount of data from HTS and combinatorial synthesis, ML methods have shown to be an eminent tool in mining chemical information from large databases to design drugs with specific properties [Lo et al., 2018]. Selecting the most appropriate HTS hits is critical to drug discovery phase [Holenz and Stoy, 2019], which would highly impact the success of clinical trials. There are multiple criteria that must be considered in the hit selection process such as potency, toxicity, permeability, solubility, selectivity at desired pharmaceutical targets and physico-chemical that impact pharmacokinetics and drug safety. Some of these criteria emerge from Absorption, Distribution, Metabolism, Excretion, and Toxicology (ADMET) properties of the compound. This very well fits into a challenging Multi-Objective Optimization (MOO) problem also known as multi-attribute optimization or Pareto optimization [Lambrinidis and Tsantili-Kakoulidou, 2018]. MOO involves finding a molecule that balances between different properties that are usually conflicting. The goal is then to find a lead among all possible ones that provides the best trade-off depending on the goal and application. [Perron et al., 2018] describes the use of deep learning to de novo design and address the MOO problem using ligand-based design methods.

The Simplified Molecular-Input Line-Entry System (SMILES), which represents molecu-lar graphs as strings of characters [Weininger, 1988] has facilitated the use of recurrent neural networks (RNN) and other deep learning methods in de novo drug design. For instance, [Arús-Pous et al., 2020] use a deep learning SMILES-based generative architec-ture that first exploits RNN that generates scaffolds and then a model to generate suitable decorations for each attachment point in the scaffold. Along similar lines one can refer to [Lim et al., 2020] and [Li et al., 2019] where graph generative neural networks (GGNN) are utilized molecular generation from scaffolds. Moreover, [Ma et al., 2015] show that deep neural networks are a better practical method for quantitative structure-activity relation-ship (QSAR) problems for predicting on-target and off-target activities in the drug discov-ery process.

One can also find traces of reinforcement learning in some recent algorithms in molecu-lar design. [Li et al., 2020] introduce an Actor-Critic deep reinforcement learning algorithm to address the MOO problem that can be potentially used in molecular design. [Olivecrona et al., 2017] provide a policy-based reinforcement learning approach to fine-tune RNNs for generating molecules. In this ap- proach, the fine-tuning of a pre-trained RNN occurs through learning an augmented episodic likelihood, a composite of prior likelihood and user-defined scoring function. [Popova et al., 2018] introduce another instance of such methods. Finally, to evaluate or compare various algorithms that exploit AI/ML or clas-sical methods for de novo molecular design, one can consult [Brown et al., 2019] or [Neil et al., 2018] where various standardized benchmarks are provided for such purpose.

6.4 Pharmacokinetics and Pharmacodynamics

Pharmacokinetics (PK) and Pharmacodynamics (PD) are two major topics that are studied and investigated at early stages of the drug development process. A very common way to describe those is that PK is about what body does to the compound and PD is what the compound under study does to the body. In other words, how body reacts to the com-pound and accepts it is related to PK and how the compound impacts the body, not only from the efficacy standpoint and its designated target, but how it impacts the heart rate, blood pressure, liver enzymes, etc. PK can be studied by four different ADME principles we discussed in the previous section. They are absorption, distribution, metabolism, and excretion. For more details on each of those principles and the role of PK [Mehrotra et al., 2007] is a good article to consult. Bioavailability, clearance, and half-life are some of the key parameters in PK and the concentration vs. time plot is one of the most important plots that is analyzed to extract some key PK properties of the compound. The goal of modeling in PK is to model the time course and availability of the drug in plasma. To model how concentration is changed over time, multi-compartment models are used. Such models contain the central compartment (measurements from blood stream representing the main body) and some other peripheral compartments (representing more slowly equilibrating tissues) [Mortensen et al., 2008]. Two compartment models are very common that are being used in practice. Concentration in different compartments is described by Ordinary Differential Equations (ODE) in these models. The PD model, on the other hand, connects the plasma concentration level to the drug effect and therefore, in the joint PK/PD models, the full picture of effect over time can be studied and right dose regimen can be extracted for further studies in early phase clinical trials.

Not surprisingly, deep neural networks have been employed in PK/PD modeling as well. [Lu et al., 2021] propose a novel PK/PD framework based on neural ordinary differential equations and show it outperforms the state-of-the-art model in temporal prediction metrics. It also enables patient response simulations for doses that have not been tested. Recently, [Liu et al., 2020] utilized RNN based on LSTM to analyze simulated PK/PD data and to capture temporal dependencies of PD profiles. DNN has been applied to assign individualized absorption models in PK analysis in [Jaber et al., 2021] with a high accuracy on the external test data. [Wenzel et al., 2019] use a multitask DNN to model ADME and toxicity data that capture hidden trends among ADME-Tox parameters in correlated data sets. With more advancement in DNN methods and the importance of PK/PD and ADME-Tox modeling in drug development, we expect more application of such approaches in this field in coming years.

6.5 Applications in Clinical Trials, Clinical Research and Healthcare

AI and in particular deep learning and reinforcement learning methods have impacted the field of medical and clinical research significantly in the past few years. There have been always deficiencies in this field such as errors in diagnosis of the disease, mistakes in treatment assignment, and in general various sources of waste in the healthcare system [Berwick and Hackbarth, 2012] that has invited AI tools to address the issues as much as possible. [Shah et al., 2019] provide a nice and high-level perspective on the role of AI/ML in clinical development and outlines strategies for modernizing the clinical development process by utilizing AI/ML based solutions. Similarly, [Woo, 2019] reviews the impact of AI/ML in clinical trials from applications of natural language processing, to help in design of clinical trials and enhancement of trial enrollment.

In the following, the contributions of DNN and RL methods in clinical research and healthcare in general are separately discussed in more detail.

6.5.1 Contribution of DNNs

The application of deep neural networks (DNNs) in clinical research is dominated by super- vised learning. Generally, there are valid concerns here such as the labeled data that are used to train DNN models may not be the ground truth as usually that may not be known and therefore those labels are biased towards a specific direction e.g., a pathologist's point of view in reading a biopsy image slide. Moreover, there are not many studies that put AI/ML method to test in a say, randomized trial. In general, the lack of clinical context is a key limitation across studies that compare human and machine performance, where the diagnosis is just done only by the data at hand without any context [Esteva et al., 2019]. Most studies that evaluate the role of AI are based on retrospective analyses that suffer from various issues [Topol, 2019]. As a result, as AI/ML enters medical research field and is embarking on an impactful role to address some of existing deficiencies and issues, a new guideline is needed to make sure the way it is done is transparent and does not cause any harm to the patients and other stake holders. More information on this can be found in [Topol, 2020].

6.5.1.1 Analyzing Medical Images

Medical Imaging is perhaps the field with the most direct application of DNN and as a result, there are many studies that evaluated the role of AI for different diagnosis purposes and as a potential replacement for human specialists. This includes analyzing X-rays, CT scans and other types of medical images by considering different statistical measures such as the Area Under the ROC Curve (AUROC), sensitivity, specificity, and other related classification measures. [Nam et al., 2019] developed a 25-layer CNN for nodule detection algorithm on chest radiographs and compare the results to human radiologists. They show the algorithm outperforms thoracic radiologists with low false positives while preserving sensitivity. Obtaining large and labeled datasets to train DNN is neither easy nor cheap in this space. [Li et al., 2018] provide a method that can work on small amount of labeled chest x-ray data that are otherwise very ex- pensive to obtain. Along similar lines, [Wang et al., 2017] present a new chest x-ray dataset by using Natural Language Processing (NLP) based text mining techniques on text radiological reports. They show commonly occurred thoracic diseases can be detected by a unified weakly-supervised multi-label image clas-sification method. Their suggested unified weakly-supervised method comprises of four major ImageNet pre-trained CNN models: AlexNet [Krizhevsky et al., 2012], GoogLeNet [Szegedy et al., 2015], VGGNet [Simonyan and Zisserman, 2014], and the ResNet [He et al., 2016]. One common theme behind application of such DNN techniques for x-rays is that although they outperform human radiologists most of the time, but their AUROC is far from optimal and therefore a fully automated DNN based classifier seems to be at early stages even for common disease patterns [Wang et al., 2017].

Pathology is another area that can benefit significantly from DNNs in diagnostic of can-cer tumors and other diseases such as Non-Alcoholic Steatohepatitis (NASH) in the liver. In fact, the speed of turning around the results from biopsy to final diagnosis, accuracy of reads and reduction in its variability can significantly improve drug development in this field. Overcoming issues that can be caused by inter- and intra-reader variability could be listed as one of the main motivations to utilize DNNs for such applications. Biopsy reads are decisive in inclusion of candidate patients in NASH clinical trials and variability in those reads between the baseline and end of treatment, as well as lack of agreement between pathologists have contributed to failure in some clinical trials. To utilize DNNs glass slides of sampled tissue that have been traditionally used for biopsy reads should be first converted to digital images by Whole-Slide Imaging (WSI) system. There is a guide-line published by Food and Drug Administration (FDA) [Office of In Vitro Diagnostics and Radiological Health, 2016] on this matter too. Adaptation of DNN in this field has not been as fast compared to other related fields such as radiology or medical imaging [Acs and Rimm, 2018]. Nonetheless, there are studies that have investigated the perfor-mance of AI/ML methods and compared them to human pathologists. [Bejnordi et al., 2017] conducted a comparison between five deep learning algorithms and 11 pathologists at detecting metastases of lymph nodes of women with breast cancer. Some of the algorithms did better than pathologists under a time constraint, which is not usually the case in real life, and had comparable performance to human pathologists in the absence of time constraints. Similar studies such as [Cruz-Roa et al., 2017] and [Yu et al., 2016] evaluated the performance of deep learning using digital pathology images in breast and lung cancer, respectively. The point in all these is that DNNs may not be still a solid replacement for human pathologists, and they are still in beginning stages, but combining human pathologist experience with AI and treating it as an assistance has proven to be useful too [Steiner et al., 2018]. FDA has already approved some proprietary algorithms in this space and the list is expanding rapidly [Topol, 2019].

Finally, a nice review on deep learning algorithms in medical image analysis and a good summary of different contributions in this field that spans from image classification and segmentation to object detection can be found in [Litjens et al., 2017].

6.5.1.2 Electronic Health Records (EHR)

With each hospitalization of a patient numerous pieces of data are generated. That is the same for clinical trials and keeping the document or patient narratives for the participants in large trials. There is potentially valuable information in all these documents that can benefit the patient and future treatments in similar disease states. Sifting through old documents, protocols, or related publications to efficiently design a trial for a specific disease state is another example of text mining that requires a lot of man hour to accomplish with a high likelihood of making errors. Automating this with a smart agent makes the process much more reliable and efficient. Natural Language Processing (NLP) and the use of RNNs is the solution here and the amount of research in the past few years on this topic has been expanding very rapidly. [Shickel et al., 2017] review recent deep learning methods on EHR data while [Rajkomar et al., 2018] show that deep learning methods can predict multiple events using EHR data without site-specific data harmonization.

6.5.1.3 Wearables and Digital Biomarkers

Wearables or wearable technology are defined as smart electronic devices that can be worn and has one or multiple sensors to perform certain measurements. Recent developments in smart watches and the boom in the use of wearable devices in general has opened new horizons in clinical world from measurement of some basic biomarkers such as heart rate or blood pressure to identifying specific patterns of behavior such as eating or sleeping. Different sensors in smart wearables are behind producing different digital biomarkers, which can then be used for various analyses. Camera, microphone, Electrocardiogram (ECG), gyroscope, accelerometer, barometer, etc. are a few examples of such sensors.

There are studies investigating the role of wearables and digital biomarkers in different disease areas. [Kourtis et al., 2019] show how different manifestations of Alzheimer's disease can be phenotyped digitally using respective sensors in wearable devices. [Beauchamp et al., 2020] investigate the use of wearables in oncology and during cancer treatment with key primary outcome of adherence. [Sathyanarayana et al., 2016] evaluate the feasibility of predicting sleep quality using activity wearable data during the day. They compare different DNN methods with traditional logistic regression in their prediction. [Siirtola et al., 2018] utilize wearable sensors' data during sleep for early detection of migraine attacks. Multiple sensors had been used to produce required data from different measurements for their modeling including accelerations, galvanic skin response, blood volume pulse, heart rate and its variability and temperature. They have used more traditional statistical methods such as Quadratic Discriminant Analysis (QDA) and Linear Discriminant Analysis (LDA) in their classifier. Another disease area that can benefit from wearable devices and measurements heart failure. For instance, wearable devices are very good tools to measure activity and capture physiological data and therefore can be used in evaluating improvements of functional capability in patients with heart failure. [DeVore et al., 2019] discuss potential applications of wearable devices in Heart Failure (HF) space and some challenges or limitations. [Pevnick et al., 2018] go into details of various wearable devices that can be adapted in HF and provide frameworks to better evaluate potentials of such devices in improving healthcare in this disease area.

More examples of applications of DNNs and in general the role of AI in healthcare can be found in [Topol, 2019].

6.5.2 Contribution of Reinforcement Learning

Intuitively, in the medical and clinical research field, RL can be applied in situations where a sequence of decisions are required to achieve a long term benefit. Unlike having a fixed treatment regime and putting that to test in a clinical trial, there is a dynamic process going on that can generate new hypotheses. Dynamic Treatment Regimes (DTR) is the term that is used for these cases [Chakraborty and Murphy, 2014]. In that article, they study techniques such as Q-learning and marginal structural models to discuss this field of research as well as Sequential Multiple Assignment Randomized Trial (SMART) designs. Chronic diseases such as cancer or Type 1 diabetes are some areas that DTR can be applied to. We briefly review these two disease states and the impact from RL in the following.

6.5.2.1 Cancer Treatment

There have been multiple studies investigating RL approaches in exploring efficient treatment strategies for those disease states. A summary of RL methods for cancer treatment regimes is provided in [Yu et al., 2019]. [Zhao et al., 2009] employ Q-learning to learn an optimal policy for clinical trials that are designed to discover individualized treatment regimes for cancer therapy. They demonstrate it outperforms approaches based on adaptive design. [Padmanabhan et al., 2017] exploit a model-free Q-learning method to develop an optimal cancer chemotherapy dosing.

6.5.2.2 Diabetes

Type 1 Diabetes Mellitus (T1DM) is another form of chronic disease that can potentially benefit from RL approaches. In particular, the concept of Artificial Pancreas (AP) [Cobelli et al., 2011, Albisser et al., 1974] that is used in blood glucose control by computing and administrating appropriate doses of insulin, which includes a Continuous Glucose Monitoring (CGM) device and an insulin pump, can be thought of as a closed-loop control system that fits well into a reinforcement learning algorithm. The blood glucose management with minimizing hypoglycemia events (an event caused by deficiency of blood glucose in blood stream that can result in dizziness, shakiness or even passing out in severe cases) involves a high between and within patient variability. Moreover, there are various parameters such as lifestyle, eating behavior, amount of exercise and many other factors that play an important role in this control problem. Therefore, a well defined model to describe the problem or a one rule fits all type of approach is almost impossible in this case and rather it a model free approach, in statistical term, tailored to each patient is what is required here. An RL-based algorithm can provide different optimal policies for different patients and be a potential solution to this problem.

There has been a lot of attention to RL approaches for tackling the aforementioned problem. For instance, [Daskalaki et al., 2013] propose an adaptive personalized algorithm based on Actor-Critic (AC) learning approach to control insulin infusion and optimize glucose regulation by providing daily updates of the Basal Rate (BR) and Insulin-To-Carbohydrate (IC) ratio. Along similar lines, [Sun et al., 2018] propose an Adaptive Basal-Bolus Algorithm (ABBA) using AC learning approach and inputs from Self Monitoring Blood Glucose (SMBG) or CGM measurements.

[Noori et al., 2017] employ an on-policy Temporal Difference (TD) based approach to tackle similar control problem and finally, [Luckett et al., 2019] propose a new method called V-learning, which is designed to find the optimal policy with minimal assumption on data that is collected by mobile technologies and suited for mobile health applications. They also apply it to estimate an optimal policy for glucose regulation in T1DM patients.

6.5.2.3 Mobile Health

In addition to the V-learning algorithm [Luckett et al., 2019] that provides an RL based solution for data collected by mobile devices, and is discussed in the previous section, there are other algorithms that consider RL based solutions for mobile health. [Lei et al., 2017] propose an online Actor- Critic contextual bandit algorithm that uses real-time data collected by a mobile device or wearables and provides personalized intervention, or as they call it Just-In-Time Adaptive Intervention (JITAI). Contextual bandits, as a powerful tool for sequential decision making, are natural framework for mobile health. [Tewari and Murphy, 2017] survey the literature on contextual bandits and discuss different challenges, e.g., initialization of the learning algorithm, computational considerations, finding interpretable policies, etc. in its application to real-world problems.

6.5.2.4 Other Medical and Healthcare Domains

Reinforcement learning has proven to be impactful in various other fields of MR and can make the process more reliable and efficient. Areas like medical diagnosis [Fakih and Das, 2006], medical image examination [Bernstein and Burnaev, 2018, Sahba et al., 2006], drug discovery [Serrano et al., 2018, Neil et al., 2018], health and lifestyle management in diabetic or obese patients [Yom-Tov et al., 2017, Forman et al., 2019], and many other examples. For more detailed information on this topic one can consult [Yu et al., 2019].

6.6 Personalized Medicine

Personalized medicine or, in general, precision health, is highly related to reinforcement learning which is one of key area of artificial intelligence. The need for evidence based personalized medicine has been appeared in an early critique of statistical methods in medicine published in 1835 [Poisson, 2001]. Until recently, with the advancement of technology to collect more granular level individual patient information including DNA sequencing, both clinicians and statisticians have seen the great needs to develop statistical methods to advance the concept of personalized solution [Longford and Nelder, 1999]. In this section, we provide some review on the personalized solution for the past, current, and discuss the challenges for the future development.

6.6.1 Subgroup Analysis and Identification, and Modern Personalized Medicine

Subgroup analysis, subgroup identification, and personalized medicine are closely related, and they can be considered as three generations of methods for personalized medicine, although their objectives could be slightly different.

The subgroup analysis is often referred to as to evaluate treatment effects on a predefined subgroup of patients based on their baseline covariate values. Those subgroups are often pre-specified, and those analysis are often written in protocol for secondary or exploratory objectives. The purposes for such analysis vary. The sponsor may use subgroup analysis as a salvage strategy for a phase III trial in case it may not meet the primary objective for all enrolled patients. It can be used to pursue an additional treatment indication for a special patient population within a large study. It can also be used to evaluate scientific hypotheses for further studies. Thus, subgroup analysis is utilized for both confirmatory and exploratory purposes.

Explicitly specifying the subgroups before conducting analysis is often challenging. The concept that figuring out subgroups from data is attractive. Retrospective data driven subgroup identification has gained significant popularity for the past decade, and various methods have been proposed to search subgroups for hypothesis generation. To highlight a few, [Su et al., 2009] propose the interaction trees method which extend the classification and regression tree (CART) by incorporating a treatment by split interaction. [Lipkovich et al., 2011] develop algorithms extending the bump hunting methods to search differential treatment effects. [Loh et al., 2015] extend their previous work to search subgroups which adjusts covariate selection bias when we have both categorical and continuous covariates. One key issue of subgroup identification is multiplicity. The total searching space is often less understood analytically which poses additional challenge to adjust p-values. Some ad hoc approaches are often adopted such as splitting data into training and testing datasets (or out of bag samples) to evaluate the estimated subgroups.

There are some fundamental challenges for subgroup identification. First, there is no unique definition of subgroups. For example, some methods are intent to maximize the treatment by covariate interaction, and some methods are searching for differential treatment effects. Second, many of those existing methods are tree-based approach, and their optimization is layer by layer. The final solution may not be the global optimal solution, and their theoretical properties are difficult to evaluate. Third, those methods only focus on treatment benefit. Consequently, those methods often face a dilemma that whether selects a small subgroup with significant treatment benefit versus a larger subgroup having moderate treatment advantage. Furthermore, the geometric shapes of subgroups are often not clearly defined. Some methods only search for a single rectangle shape subgroup, and some methods allow multiple half open spaces.

The main purpose of subgroup identification is to maximize patient benefit because we believe that patients in such subgroups can achieve better outcomes when taking treatment. By viewing subgroup identification as an outcome optimization, we form a new framework under the individualized treatment recommendation (ITR). ITR is a reinforcement learning based approach for personalized medicine and it gained tremendous popularity recently. The method considers each previous observation as a small experiment trying different treatment while observing some reward. Then, the algorithm is to figure out a treatment assignment rules in a defined functional space (e.g., linear models or tree models) to maximize patient's benefit [Qian and Murphy, 2011]. The method and framework also have significant benefit over the traditional methods that it can handle both randomized control trials as well as observational studies by adjusting the confounders through inverse probability weighting scheme or doubly robust methods.

Following the work by [Qian and Murphy, 2011; Zhao et al., 2012; Zhang et al., 2012], [Fu et al., 2016] connect subgroup identification problems in pharmaceutical setting with personalized solution methods in academic exercise. They coin the acronym ITR from traditional individualized treatment rule to Individualized Treatment Recommendation to increase broad medical acceptance. Their paper also proves that for all subgroup identification related methods, it is important to remove the intercept and covariate effects to increase numerical performance which is similar to centralizing covariate matrix before fitting a linear model. Their method uses a comprehensive search scheme to maximize a single objective function within a 3-layer tree structure. The authors argue that this setting satisfied majority of the clinical need. An R and C++ implementation of this method can be found at https://github.com/fuhaoda/ITR. [Zhao et al., 2012] make a connection that optimizing the patient outcome can be formulated as a weighted classification problem. This insightful connection links the field of machine learning with personalized medicine and opens many possibilities. For example, they modify support vector machine for ITR, and [Zhang et al., 2020; Qi et al., 2020] generalize the idea into multicategory treatments with geometric interpretation. [Zhang et al., 2020] is also the first paper to prove a method with Fisher's consistency in selecting an optimal treatment among multi-category choices. [Liang et al., 2018] modify deep learning method by a weighted softmax loss function, so that we can enjoy the deep learning architect for more complicated personalized medicine settings when data set are large. [Doubleday et al., 2018] extend random forest methods for personalized solution and proposed corresponding variable importance in ITR setting. In practice, people may not only care about maximizing treatment efficacy and patients are equally care about drug safety. Therefore, in many situations, both have to be considered. However, the treatment recommendation is a ranking problem which can only be done in a one dimension (directly). In general, we have 3 ways to handle multiple responses. The first approach is the clinical utility index approach so that we can maximize a weighted outcome. The second approach is a constraint optimization approach while we can control safety while maximizing patients benefit [Wang et al., 2018b]. The third approach is to estimate an efficacy-safety trade off through data. In the next sessions we will discuss further opportunities and challenges.

6.6.2 Future Research in Personalized Medicine

The ITR reframed the traditional subgroup identification problems and shades new lights on personalized medicine. It connects with machine learning through a weighted classification problem. This approach has also been studied independently in computer science and it was referred to as contextual based bandit problem [Li et al., 2010]. The solution belongs to a single step off policy reinforcement learning [Sutton and Barto, 2020]. It is worth to note that the reinforcement learning algorithms are key algorithms in the field of artificial intelligence. As mentioned in Section 6.2, Google's DeepMind has used reinforcement learning algorithm developed Alpha Go and Alpha Zero to beat the best human Go game player in 2016. Applying those algorithms into medical field is not straightforward, and there are a few challenging issues. One question is how we can continue to improve the recommendation engine. Once the ITR algorithm is obtained from a training dataset, it will be a deterministic function conditional on patient's covariate information. To continue to improve the algorithms, some randomness for treatment exploration must be introduced. The epsilon-greedy algorithm, Thompson sampling, and upper confidence bounds are three popular choices. However, in medicine field, it may not be ethnical to allow patients to try some solutions which are known to be risky. Therefore, research on how to balance and quantify individual risk, and build it into exploration phase are needed.

The reinforcement learning framework greatly extend the personalized medicine from a single decision point to multi-stage personalized interventions. For chronic disease, patients often have to switch or intensity their treatments. Dynamic treatment regime [Murphy, 2003] provides statistical interpretation of reinforcement learning. The Q-learning methods based on Bellman equations are popular approaches. SMART and Micro-randomization trials provide a way to formally study and develop algorithms for personalized solution [Klasnja et al., 2015]. Recently, [Luckett et al., 2019] extend the traditional dynamic treatment regime from a few stage-wise decisions into almost continuous horizon for mobile health.

Besides adopting reinforcement learning approaches into personalized medicine areas, there are other unique challenges in medical field. For example, the diagnostic cost constraints are often raised. Suppose we only have $100 to diagnose a sub phenotype for better personalized intervention. We can either choose 10 low-cost biomarkers or measure two expensive lab tests. Under such constraint, how can we maximize our diagnostic accuracy? The cost can be generalized to convenient cost. For instance, in mobile health it is unrealistic to force patients to wear 10+ sensors for personalized interventions. How can we select the most relevant devices based on different patient profile to achieve adequate diagnostic accuracy? With the advancement in device and technology, we can collect more data to better quantify individual patients. Those data provide great opportunity to generate actionable insights to improve patient outcomes.

It has been a journey from the first documented controlled clinical trial in The Bible to the gold standard randomized one today. And this journey is continued to the 21st century as personalized medicine. Personalized medicine starts as subgroup analysis to artificial intelligence-based reinforcement learning ITR algorithms. We are confident that this data-driven medical decision-making will continue to be a key topic in medical research and a crucial path to improve patient outcomes.

6.7 Drug Manufacturing and Quality Control

Manufacturing and packaging in pharmaceutical industry is a crucial step, where investments on research and development during clinical trials of an approved drug will be paid off by making it available to the public. High quality standards are definitely a requirement at this step. FDA has also issued a guidance [FDA, 2004] onto address issues and questions on innovative manufacturing.

The use of machine learning and statistical modeling in this field has been increased over the past 20 years [Guerra and Glassey, 2018], where they have been utilized in different applications such as predicting chemical deterioration of the compound, managing distribution of products, etc. In a recent work, [Du Plessis, 2020] discuss the role reinforcement learning approach for inventory and supply chain management in pharmaceutical industry. Or [Poongodi et al., 2020] studied the role of Internet of Things (IoT) in drug manufacturing handling various environmental conditions in the process.

However, it would be also interesting to focus on quality control side of the story, where the goal is to detect faults or defects in packaging from images. This is where deep learning methods have proven to be advantageous. This perhaps is one of the main contributions of DNN in manufacturing and quality control. The challenge in this area is the computational time and data processing. The speed of process on production line is usually high and a procedure that can produce output in a faster time is preferred. As a result, a pre-processing in combination with the use of light-weight CNN can be a potential solution to this problem [Malesa and Rajkiewicz, 2021; Weimer et al., 2016]. Usually, these models are pre-trained on a large dataset of images such as ImageNet [Deng et al., 2009], and then will be fine-tuned to a specific application using transfer learning, where the final layers are re-trained on images specific to the application. [Wang et al., 2018a] provides a comprehensive review on existing deep learning methods in manufacturing and quality control.

6.8 Discussion

After briefly discussing the AI/ML topic and different branches of modern ML algorithms (deep learning, reinforcement learning, etc.), we provided a comprehensive review of such methods and how they are employed in drug development, clinical practice, and medical research in general. Evidently, these algorithms have gained a lot of momentum in the past few years and got improved significantly from technical performance point of view as well as computational efficiency. It is almost impossible to imagine complete absence of new AI/ML algorithms in all the aspects of this industry. In fact, it seems unavoidable to adopt such methods to keep up with the pace of new advancements in science and engineering and get closer to the desired outcome more efficiently. We saw in previous sections that CNNs and NLPs that are based on RNNs are the most common algorithms employed in clinical settings due to their high adaptability and wide range of applications. Modern AI/ML methods have undoubtedly opened new doors in science and have conquered territories unbeknownst to humans. Google's Deep mind AlphaFold 2, a highly accurate protein structure prediction [Jumper et al., 2021], is an epitome of such statement. An algorithm that, according to some scientists, is a game changer and has solved a 50-year-old protein folding problem [Service, 2020].

Having said that, there are some limitations in the use of modern AI/ML methods. Applicability of such algorithms highly depends on the problem and its purpose. The minimum reliability required in the application or the cost of making mistakes in the process are common factors that can limit the use of AI models and determine how aggressive we are allowed to be in replacing humans with AI. The higher the cost of making mistakes, the more conservative we ought to be. For instance, as we discussed in Section 6.5, a full replacement of a human pathologist or radiologist with a state-of-the-art computer vision algorithm still seems nonviable. While statistical measures of evaluating such algorithms look promising, the settings under which they are tested are still more ideal than that in real world [Topol, 2019]. The cost of a misdiagnosis in this example can be detrimental and even as high as a human life. As a result, although an AI system can provide guidance and help a human pathologist or radiologist, it not ready to fully replace the specialist just yet.

Another limitation of most of AI/ML algorithms is requirement of large datasets to train the model. That is why such methods are usually called data thirsty. Moreover, the computational power needed for training such models is not cheap. Therefore, it is usually better to use relevant pre-trained models and only fine tuning it for a specific application. This is related to the concept of transfer learning, which is very common in situations where the model suffers from insufficient training data [Bozinovski and Fulgosi, 1976; Bozinovski, 2020; Pan and Yang, 2009]. Details on how it is applied in deep neural network and the concept of deep transfer learning is discussed in [Tan et al., 2018]. This concept then evolved into multi-task learning, a powerful tool for improving generalization performance by leveraging domain- specific knowledge [Caruana, 1997].

There is no doubt that the modern AI/ML is gaining more attention than ever before. Although they are associated with limitations, its key impact on drug development industry and healthcare in general should not be overlooked. Rather, it must be leveraged in full capacity to help and make life better for patients around the world. We are now seeing more important roles for AI/ML models to play in this field, especially drug discovery, in an almost day-by-day basis. We expect the trend to stay like this or even more upward for years to come. This, indeed, can be considered another small step towards artificial general intelligence (AGI).

References

Acs, B. and Rimm, D. L. (2018). Not just digital pathology, intelligent digital pathology. *JAMA oncology*, 4(3):403–404.

Agarwal, A., Hsu, D., Kale, S., Langford, J., Li, L., and Schapire, R. (2014). Taming the monster: A fast and simple algorithm for contextual bandits. In *International Conference on Machine Learning*, pages 1638–1646. PMLR.

Agrawal, S. and Goyal, N. (2012). Analysis of thompson sampling for the multi-armed bandit problem. In *Conference on learning theory*, pages 39–1. JMLR Workshop and Conference Proceedings.

Albisser, A. M., Leibel, B., Ewart, T., Davidovac, Z., Botz, C., Zingg, W., Schipper, H., and Gander, R. (1974). Clinical control of diabetes by the artificial pancreas. *Diabetes*, 23(5):397–404.

Arús-Pous, J., Patronov, A., Bjerrum, E. J., Tyrchan, C., Reymond, J.-L., Chen, H., and Engkvist, O. (2020). Smiles-based deep generative scaffold decorator for de-novo drug design. *Journal of cheminformatics*, 12:1–18.

Bahdanau, D., Cho, K., and Bengio, Y. (2014). Neural machine translation by jointly learning to align and translate. *arXiv preprint arXiv:1409.0473*.

Beauchamp, U. L., Pappot, H., and Holländer-Mieritz, C. (2020). The use of wearables in clinical trials during cancer treatment: Systematic review. *JMIR mHealth and uHealth*, 8(11):e22006.

Bejnordi, B. E., Veta, M., Van Diest, P. J., Van Ginneken, B., Karssemeijer, N., Litjens, G., Van Der Laak, J. A., Hermsen, M., Manson, Q. F., Balkenhol, M., et al. (2017). Diagnostic assessment of deep learning algorithms for detection of lymph node metastases in women with breast cancer. *Jama*, 318(22):2199–2210.

Bernstein, A. and Burnaev, E. (2018). Reinforcement learning in computer vision. In *Tenth International Conference on Machine Vision (ICMV 2017)*, volume 10696, page 106961S. International Society for Optics and Photonics.

Berwick, D. M. and Hackbarth, A. D. (2012). Eliminating waste in us healthcare. *Jama*, 307(14):1513–1516.

Bozinovski, S. (2020). Reminder of the first paper on transfer learning in neural networks, 1976. *Informatica*, 44(3).

Bozinovski, S. and Fulgosi, A. (1976). The influence of pattern similarity and transfer learning upon training of a base perceptron b2. In *Proceedings of Symposium Informatica*, pages 3–121.

Brown, N., Fiscato, M., Segler, M. H., and Vaucher, A. C. (2019). Guacamol: benchmarking models for de novo molecular design. *Journal of chemical information and modeling*, 59(3):1096–1108.

Caruana, R. (1997). Multitask learning. *Machine learning*, 28(1):41–75.

Chakraborty, B. and Murphy, S. A. (2014). Dynamic treatment regimes. *Annual review of statistics and its application*, 1:447–464.

Chapelle, O. and Li, L. (2011). An empirical evaluation of thompson sampling. *Advances in neural information processing systems*, 24:2249–2257.

Chen, T. and Guestrin, C. (2016). Xgboost: A scalable tree boosting system. In *Proceedings of the 22nd acm sigkdd international conference on knowledge discovery and data mining*, pages 785–794.

Cho, K., Van Merriënboer, B., Bahdanau, D., and Bengio, Y. (2014). On the properties of neural machine translation: Encoder-decoder approaches. *arXiv preprint arXiv:1409.1259*.

Chu, W., Li, L., Reyzin, L., and Schapire, R. (2011). Contextual bandits with linear payoff functions. In *Proceedings of the Fourteenth International Conference on Artificial Intelligence and Statistics*, pages 208–214. JMLR Workshop and Conference Proceedings.

Chung, J., Gulcehre, C., Cho, K., and Bengio, Y. (2014). Empirical evaluation of gated recurrent neural networks on sequence modeling. *arXiv preprint arXiv:1412.3555*.

Cobelli, C., Renard, E., and Kovatchev, B. (2011). Artificial pancreas: past, present, future. *Diabetes*, 60(11):2672–2682.

Collobert, R., Weston, J., Bottou, L., Karlen, M., Kavukcuoglu, K., and Kuksa, P. (2011). Natural language processing (almost) from scratch. *Journal of machine learning research*, 12:2493–2537.

Cruz-Roa, A., Gilmore, H., Basavanhally, A., Feldman, M., Ganesan, S., Shih, N. N., Tomaszewski, J., González, F. A., and Madabhushi, A. (2017). Accurate and reproducible invasive breast cancer detection in whole-slide images: A deep learning approach for quantifying tumor extent. *Scientific reports*, 7(1):1–14.

Daskalaki, E., Diem, P., and Mougiakakou, S. G. (2013). Personalized tuning of a reinforcement learning control algorithm for glucose regulation. In *2013 35th Annual international conference of the IEEE engineering in medicine and biology society (EMBC)*, pages 3487–3490. IEEE.

Deng, J., Dong, W., Socher, R., Li, L.-J., Li, K., and Fei-Fei, L. (2009). Imagenet: A large-scale hierarchical image database. In *2009 IEEE conference on computer vision and pattern recognition*, pages 248–255. Ieee.

DeVore, A. D., Wosik, J., and Hernandez, A. F. (2019). The future of wearables in heart failure patients. *JACC: Heart failure*, 7(11):922–932.

Doubleday, K., Zhou, H., Fu, H., and Zhou, J. (2018). An algorithm for generating individualized treatment decision trees and random forests. *Journal of computational and graphical statistics*, 27(4):849–860.

Du Plessis, M. (2020). Reinforcement learning for inventory management in information-sharing pharmaceutical supply chains. PhD thesis, Stellenbosch: Stellenbosch University.

El Hihi, S. and Bengio, Y. (1996). Hierarchical recurrent neural networks for long-term dependencies. In *Advances in neural information processing systems*, pages 493–499.

Esteva, A., Robicquet, A., Ramsundar, B., Kuleshov, V., DePristo, M., Chou, K., Cui, C., Corrado, G., Thrun, S., and Dean, J. (2019). A guide to deep learning in healthcare. *Nature medicine*, 25(1):24–29.

Fakih, S. J. and Das, T. K. (2006). Lead: A methodology for learning efficient approaches to medical diagnosis. *IEEE transactions on information technology in biomedicine*, 10(2):220–228.

Fan, J. and Lv, J. (2008). Sure independence screening for ultrahigh dimensional feature space. *Journal of the royal statistical society: Series B (statistical methodology)*, 70(5):849–911.

FDA et al. (2004). Guidance for industry, pat-a framework for innovative pharmaceutical development, manufacturing and quality assurance. http://www. fda. gov/cder/guidance/published. html.

Forman, E. M., Kerrigan, S. G., Butryn, M. L., Juarascio, A. S., Manasse, S. M., Ontañón, S., Dallal, D. H., Crochiere, R. J., and Moskow, D. (2019). Can the artificial intelligence technique of reinforcement learning use continuously-monitored digital data to optimize treatment for weight loss? *Journal of behavioral medicine*, 42(2):276–290.

Fu, H., Zhou, J., and Faries, D. E. (2016). Estimating optimal treatment regimes via sub-group identification in randomized control trials and observational studies. *Statistics in medicine*, 35(19):3285–3302.

Guerra, A. C. and Glassey, J. (2018). Machine learning in biopharmaceutical manufacturing. *European pharmaceutical review*, 23(4):62–65.

He, K., Zhang, X., Ren, S., and Sun, J. (2016). Deep residual learning for image recognition. In *Proceedings of the IEEE conference on computer vision and pattern recognition*, pages 770–778.

Hochreiter, S. and Schmidhuber, J. (1997). Long short-term memory. *Neural computation*, 9(8): 1735–1780.

Holenz, J. and Stoy, P. (2019). Advances in lead generation. *Bioorganic & medicinal chemistry letters*, 29(4):517–524.

Jaber, M. M., Yaman, B., Sarafoglou, K., and Brundage, R. C. (2021). Application of deep neural networks as a prescreening tool to assign individualized absorption models in pharmacokinetic analysis. *Pharmaceutics*, 13(6):797.

Jumper, J., Evans, R., Pritzel, A., Green, T., Figurnov, M., Ronneberger, O., Tunyasuvunakool, K., Bates, R., Žídek, A., Potapenko, A., et al. (2021). Highly accurate protein structure prediction with alphafold. *Nature*, 596(7873):583–589.

Kim, Y., Denton, C., Hoang, L., and Rush, A. M. (2017). Structured attention networks. *arXiv preprint arXiv:1702.00887*.

Klasnja, P., Hekler, E. B., Shiffman, S., Boruvka, A., Almirall, D., Tewari, A., and Murphy, S. A. (2015). Microrandomized trials: An experimental design for developing just-in-time adaptive interventions. *Health psychology*, 34(S):1220.

Kourtis, L. C., Regele, O. B., Wright, J. M., and Jones, G. B. (2019). Digital biomarkers for alzheimers disease: the mobile/wearable devices opportunity. *NPJ digital medicine*, 2(1):1–9.

Krizhevsky, A., Sutskever, I., and Hinton, G. E. (2012). Imagenet classification with deep convolutional neural networks. *Advances in neural information processing systems*, 25:1097–1105.

Lambrinidis, G. and Tsantili-Kakoulidou, A. (2018). Challenges with multi-objective qsar in drug discovery. *Expert opinion on drug discovery*, 13(9):851–859.

LeCun, Y., Bengio, Y., and Hinton, G. (2015). Deep learning. *Nature*, 521(7553):436–444.

Lei, H., Tewari, A., and Murphy, S. A. (2017). An actor-critic contextual bandit algorithm for personalized mobile health interventions. *arXiv preprint arXiv:1706.09090*.

Li, K., Zhang, T., and Wang, R. (2020). Deep reinforcement learning for multiobjective optimization. *IEEE transactions on cybernetics*, 51(6):3103–3114.

Li, L., Chu, W., Langford, J., and Schapire, R. E. (2010). A contextual-bandit approach to personalized news article recommendation. In *Proceedings of the 19th international conference on World Wide Web*, pages 661–670.

Li, Q., Cai, W., Wang, X., Zhou, Y., Feng, D. D., and Chen, M. (2014). Medical image classification with convolutional neural network. In *2014 13th international conference on control automation robotics & vision (ICARCV)*, pages 844–848. IEEE.

Li, Y. (2017). Deep reinforcement learning: An overview. *arXiv preprint arXiv:1701.07274*.

Li, Y., Hu, J., Wang, Y., Zhou, J., Zhang, L., and Liu, Z. (2019). Deepscaffold: A comprehensive tool for scaffold-based de novo drug discovery using deep learning. *Journal of chemical information and modeling*, 60(1):77–91.

Li, Z., Wang, C., Han, M., Xue, Y., Wei, W., Li, L.-J., and Fei-Fei, L. (2018). Thoracic disease identification and localization with limited supervision. In *Proceedings of the IEEE Conference on Computer Vision and Pattern Recognition*, pages 8290–8299.

Liang, M., Ye, T., and Fu, H. (2018). Estimating individualized optimal combination therapies through outcome weighted deep learning algorithms. *Statistics in medicine*, 37(27):3869–3886.

Lim, J., Hwang, S.-Y., Moon, S., Kim, S., and Kim, W. Y. (2020). Scaffold-based molecular design with a graph generative model. *Chemical science*, 11(4):1153–1164.

Lipkovich, I., Dmitrienko, A., Denne, J., and Enas, G. (2011). Subgroup identification based on differential effect search—a recursive partitioning method for establishing response to treatment in patient subpopulations. *Statistics in medicine*, 30(21):2601–2621.

Litjens, G., Kooi, T., Bejnordi, B. E., Setio, A. A. A., Ciompi, F., Ghafoorian, M., Van Der Laak, J. A., Van Ginneken, B., and Sánchez, C. I. (2017). A survey on deep learning in medical image analysis. *Medical image analysis*, 42:60–88.

Liu, X., Liu, C., Huang, R., Zhu, H., Liu, Q., Mitra, S., and Wang, Y. (2021). Long short-term memory recurrent neural network for pharmacokinetic-pharmacodynamic modeling. *International journal of clinical pharmacology and therapeutics*, 59(2):138–146.

Lo, Y.-C., Rensi, S. E., Torng, W., and Altman, R. B. (2018). Machine learning in chemoinformatics and drug discovery. *Drug discovery today*, 23(8):1538–1546.

Loh, W.-Y., He, X., and Man, M. (2015). A regression tree approach to identifying subgroups with differential treatment effects. *Statistics in medicine*, 34(11):1818–1833.

Longford, N. T. and Nelder, J. A. (1999). Statistics versus statistical science in the regulatory process. *Statistics in medicine*, 18(17-18):2311–2320.

Lu, J., Bender, B., Jin, J. Y., and Guan, Y. (2021). Deep learning prediction of patient response time course from early data via neural-pharmacokinetic/pharmacodynamic mod- elling. *Nature machine intelligence*, 1–9.

Luckett, D. J., Laber, E. B., Kahkoska, A. R., Maahs, D. M., Mayer-Davis, E., and Kosorok, M. R. (2019). Estimating dynamic treatment regimes in mobile health using v-learning. *Journal of the american statistical association*.

Ma, J., Sheridan, R. P., Liaw, A., Dahl, G. E., and Svetnik, V. (2015). Deep neural nets as a method for quantitative structure–activity relationships. *Journal of chemical information and modeling*, 55(2):263–274.

Malesa, M. and Rajkiewicz, P. (2021). Quality control of pet bottles caps with dedicated image cali- bration and deep neural networks. *Sensors*, 21(2):501.

Mehrotra, N., Gupta, M., Kovar, A., and Meibohm, B. (2007). The role of pharmacokinetics and pharmacodynamics in phosphodiesterase-5 inhibitor therapy. *International journal of impotence research*, 19(3):253–264.

Mnih, V., Badia, A. P., Mirza, M., Graves, A., Lillicrap, T., Harley, T., Silver, D., and Kavukcuoglu, K. (2016). Asynchronous methods for deep reinforcement learning. In *International conference on machine learning*, pages 1928–1937. PMLR.

Mnih, V., Kavukcuoglu, K., Silver, D., Rusu, A. A., Veness, J., Bellemare, M. G., Graves, A., Riedmiller, M., Fidjeland, A. K., Ostrovski, G., et al. (2015a). Human-level control through deep reinforce- ment learning. *nature*, 518(7540):529–533.

Mortensen, S., Jónsdóttir, A. H., Klim, S., and Madsen, H. (2008). Introduction to pk/pd modelling.

Mullard, A. (2018). 2017 fda drug approvals. *Nature reviews drug Discovery*, 17(2):81–86.

Murphy, S. A. (2003). Optimal dynamic treatment regimes. *Journal of the royal statistical society: Series B (statistical methodology)*, 65(2):331–355.

Nam, J. G., Park, S., Hwang, E. J., Lee, J. H., Jin, K.-N., Lim, K. Y., Vu, T. H., Sohn, J. H., Hwang, S., Goo, J. M., et al. (2019). Development and validation of deep learning–based automatic detec- tion algorithm for malignant pulmonary nodules on chest radiographs. *Radiology*, 290(1): 218–228.

Narisetty, N. N. and He, X. (2014). Bayesian variable selection with shrinking and diffusing priors. *The annals of statistics*, 42(2):789–817.

Neil, D., Segler, M., Guasch, L., Ahmed, M., Plumbley, D., Sellwood, M., and Brown, N. (2018). Exploring deep recurrent models with reinforcement learning for molecule design. In *ICLR 2018 Conference*. ICLR.

Nikooienejad, A., Wang, W., and Johnson, V. E. (2016). Bayesian variable selection for binary outcomes in high-dimensional genomic studies using non-local priors. *Bioinformatics*, 32(9):1338–1345.

Nikooienejad, A., Wang, W., and Johnson, V. E. (2020). Bayesian variable selection for survival data using inverse moment priors. *The annals of applied statistics*, 14(2):809.

Noori, A., Sadrnia, M. A., et al. (2017). Glucose level control using temporal difference methods. In *2017 Iranian Conference on Electrical Engineering (ICEE)*, pages 895–900. IEEE.

Office of In Vitro Diagnostics and Radiological Health (2016). Technical performance assessment of digital pathology whole slide imaging devices. In *Guidance for industry and food and drug admin- istration staff*, pages 1–27. FDA.

Olivecrona, M., Blaschke, T., Engkvist, O., and Chen, H. (2017). Molecular de-novo design through deep reinforcement learning. *Journal of cheminformatics*, 9(1):1–14.

Padmanabhan, R., Meskin, N., and Haddad, W. M. (2017). Reinforcement learning-based control of drug dosing for cancer chemotherapy treatment. *Mathematical biosciences*, 293:11–20.

Pan, S. J. and Yang, Q. (2009). A survey on transfer learning. *IEEE Transactions on knowledge and data engineering*, 22(10):1345–1359.

Perron, Q., Hoffmann, B., Tajmouati, H., Fourcade, R., Do Huu, N., Skiredj, A., and Gaston-Mathé, Y. (2018). Deep learning applied to ligand-based de novo design: A real-life lead optimization case study. In *Presented at the XXV EFMC International Symposium on Medicinal Chemistry*.

Pevnick, J. M., Birkeland, K., Zimmer, R., Elad, Y., and Kedan, I. (2018). Wearable technology for cardiology: an update and framework for the future. *Trends in cardiovascular medicine*, 28(2):144–150.

Poisson, M. (2001). Statistical research on conditions caused by calculi by doctor civiale. *International journal of epidemiology*, 30(6):1246–1249.

Poongodi, T., Agnesbeena, T. L., Janarthanan, S., and Balusamy, B. (2020). Accelerating data acquisition process in the pharmaceutical industry using internet of things. In *An Industrial IoT Approach for Pharmaceutical Industry Growth*, pages 117–152. Elsevier.

Popova, M., Isayev, O., and Tropsha, A. (2018). Deep reinforcement learning for de novo drug design. *Science advances*, 4(7):eaap7885.

Qi, Z., Liu, D., Fu, H., and Liu, Y. (2020). Multi-armed angle-based direct learning for estimating optimal individualized treatment rules with various outcomes. *Journal of the American statistical association*, 115(530):678–691.

Qian, M. and Murphy, S. A. (2011). Performance guarantees for individualized treatment rules. *Annals of statistics*, 39(2):1180.

Rajkomar, A., Oren, E., Chen, K., Dai, A. M., Hajaj, N., Hardt, M., Liu, P. J., Liu, X., Marcus, J., Sun, M., et al. (2018). Scalable and accurate deep learning with electronic health records. *NPJ digital medicine*, 1(1):1–10.

Réda, C., Kaufmann, E., and Delahaye-Duriez, A. (2020). Machine learning applications in drug development. *Computational and structural biotechnology journal*, 18:241–252.

Roberts, D. A., Yaida, S., and Hanin, B. (2021). The principles of deep learning theory. *arXiv preprint arXiv:2106.10165*.

Sahba, F., Tizhoosh, H. R., and Salama, M. M. (2006). A reinforcement learning framework for medical image segmentation. In *The 2006 IEEE International Joint Conference on Neural Network Proceedings*, pages 511–517. IEEE.

Sainath, T. N., Kingsbury, B., Mohamed, A.-r., Dahl, G. E., Saon, G., Soltau, H., Beran, T., Aravkin, A. Y., and Ramabhadran, B. (2013). Improvements to deep convolutional neural networks for lvcsr. In *2013 IEEE workshop on automatic speech recognition and understanding*, pages 315–320. IEEE.

Sathyanarayana, A., Joty, S., Fernandez-Luque, L., Ofli, F., Srivastava, J., Elmagarmid, A., Arora, T., and Taheri, S. (2016). Sleep quality prediction from wearable data using deep learning. *JMIR mHealth and uHealth*, 4(4):e125.

Schneider, P., Walters, W. P., Plowright, A. T., Sieroka, N., Listgarten, J., Goodnow, R. A., Fisher, J., Jansen, J. M., Duca, J. S., Rush, T. S., et al. (2020). Rethinking drug design in the artificial intelligence era. *Nature reviews drug discovery*, 19(5):353–364.

Serrano, A., Imbernón, B., Pérez-Sánchez, H., Cecilia, J. M., Bueno-Crespo, A., and Abellán, J. L. (2018). Accelerating drugs discovery with deep reinforcement learning: An early approach. In *Proceedings of the 47th International Conference on Parallel Processing Companion*, pages 1–8.

Service, R. F. (2020). 'the game has changed.' AI triumphs at protein folding. *Science*, 370(6521): 1144–1145

Shah, P., Kendall, F., Khozin, S., Goosen, R., Hu, J., Laramie, J., Ringel, M., and Schork, N. (2019). Artificial intelligence and machine learning in clinical development: a translational perspective. *NPJ digital medicine*, 2(1):1–5.

Shickel, B., Tighe, P. J., Bihorac, A., and Rashidi, P. (2017). Deep ehr: a survey of recent advances in deep learning techniques for electronic health record (ehr) analysis. *IEEE journal of biomedical and health informatics*, 22(5):1589–1604.

Shin, M., Bhattacharya, A., and Johnson, V. E. (2018). Scalable bayesian variable selection using nonlocal prior densities in ultrahigh-dimensional settings. *Statistica sinica*, 28(2):1053.

Siirtola, P., Koskimäki, H., Mönttinen, H., and Röning, J. (2018). Using sleep time data from wearable sensors for early detection of migraine attacks. *Sensors*, 18(5):1374.

Silver, D., Hubert, T., Schrittwieser, J., Antonoglou, I., Lai, M., Guez, A., Lanctot, M., Sifre, L., Kumaran, D., Graepel, T., et al. (2018). A general reinforcement learning algorithm that masters chess, shogi, and go through self-play. *Science*, 362(6419):1140–1144.

Simonyan, K. and Zisserman, A. (2014). Very deep convolutional networks for large-scale image recognition. *arXiv preprint arXiv:1409.1556*.

Steiner, D. F., MacDonald, R., Liu, Y., Truszkowski, P., Hipp, J. D., Gammage, C., Thng, F., Peng, L., and Stumpe, M. C. (2018). Impact of deep learning assistance on the histopathologic review of lymph nodes for metastatic breast cancer. *The American journal of surgical pathology*, 42(12):1636.

Su, X., Tsai, C.-L., Wang, H., Nickerson, D. M., and Li, B. (2009). Subgroup analysis via recursive partitioning. *Journal of machine learning research*, 10(2).

Sun, Q., Jankovic, M. V., Budzinski, J., Moore, B., Diem, P., Stettler, C., and Mougiakakou, S. G. (2018). A dual mode adaptive basal-bolus advisor based on reinforcement learning. *IEEE journal of biomedical and health informatics*, 23(6):2633–2641.

Sutskever, I. (2013). *Training recurrent neural networks*. University of Toronto, Toronto, Canada.

Sutskever, I., Vinyals, O., and Le, Q. V. (2014). Sequence to sequence learning with neural networks. In *Advances in neural information processing systems*, pages 3104–3112.

Sutton, R. S. and Barto, A. G. (2020). *Reinforcement learning: An introduction*. MIT press, second edition.

Szegedy, C., Liu, W., Jia, Y., Sermanet, P., Reed, S., Anguelov, D., Erhan, D., Vanhoucke, V., and Rabinovich, A. (2015). Going deeper with convolutions. In *Proceedings of the IEEE conference on computer vision and pattern recognition (CVPR)*.

Taigman, Y., Yang, M., Ranzato, M., and Wolf, L. (2014). Deepface: Closing the gap to human-level performance in face verification. In *Proceedings of the IEEE conference on computer vision and pattern recognition*, pages 1701–1708.

Tan, C., Sun, F., Kong, T., Zhang, W., Yang, C., and Liu, C. (2018). A survey on deep transfer learning. In *International conference on artificial neural networks*, pages 270–279. Springer.

Tewari, A. and Murphy, S. A. (2017). From ads to interventions: Contextual bandits in mobile health. In *Mobile Health*, pages 495–517. Springer.

Topol, E. J. (2019). High-performance medicine: the convergence of human and artificial intelligence. *Nature medicine*, 25(1):44–56.

Topol, E. J. (2020). Welcoming new guidelines for ai clinical research. *Nature medicine*, 26(9):1318–1320.

Tsehay, Y. K., Lay, N. S., Roth, H. R., Wang, X., Kwak, J. T., Turkbey, B. I., Pinto, P. A., Wood, B. J., and Summers, R. M. (2017). Convolutional neural network based deep-learning architecture for prostate cancer detection on multiparametric magnetic resonance images. In *Medical imaging 2017: Computer-aided diagnosis*, volume 10134, page 1013405. International Society for Optics and Photonics.

Vaswani, A., Shazeer, N., Parmar, N., Uszkoreit, J., Jones, L., Gomez, A. N., Kaiser, Ł., and Polosukhin, I. (2017). Attention is all you need. In *Advances in neural information processing systems*, pages 5998–6008.

Wang, X., Peng, Y., Lu, L., Lu, Z., Bagheri, M., and Summers, R. M. (2017). Chestx-ray8: Hospital-scale chest x-ray database and benchmarks on weakly-supervised classification and localization of common thorax diseases. In *Proceedings of the IEEE conference on computer vision and pattern recognition*, pages 2097–2106.

Wang, Y., Fu, H., and Zeng, D. (2018b). Learning optimal personalized treatment rules in consideration of benefit and risk: with an application to treating type 2 diabetes patients with insulin therapies. *Journal of the American statistical association*, 113(521):1–13.

Weimer, D., Scholz-Reiter, B., and Shpitalni, M. (2016). Design of deep convolutional neural network architectures for automated feature extraction in industrial inspection. *CIRP annals*, 65(1):417–420.

Weininger, D. (1988). Smiles, a chemical language and information system. 1. introduction to methodology and encoding rules. *Journal of chemical information and computer sciences*, 28(1):31–36.

Wen, M., Zhang, Z., Niu, S., Sha, H., Yang, R., Yun, Y., and Lu, H. (2017). Deep-learning-based drug–target interaction prediction. *Journal of proteome research*, 16(4):1401–1409.

Wenzel, J., Matter, H., and Schmidt, F. (2019). Predictive multitask deep neural network models for adme-tox properties: learning from large data sets. *Journal of chemical information and modeling*, 59(3):1253–1268.

Woo, M. (2019). An ai boost for clinical trials. *Nature*, 573(7775):S100–S100.

Woodroofe, M. (1979). A one-armed bandit problem with a concomitant variable. *Journal of the American Statistical Association*, 74(368):799–806.

Yang, R. and Yu, Y. (2021). Artificial convolutional neural network in object detection and semantic segmentation for medical imaging analysis. *Frontiers in oncology*, 11:573.

Yom-Tov, E., Feraru, G., Kozdoba, M., Mannor, S., Tennenholtz, M., and Hochberg, I. (2017). Encouraging physical activity in patients with diabetes: intervention using a reinforcement learning system. *Journal of medical internet research*, 19(10):e338.

You, J., McLeod, R. D., and Hu, P. (2019). Predicting drug-target interaction network using deep learning model. *Computational biology and chemistry*, 80:90–101.

Yu, C., Liu, J., and Nemati, S. (2019). Reinforcement learning in healthcare: A survey. *arXiv preprint arXiv:1908.08796*.

Yu, K.-H., Zhang, C., Berry, G. J., Altman, R. B., Ré, C., Rubin, D. L., and Snyder, M. (2016). Predicting non-small cell lung cancer prognosis by fully automated microscopic pathology image features. *Nature communications*, 7(1):1–10.

Zeng, X., Zhu, S., Lu, W., Liu, Z., Huang, J., Zhou, Y., Fang, J., Huang, Y., Guo, H., Li, L., et al. (2020). Target identification among known drugs by deep learning from heterogeneous networks. *Chemical science*, 11(7):1775–1797.

Zhang, B., Tsiatis, A. A., Davidian, M., Zhang, M., and Laber, E. (2012). *Estimating optimal treatment regimes from a classification perspective. Stat*, 1(1):103–114.

Zhang, C., Chen, J., Fu, H., He, X., Zhao, Y.-Q., and Liu, Y. (2020). Multicategory outcome weighted margin-based learning for estimating individualized treatment rules. *Statistica sinica*, 30:1857.

Zhao, Y., Kosorok, M. R., and Zeng, D. (2009). Reinforcement learning design for cancer clinical trials. *Statistics in medicine*, 28(26):3294–3315.

Zhao, Y., Zeng, D., Rush, A. J., and Kosorok, M. R. (2012). Estimating individualized treatment rules using outcome weighted learning. *Journal of the American Statistical Association*, 107(499):1106–1118.

Zou, H. (2006). The adaptive lasso and its oracle properties. *Journal of the American Statistical Association*, 101(476):1418–1429.

Zou, H. and Hastie, T. (2005). Regularization and variable selection via the elastic net. *Journal of the Royal Statistical Society: Series B (statistical methodology)*, 67(2):301–320.

7

Challenges in Cancer Clinical Trials

Fan Xia[1], Xiao Lin[2], and Xiang Guo[2]

[1]CSPC Pharmaceutical Group Limited, Shanghai, China

[2]BeiGene, Beijing, China

CONTENTS

DOI: 10.1201/9781003107323-7

Innovative methodologies are always proposed for and applied to the development of oncology therapies, not only because cancer is a major cause of death and reduced life expectancy with high unmet medical needs, but also due to the complexity of cancer pathogenesis which demands innovative approaches to mitigate risk and optimize resources. In the past few years, we have seen a rapid increase in the total number of oncology clinical trials (Iqvia 2019). With the significant resource put into, the standard of care for cancer patients and competitive landscape are shifting rapidly, so the challenges in oncology drug development are foreseeable.

Challenges can range from patient enrollment, target population, treatment regimens, regulatory negotiation and so on. In this chapter, we will focus on below challenges that may be more commonly occurred. In Section 7.1, endpoints used in oncology clinical trials will be introduced, with the focus on surrogate endpoints and regulator's attitude to surrogate endpoints. Since time-to-event endpoints are usually regarded as primary endpoints in oncology, basic concepts will firstly be introduced in Section 7.2 and then followed by the considerations if proportional hazards assumption does not hold. The challenges in competing risk and applying estimand framework were also included in this section. Then some hot topics covering early-phase to late-phase drug development are presented in Section 7.3, together with authors' thinking behind these topics. Topics include dose-finding method to find optimal biological dose which is expected in immunotherapy or target therapy development, use of historical data to bring more information at an early stage to support decision-making, application of platform design and master protocol for an efficient and collaborative development strategy, adaptive design in confirmatory study to increase trial success probability and methodology used to handle treatment switching. In Section 7.4, regulatory risk and guidance related to oncology development will be summarized. Two case studies will be provided in Section 7.5 to give a direct impression of how the innovative methods were used in real clinical studies.

7.1 Endpoints for Cancer Clinical Trials

7.1.1 Overview of Endpoints for Regulatory Approval

In clinical trials, an endpoint is selected on a clinical and regulatory basis to evaluate the safety and provide evidence for the effect of an investigated medical product. In late phase confirmatory trials, the selection of trial primary endpoint(s) is an essential part of study design and is especially critical to establish quality and substantial evidence of effectiveness US Food and Drug Administration (FDA) (2019a).

For cancer treatment, the primary endpoint(s) of efficacy studies generally relates to an improvement in symptoms, decreased process of decrease worsening, or prolongation of survival. Regulatory authorities not only have made general recommendations for the clinical trial endpoints used to support marketing approval (US Food and Drug Administration (FDA) 2018a) but also have shared specific considerations for endpoints used in specific disease areas (US Food and Drug Administration (FDA) 2014, US Food and Drug Administration(FDA) 2015b, European Medicines Agency (EMA) 2018, US Food and Drug Administration (FDA) 2018b). Regarding Time-To-Event (TTE) endpoints, which are usually used as primary endpoint(s) in late-phase oncology trials, efforts (DATECAN) have been made to standardize the definitions by a joint research organization (Bellera et al. 2013). The DATECAN (Definitions for the Assessment of Time-To-Event Endpoints in CANcer) initiative aims to provide recommendations for definitions of common TTE endpoints and help researchers to compare results across clinical trials more easily. The DATECAN initiatives have published guidelines in breast cancer, Gastrointestinal Stromal Tumors (GIST), pancreatic cancer and etc. (Bonnetain et al. 2014, Bellera et al. 2015, Gourgou-Bourgade et al. 2015). By reviewing the regulatory and industrial efforts, Table 7.1 summarized commonly used endpoints in cancer clinical trials, including regulatory considerations, study design recommendations, and analytic properties (also refer to Wilson et al. 2015, US Food and Drug Administration (FDA) 2018a).

Overall Survival (OS) is undisputed a precise and objective measure and is acknowledged as "gold-standard" measurement of cancer treatment benefit. However, with the increased life expectancy of cancer patients and accelerated development of innovative medicine against cancer, the challenges, including requiring long observation period and confounding from subsequent treatments, have increased with designing and analyzing OS studies. Therefore, though it is usually considered as an essential or important endpoint for many progressive cancers, OS is more often applied as a primary endpoint in advanced cancer late-line studies.

The increased challenges with OS as primary endpoint have created needs for potentially faster clinical trial conduction and approval process based on "surrogate" endpoints for OS. The surrogate endpoints are often relatively easy to measure, available over a shorter observation period, and meanwhile allow clinical meaningful inspection of treatment effect as a "surrogate" for true measure of clinical benefit through OS (US Food and Drug Administration (FDA) 2018a, 2018d). The clinical endpoints such as Objective Response Rate (ORR), Progression-Free Survival (PFS), Disease-Free Survival (DFS), and etc., are commonly adopted as surrogate endpoints for cancer clinical trials. In addition, pathologic endpoint like pathological Complete Response (pCR) for neoadjuvant treatment of early-stage breast cancer (European Medicines Agency (EMA) 2014, US Food and Drug Administration (FDA) 2020b) and biomarkers like plasma testosterone levels for advanced prostate cancer (US Food and Drug Administration (FDA)2019b) have also been accepted as validated surrogate endpoints to support accelerated approval of drugs. The FDA's surrogate endpoint table (US Food and Drug Administration (FDA) 2020a) provides valuable information to drug developers on endpoints that may be considered and discussed with FDA for individual development programs. Examples of recent approvals based on surrogate endpoints are available in Blumenthal et al. (2017).

Despite the attractive advantages of using surrogate endpoints to accelerate cancer drug development process, the potential perils of using a surrogate shall also be noticed (Kemp and Prasad 2017). Firstly, the surrogate endpoints currently used in cancer clinical trials are generally based on tumor image assessment, pathological tests, or laboratory tests. These endpoints are therefore potentially subject to assessment bias, especially in open-label studies. Secondly, the evaluation and validation of surrogate endpoints is challenging and often controversial from a statistical perspective, which will be further discussed in Section 7.1.2. Nevertheless, the reality is that many surrogate endpoints have already been used in clinical practice. Thirdly, it is important to note that a surrogate endpoint may be valid for a particular indication (e.g., non-small-cell lung cancer) or type of treatment (e.g., cytotoxic agents) but not for other indications (e.g., small cell lung cancer) or other types of treatment (e.g., cancer immunotherapy).

TABLE 7.1

Commonly Used Endpoints for Regulatory Approval of Cancer Drugs

Type of Endpoint	Regulatory Considerations	Study Design Recommendations	Analytic Properties	
			Advantages	Dis-advantages
Overall Survival (OS) — Clinical Endpoint and direct measure of benefit	Regular Approval	Randomized. Open-label design is accepted. Usually in advanced or metastatic disease stage	• Acknowledged as "gold-standard" evidence: • Easily and precisely measured; • objective and no assessment bias	• Include non-cancer deaths; • Result in large sample size and/or long follow-up; • Can be confounded by subsequent treatment(s), especially treatment crossover.
Endpoints measuring improvement in symptoms (patient-reported outcomes, PRO)		Randomized. Blinding is essential	• Patient perspectives of clinical benefit; • Can be assessed earlier, i.e., short-term trials	• Blinding is essential. • Balanced timing of assessments among arms is critical • Data are often missing or incomplete; • Clinical relevance of small changes is unknown; • Lack of validated instruments for many disease settings; • Definitions vary among studies
Complete Response or Objective Response Rate (ORR) — Clinical Endpoint and as Surrogate Endpoint	Accelerated approval (AA) or Regular approval	Randomized or single-arm settings; Blinding is recommended in randomized setting Independent blinded review is essential	• Can be assessed earlier and with smaller sample size compared with survival studies; • Effect on tumor attributable to drug(s), not natural history	• Definitions vary among studies • Frequent radiological or other assessments. • Not a comprehensive measurement of benefit. For example, do not include treatment benefit on disease control and duration of response. • May not always correlate with survival

(Continued)

TABLE 7.1

Commonly Used Endpoints for Regulatory Approval of Cancer Drugs *(Continued)*

	Type of Endpoint	Regulatory Considerations	Study Design Recommendations	Analytic Properties	
				Advantages	Dis-advantages
Endpoints measuring decreased time in disease recurrent or worsening, such as Progression-Free Survival (PFS); Time to Progression (TTP); Disease Free Survival (DFS) or Event Free Survival (EFS), etc.	Clinical Endpoint and as Surrogate Endpoint	Accelerated Approval (AA) or Regular Approval	• Randomized; • Blinding is recommended; • Independent blinded review is recommended, especially in open-label setting *Note: PFS/TTP is usually used in advanced or metastatic disease setting; DFS is usually used in adjuvant setting*	• Smaller sample size and shorter follow-up time compared with OS trial • Not affected by subsequent treatment(s) • Generally objective and quantitative *for PFS only; compared with ORR, include clinical benefit of stable disease*	• Potentially subject to assessment bias, particularly in open-label studies • Definitions, especially on censoring rules, may vary among studies • Balanced timing of assessments among treatment arms is critical • May not always as good surrogate endpoint of OS • Frequent radiological assessments may be needed in some disease settings for tumor assessment-based endpoints (such as PFS)

Patient Reported Outcome (PRO) provide patient's perspectives of the clinical benefit. In cancer trials, the use of PRO endpoint(s) as the primary endpoint(s) (e.g., for painful conditions) or as secondary endpoint(s) has become a prominent topic in cancer research, as patients with progression of cancer frequently experience multiple symptoms, economic burden, long-term health-care management problems and lack of emotional well-being. Lipscomb et al. (2007) discussed specific administrative policies and management procedures to improve PRO data collection, analysis, and dissemination of findings in cancer trials. The Patient-Centered Outcome Research Institutes (PCORI) suggested methodology standards in November 2013 for design and conduct in patient-centered comparative effective research. The widely used PRO instrument include the FACT (Cella et al. 1993) and FACT-G (Overcash et al. 2001), which are used to assess functional and symptom outcomes, and EORTC-QLQ (Aaronson et al. 1993), which is used to assess cancer-specific quality of life outcomes. Meanwhile, other various PRO instruments have also been proposed. To select the appropriate PRO instruments, the most important criteria include reliability, validity and responsiveness to changes over time (Turner et al. 2007, Patrick et al. 2011).

7.1.2 Surrogate Endpoint Validation

The use of surrogate endpoint requires rigorous evidence-based justification. A "perfect" surrogate endpoint, as described by Prentice (1989) is "a response variable for which a test of null hypothesis of no relation to the treatment groups under comparison is also a valid test of the corresponding null hypothesis based on the true endpoint". Given that

1. treatment (Z) has a significant impact on both the surrogate endpoint (S) and the true endpoint (T), i.e., $f(S|Z) \neq f(S)$; $f(T|Z) \neq f(T)$,
2. and the surrogate endpoint significantly impact the true endpoint T, $f(T|S) \neq f(T)$, the Prentice rule particularly requires:
3. the failure rate for true endpoint to be independent of treatment conditional on the surrogate endpoint (S), expressed by $f(T|S, Z) \equiv f(T|S)$).

The Prentice definition, which actually requires that the full effect of treatment upon the true endpoint is captured by the surrogate endpoint, has been criticized as too strict (Fleming and Powers 2012). To overcome the limitation, several practical definitions of surrogate endpoint and corresponding surrogate endpoint validation methods have been proposed (De Gruttola et al. 2001, Weir and Walley 2006). Of special interest was the meta-analytic methods, which combine information from multiple studies with reliable estimates of treatment effect to explore the causal relationship between the surrogate endpoint and the true endpoint (Daniels and Hughes 1997, Buyse et al. 2000, Gail et al. 2000). Taking the most popular Buyse et al. (2000) approach of the class as an example, suppose we have data from N trials in which n_i patient is enrolled in the ith trial, the two-stage random-effect representation of Buyse et al. (2000) approach is:

$$S_{ij} \mid Z_{ij} = \mu_s + m_{si} + \alpha Z_{ij} + a_i Z_{ij} + \varepsilon_{Sij}$$

$$T_{ij} \mid Z_{ij} = \mu_T + m_{Ti} + \beta Z_{ij} + b_i Z_{ij} + \varepsilon_{Tij},$$

where μ_s and μ_T are fixed intercepts, α and β are the fixed effects of treatment Z on the surrogate endpoint S and true endpoint T, respectively, m_{si} and m_{si} are random intercepts,

a_i and b_i are the random effects of treatment Z on the endpoints S and T in trial i, respectively, and ε_{Sij} and ε_{Tij} are the error terms in the randomize-effects model. After fitting the two-stage model, surrogacy can be assessed by coefficients of determination at individual level ($R^2_{ind} = R^2_{\varepsilon_{Ti}|\varepsilon_{Si}}$) and at trial level ($R^2_{trial} = R^2_{b_i|a_i}$). Regulatory authorities have typically required verification of a surrogate endpoint both at the individual and trial level.

Despite the benefit that using surrogate endpoint may facilitate accelerated regulatory approval based on smaller and/or shorter clinical trials, we need also to evaluate the potential limitations and risks. Firstly, regulatory approval, especially the full regulatory approval that do not entail further post-approval commitments for efficacy, based on a surrogate endpoint (such as PFS) may limit insights about long-term efficacy (such as on OS), and may also lead to less reliable assurances about safety given the smaller number of patients exposed and shorter follow-up time. Secondly, as mentioned earlier, the strength of surrogacy depends on many factors such as the disease, the treatment setting, and the heterogeneity of the underlying patient population, while the use of a weak surrogate endpoint can increase false decision-making probability. Especially, the checkpoint inhibitors are becoming standard of care therapy for many disease treatment settings, which have a unique mechanism of action that differs from chemotherapy or targeted therapies. For the development of checkpoint inhibitors, factors such as pseudoprogression, delayed but durable treatment effect, heterogeneity among patient biomarker subsets etc., will introduce uncertainty to the surrogacy between commonly used surrogate endpoints (e.g., PFS and ORR) and OS. Based on systematic literature review of published evidence (Branchoux et al. 2019), meta-analysis indicates that there is insufficient data to support validated surrogate endpoint for OS for patients treated with immune-checkpoint inhibitors. Adequate surrogacy assessment of promising composite endpoints which consider a duration component is encouraged. As a conclusion, surrogate endpoints should be evaluated specifically in a case-by-case scenario.

7.1.3 Imaging Endpoints Assessment Criteria and Process Standards

Endpoints like PFS and ORR are based on tumor response measurements from imaging data. For assessment of imaging-based tumor response data, standard response criteria have been proposed. For solid tumors, the Response Evaluation Criteria in Solid Tumor (RECIST) has been uniformly adopted to evaluate tumor changes, to suggest overall response destinations at each tumor imaging assessment, and finally to conclude the Best Overall Response (BOR) level achieved. The RECIST was first published in 2000 (Therasse et al. 2000) and the latest revision was made in 2009 as version v1.1 (Eisenhauer et al. 2009). For lymphoma staging and tumor response evaluation, the LUGANO classification criteria (Cheson et al. 2014), which incorporates PET-CT as a standard component for FDG-avid lymphomas while retaining CT evaluation for other lymphomas subtypes, is the most commonly used criteria in clinical practice. Recently, both RECIST and LUGONA criteria have been adapted for immune-based treatment (Cheson et al. 2016, Seymour et al. 2017).

When imaging is used to assess a trial primary endpoint(s) or a component, both FDA and NMPA recommend utilizing standard processes for imaging acquisition, quality control and monitoring, review and interpretation, re-review and modification, as well as utilizing standardized evaluation criteria for consistent disease response assessment (US Food and Drug Administration (FDA) 2018e, National Medical Products Administration (NMPA) 2020).

Especially, to reduce variability in endpoint measurements and to maintain trial integrity, heath authorities usually recommend or require to apply Independent Central Review (ICR) for image data interpretation. ICR is the process by which all image data and selected clinical data acquired as part of a clinical protocol are submitted to a centralized facility and reviewed by independent physicians (radiologists and clinicians) who are not involved in the treatment of the patients. ICR is advocated by regulatory authorities to enhance the credibility of image interpretation and to better ensure consistency of image assessments in scenarios where the endpoint(s) depending on medical imaging assist in critical regulatory decision and meanwhile assessment bias is anticipated. This includes single-arm studies or open-label randomized studies, studies with imaging acquisition or interpretation variability anticipated, and studies with complicated measuring criteria. Once ICR is adopted, ICR image readers are expected to be blinded to patient treatment data to avoid assessment bias. Blinding may include the treatment arm (or any data that might un-blind the treatment arm), and/or any other clinical data information that may influence independent readers, such as the total number of exams for a patient (to exclude progression bias), the results or assessments of other reviewers participating in the review process (except during adjudication), imaging exam date, and etc. (Ford et al. 2009). Besides blinding, development of ICR charter, which outlines the ICR design, criteria, methodology, image review system, recording of review results, assessment of reviewer performance etc. has also been suggested by both FDA and NMPA to standardize the ICR process and increase ICR review robustness and accuracy.

7.2 Cancer Trials with Time-to-Event Endpoints

7.2.1 Basic Concepts and Conventional Statistical Techniques

TTE endpoints are usually used as the primary endpoints in randomized cancer clinical trials. This typically includes OS, PFS, Disease Free Survival (DFS) etc. A TTE endpoint is defined as time to occurrence of any well-defined event. For example, the event can be "death from any cause" for OS and "disease objective progression or death as whichever occurs first" for PFS.

7.2.1.1 Censoring

The application of statistical techniques to analyze TTE data is usually complicated by censoring. On one hand, clinical trials are conducted within a limited follow-up period and the interested event(s) may not be observed when reaching clinical cutoff date (such censoring is usually referred to as "administrative censoring"). On the other hand, the occurrence of "intercurrent events" (refer to Figure 7.1 for the illustration and Section 7.2.4 for the definition), such as patients' use of non-protocol anti-cancer therapy, may also lead to censoring at the standard definitions of many common endpoints such as PFS and DFS.

Censoring can be seen as a form of missing data. Censoring may or may not relate to the event process, corresponding to "informative censoring" and "non-informative censoring", respectively (Ranganathan and Pramesh 2012). By analogy with "missing at random", non-informative censoring assumes that the patients with censored observations have the same risk of experiencing an event with the non-censored patients who have not

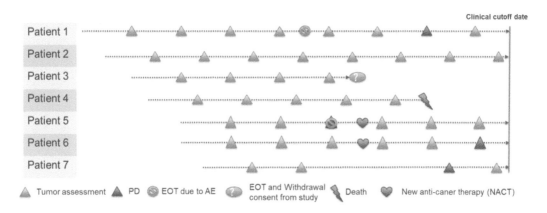

FIGURE 7.1
Journeys of seven patients illustrating the difficulty to define the treatment effect on PFS due to occurrence of different types of "intercurrent events" between the patient randomization and the clinical cut-off date.

yet experienced event. By contrast, informative censoring indicates that the probability of an individual being censored relates to probability that the individual has an event. Conventional statistical methods for analyzing TTE data usually assumes non-informative censoring, though this may not be true in practice. Specially, imbalanced pattern of informative censoring between treatment arms may result in analysis bias in the application of the conventional TTE analyses (Templeton et al. 2020). For example, if a patient in the control arm dropped out from the study because of disease worsening, the patient tends to have shorter OS than the non-censored patients of the same follow-up duration. The classic TTE analysis methods which "estimate" the patient's future OS risk by the non-censored patients at the time point may mislead the analysis results by over-estimating the OS in the control arm. In clinical trials, censoring except for administrative censoring is likely to be informative while cannot be easily identified and fixed through statistical analysis. Therefore, it is important to minimize non-administrative censoring, transparently report numbers of censoring and reasons for each of the treatment arms, and report results of supplementary analysis accounting for different rules of handing censoring when necessary.

Depending on the censoring scheme, there are right censoring, left censoring, and interval censoring. By the definition, OS data is right-censored data and meanwhile, PFS data are by nature interval-censored data considering the trial visit schedule (Panageas et al. 2007). It is common practice to employ the right censoring techniques to analyze interval-censored data when the trial is randomized and have balanced and consistent surveillance intervals, though statistical techniques for analyzing interval data have been proposed back to 1976 (Turnbull 1976).

7.2.1.2 Kaplan-Meier Estimation, Log-Rank Test and Cox Regression

In clinical trials, the classic statistical techniques in analyzing right-censored TTE data are commonly based on the non-parametric Kaplan Meier (KM) product limit estimation of survival function or the semi-parametric Cox proportional hazards regression (short as Cox method in below sections).

In data analysis and reporting perspectives, the KM method provides non-parametric estimators of survival function for all time points less than the study largest observation

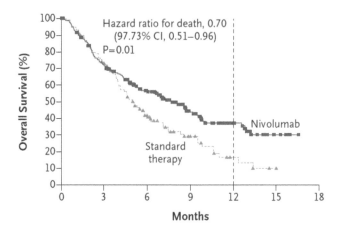

FIGURE 7.2
Kaplan–Meier curves for overall survival from Checkmate-141 study, which exhibits delayed treatment effect characteristic. (Source: Ferris, Blumenschein et al. 2016. N Engl J Med, 375(19):1856–1867.)

time. KM method is commonly applied to generate estimators of median survival time and event-free survival rates by landmark time points. In terms of comparing the difference between survival curves fitted by KM estimates, hypothesis testing is typically based on Log-Rank test.

$$\text{Log-Rank test statistic: } Z = \frac{\sum_{j=1}^{J}(D_{1j} - D_j R_{1j} / R_j)}{\sqrt{\sum_{j=1}^{J} R_{1j} R_{2j} D_j (R_j - D_j) / [R_j^2 (R_j - 1)]}},$$

where $j = 1, \ldots, J$ is the *jth* event time; R_{1j}, R_{2j} and R_j are the patients at risk at the time j for the treatment, control arms and at the study level, respectively; D_{1j} and D_j are the patients having had events at the time j for treatment arm and at the study level, respectively. Under the null hypothesis of identical survival function between arms, the Log-rank test statistic Z follows normal distribution approximately. In terms of treatment effect estimation, hazard ratio, which describes the relative risk based on comparison of hazard rates, is usually used to quantify the treatment effect and is produced by Cox method based on proportional hazard assumption. Proportional hazard assumption indicates that the hazard ratio for any two individuals is constant over time.

In the study design perspective, sample size calculation for survival trials is largely based on normal approximation to log-rank test statistics with assuming exponential survival function(s) for each treatment arm. The number of events rather than the number of patients determine the study power and is firstly calculated. The number of patients is then determined considering study enrollment rates and follow-up time. There are copious formulas around as references (Lachin and Foulkes 1986, Lakatos 1988).

However, these conventional methods present many challenges. Firstly, Non-Proportional Hazards (NPH), which are against the assumptions required by proportional hazards methods, are common rather than exceptional in cancer trials. Secondly, patients may experience competing risks with high frequency, which may prevent an event of interest from ever happening. These controversial issues, together with the latest methodology innovation or industrial consensus, will be discussed in Section 7.2.2 and 7.2.3, respectively.

7.2.2 Non-Proportional Hazards (NPH) and Statistical Considerations

There are various types of NPH in actual trials, in which the underlying hazard ratios between arms are non-constant over time and may of different patterns. For example, in the IPASS study (Mok et al. 2009), the OS Kaplan-Meier curves crossed; in the E2100 study (Miller et al. 2007), the PFS Kaplan-Meier curves separate at initial time but the gap narrows with time. By contrast, the delayed separation and long-term survival have been more frequently observed in cancer immunotherapy trials. An example of this phenomenon appears in CheckMate141 study (Figure 7.2, Ferris et.al. 2016).

There could be multiple reasons related to the NPH patterns. It may take time for the treatment to measurably impact progression or survival due to the mechanism of action of the treatment drugs (e.g., checkpoint inhibitors). Also, heterogeneity between subgroups of patients may increase variation in the survival curves. Furthermore, treatment switching may also lead to NPH in overall survival analysis.

The occurrence of NPH weakens the performance of widely used statistical methods as mentioned above and raises challenges for interpretations of the classic estimators. For example, the log-rank test which is most powerful when proportional hazard assumption holds will lose power in the presence of NPH (though still valid), and the hazard ratio estimated through Cox method may not be an intuitive measurement of the treatment difference between groups.

Recognizing the challenges, FDA had initiated a cross-pharma working group with pharmaceutical companies to systematically review the strengths and limitations of available methods and to identify appropriate alternative statistical tests and summary measures under NPH conditions. The working group has publicly presented their work at a Duke–US FDA workshop (Duke and FDA 2018) and has proposed a new method called "MaxCombo". Achievements from this working group have also been presented in Roychoudhury et al. (2019) and Lin et al.(2020).

7.2.2.1 Hypothesis Testing under NPH

In order to increase test power under NPH, Weighted Log-Rank Test (WLR) can be used. The WLR test has been proposed by Fleming and Harrington (1991) to incorporate a weight function. The general formula of weighted log-rank test statistics $G^{\rho,\gamma}$ is defined as below:

$$G^{\rho,\gamma} = \frac{\sum_{j=1}^{J} W_j (D_{1j} - D_j R_{1j} / R_j)}{\sqrt{\sum_{j=1}^{J} W_j^2 R_{1j} R_{2j} D_j (R_j - D_j) / [R_j^2 (R_j - 1)]}},$$

where $W_j = S(t_j)^\rho (1 - S(t_j))^\gamma$ is the weight function based on observed survival, $S(t)$ is the survival function, ρ and γ are parameters determining the shape of the weight function. Taking $\rho = 0,1$ and $\gamma = 0,1$ as example, WLR test can be used for below scenarios with test statistics as

- $G^{0,0}$, which becomes the standard log-rank test
- $G^{1,0}$, which weights the early portions of survival curves

- $G^{0,1}$, which weights the late portions of survival curves and has been accordingly suggested for situations in which the treatment effect potentially be delayed (Fine 2007)
- $G^{1,1}$, which weights the middle portions of survival curves.

To provide a robust power under different NPH scenarios, various combination tests have been proposed (Lee 2007, Yang and Prentice 2010, Karrison 2016, Roychoudhury et al. 2019). The "MaxCombo" test proposed by the NPH cross-pharma working group (Duke and FDA 2018), which takes the largest absolute values of $G^{0,0}$, $G^{1,0}$, $G^{0,1}$ and $G^{1,1}$ test statistics, was demonstrated to be more powerful compared to log-rank test in the presence of NPH while maintaining similar efficiency (though slightly lower) compared to log-rank test when PH assumption holds. However, as discussed in Korn and Freidlin (2018) which using Keynote-042 study (Mok et al. 2019) as an example, these maximum tests (including MaxCombo) can be problematic by rejecting the null hypothesis both in favor of the experimental treatment and in favor of control treatment on the same data.

The other commonly used methods for hypothesis testing are KM based tests, particularly the approach based on Restricted Mean Survival Time (RMST) (Karrison 1987, Royston and Parmar 2011, Uno et al. 2014, Tian et al. 2018). The RMST test is based on the area between the KM curves of the treatment and control arms up to a pre-specified time τ. However, the power of the RMST test depends on the chosen of τ and therefore, τ needs to be pre-specified to avoid exaggerating the statistical significance. Unfortunately, to date, there has not been a consensus criterion to define the proper τ (Li et al. 2019).

7.2.2.2 Summary Measures for Treatment Effect under NPH

KM curves for the experimental and control arms offer a comprehensive display of the treatment effect. In terms of summarizing the treatment effect with a single estimator, the RMST-based approach can be interpreted as "difference in life expectancy up to time τ" and is commonly presented. Meanwhile, the weighted hazard ratio estimated from weighted Cox regression with the weight chosen by the MaxCombo test may also complement the standard hazard ratio.

7.2.2.3 Study Design Considerations: Sample Size and Analysis Timing

For the log-rank test based design, it is important to have a careful look into the possible treatment effect pattern under a reasonable hypothesis and to conduct statistical simulation accordingly to ensure that the sample size and follow-up time will provide adequate power for the most likely treatment effect pattern. When there exist concerns of delayed treatment effect, log-rank test based designs with slightly inflated sample size (Hoering et al. 2017), additional follow-up time for higher data maturity at time of analysis (e.g., data maturity = number of events/number of patients) (Chen 2013) can provide robust power. For the implementation of the MaxCombo test-based design, the sample size calculation requires statistical simulation considering there is no closed-form of the test statistic. Lin et al. (2020) proposed a two-step iterative procedure for such a purpose.

Under NPH, planning interim analyses with log-rank based design could be controversial. In the presence of diminishing treatment effect, the statistical significance of treatment effect is maximized at an earlier stage while interim efficacy analysis based on the low fraction of information or aggressive alpha spending approach (e.g., the Pocock method,

(Pocock 1977)) is generally not accepted by healthy authorities for primary endpoint. In the presence of delayed treatment effect, implementation of interim efficacy analysis with shorter follow-up may have smaller success probability for a positive outcome whereas interim efficacy analysis with longer follow-up time may not be operational appealing given it being close to final analysis. On the other hand, futility interim analysis could increase the chance of terminating the study early and erroneously discarding an active agent (Chen 2013). Modified rules for futility monitoring may need to be considered in the case of NPH (Korn and Freidlin 2018). For MaxCombo based design, extensions in group sequential framework have been proposed in recent with a simulation-free approach (Wang et al. 2019).

7.2.3 Competing Risks and Models

Many commonly used TTE endpoints in oncology trials are "composite" endpoints where different events are encompassed. For example, an event of PFS is a composition of "disease progression" and "death without diagnosed progression", and the event of OS is actually a composition of "cancer-specific death" and "non-cancer death". Assuming every patient will experience an event with adequate follow-up, the standard statistical techniques as described in previous sections are applicable to such "composite" endpoints with focusing on time to occurrence of any risks as which occur first.

When the interest is on a specific type of event, for example, the "cancer-specific death", the other type(s) of event(s), such as "non-cancer death", become "competing risk(s)" as the occurrence of such event(s) preclude the observation of the event of interest. Marginal survival estimate in the scenario based on naïve KM estimate treating the competing event(s) as censoring event(s) are valid only under strong assumption of independence of the (latent) failure times between event process of interest and the competing event process(es), and such assumption often does not hold in actual trials (Putter et al. 2007). The competing risk challenge is relevant particularly in trials for indolent cancers or in patients with clinically significant comorbidity, who may also fail with high probability from causes unrelated to cancer or event of interest. Examples appear in the below references (Albertsen et al. 1998, Berry et al. 2010, Shen et al. 2015, de Glas et al. 2016).

Putter et al. (2007) provided a comprehensive tutorial on statistical methods in analyzing competing risks with an emphasis on practical issues in clinical trials, and Koller et al. (2012) discussed the translational aspects of competing risks to clinical research. In the book, we restrict our short overview of common concepts and practical statistical methods regarding competing risk problems based on simplex scenarios of two competing risks.

Suppose a patient may fail due to event of interest ($K = 1$) and the competing event ($K = 2$), and the potential unobservable time to occurrence of the two risks are X_1 and X_2, respectively. Let $T = min(X_1, X_2)$ as the observed time to first failure and define an indicator δ which takes value of 1 or 2 based on the observed event type. Formulate the competing risk problem as a multi-state model as presented in Figure 7.3, where the cause-specific hazards are defined as

$$\lambda_i(t) = \lim_{\Delta t \to 0} \frac{P(t \leq T < t + \Delta t, \delta = i \,|\, T > t)}{\Delta t}, i = 1 \text{ or } 2,$$

and tell us the rates at which patients who have not yet experience any of the events will experience the ith competing cause of failure in the interval $[t, t + \Delta t]$.

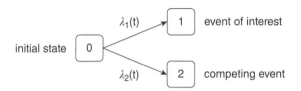

FIGURE 7.3
Competing risks as multistate model with cause-specific hazards $\lambda_1(t), \lambda_2(t)$.

On the other hand, in clinical research of competing risks, we are more often interested in the failure/survival probabilities that summarize our knowledge about the likelihoods of occurrence of each event. The cause-specific probability of failure by time t, referred as Cumulative Incidence Function (CIF) is expressed by $F_i(t) = \Pr(T \le t, \delta = i)$ for $i = 1$ *or* 2. The Aalen-Johansen (A-J) estimator (Aalen and Johansen 1978) provides the nonparametric estimator of the CIF. For cause i ($i = 1$ *or* 2), the A-J estimator can be calculated by

$$\sum_{l \le t} \hat{S}(l) \times \frac{\text{Number of patients experienced event with cause } i \text{ at time } l}{\text{Number of patients without any events and not yet censored before time } l}$$

where $\hat{S}(l)$ is the KM estimator of being free of any events before time t. To reflect the covariate effect, such as treatment effect, on cause-specific survival probability, semiparametric proportional hazards model proposed by Fine and Gray (1999) are commonly applied to estimate the sub-distribution hazard. More practical details of this topic can be referred to Putter et al. (2007).

7.2.4 Estimand for Cancer Trials with Time-to-Event Endpoints

In November 2019, the ICH E9 (R1) addendum on estimands and sensitivity analysis in clinical trials has come to effect. The addendum aims to align the clinical trial objectives with the quantification of treatment effect, and define "estimand" through population, variable, intervention effect (i.e., how intercurrent events are reflected in clinical questions), and population-level summary for the variable. For addressing intercurrent events, five analysis strategies including treatment policy strategy, hypothetical strategies, composite variable strategies, while on treatment strategies, and principal stratum strategies have been proposed.

For cancer trials with TTE endpoint, the cross-pharma Estimands in Oncology Scientific Working Group (SWG, http://www.oncoestimand.org) have attempted to connect the five analysis strategies in the estimand framework with the common definitions of TTE endpoints involving censoring. The SWG suggests that the heterogeneity in TTE endpoint definitions implicate heterogeneities in the strategies dealing with intercurrent events and thus heterogeneities in the estimands. Rufibach (2019) presented the efforts and illustrated them with actual trial examples. Degtyarev et al. (2019) reviewed the relationship between patient journeys and treatment effects and illustrated with examples how the estimand framework can structure discussions among interdisciplinary teams about the design and interpretation of oncology trials.

To illustrate the estimand challenge, we restrict our focus as well to a PFS example where the intercurrent event addressed here is the start of a New Anticancer Therapy (NACT) before the assessment of tumor progression. The FDA guidance on clinical trial endpoints for NSCLC (US Food and Drug Administration (FDA) 2015a) recommends different censoring schemes for handling NACT for PFS analysis. Meanwhile, in the estimand framework, these rules result in different estimands (Table 7.2).

Experience with the estimand framework in oncology research is still limited. However, considerations around diverse intercurrent events and their impact on trial endpoints are not new to the oncology community. In this aspect, the estimand framework is not introducing new complexity but offers a common language to discuss existing complexities with all stakeholders (Degtyarev et al. 2019)

TABLE 7.2

Rules of Handling NACT in PFS Analysis Result in Different Estimand

	Estimand Attributes				Analysis Rules of Handling NACT
Estimand	Population	Variable (Endpoint)	Analysis Strategy of Handling Intercurrent Event NACT	Summary Measure	Handling of Intercurrent event for analysis
Estimand 1	Intent-to-treat (ITT) population	**PFS** based on progression or death, whichever occurs first	**Treatment policy:** • Believe progression is a relevant value for treatment effect though NACT happened in between • The observation for the variable (PFS) is used regardless of whether the NACT occurs	Hazard Ratio	*Event* occurrence on the date of documented progression with protocol specified continued follow-up in all treatment arms.
Estimand 2			**Hypothetical policy:** • Consider the variable in which the NACT would not occur • The observation for the variable up to occurrence of NACT		*Censored* on the date of last tumor assessment with documented non-progression before initialization of NACT.
Estimand 3		**Event-Free Survival** (EFS) based on progression, death or use of NACT as event (whichever first)	**Composite policy:** make the intercurrent event part of a composite endpoint by counting it an event defining the endpoint		*Event* occurrence on the date of initialization of NACT

7.3 Novel Challenging Issues in Cancer Drug Development

7.3.1 Finding the Optimal Biological Dose (OBD)

In the dose-finding studies of cytotoxic agents, the Dose-Related Toxicity (DLT) increases with dose level and meanwhile is regarded as a surrogate endpoint for efficacy. Therefore, the goal of such dose-finding studies is to find the Maximum Toxicity Dose (MTD) within a limited sequence of candidate doses. The usual measure(s) are the toxic effects using standard criteria. In this framework, a series of rule-based or model-based dose-escalation methods for identifying MTD have been proposed for Phase I study (Storer 1989, O'Quigley et al. 1990, Neuenschwander et al. 2008).

In the new era of innovative drug development with non-cytotoxic agents such as Molecularly Targeted Therapeutics (MTT) and cancer immunotherapy, the investigated agents may be devoid of traditional toxic effects and may have effects only in biomarker defined subpopulations. The wide therapeutic window, flat dose-toxicity curve, and maybe non-monotone dose-efficacy curve raise challenges to the traditional identification of MTD. Optimal Biologic Dose (OBD) was proposed and was defined as the *minimum* dose level that produces a desirable biologic outcome and satisfies safe tolerance in the pre-defined proportion of patients. In this background, statistical methods have been proposed for finding OBD, in which defining the endpoint/biomarker to assess the biologic effect in real-time or within a short follow-up time is the most challenging task (refer to Chapter 3 of this book for technical details regarding identifying predictive biomarker).

Assuming there exist a valid assay that is able to provide short-time response results to assess the biological effect of the investigated agent, Hunsberger et al. (2005) proposed "proportion 4/6" and "proportion 5/6" designs to mimic the 3+3 design and guide dose escalation based on response rate. Zhang et.al. (2006) proposed a continuation-ratio model for trinomial outcome (no response/success/toxic) combing toxicity and efficacy assessment simultaneously. At the same time, several Phase I/II methods have been proposed to allow for including both efficacy and toxicity in dose finding (Hoering et al. 2011, Hoering et al. 2013, Zang and Lee 2014, Wages and Tait 2015). Especially, Zang and Lee (2014) described several adaptive designs on logistic or isotonic regression to model the dose-efficacy curve.

With all these past efforts, the development of OBD dose finding methods remains an active area of research, especially in the presence of new challenges such as delayed response for cancer immunotherapies and finding OBD for combination of biologic agents.

7.3.2 Use of Historical Data

The use of historical information is not a new concept, which has been discussed in ICH E10 back to 2001 for its validity of inference in particular situations (such as when there are ethical concerns in recruiting patients for control arms) but also for its caveats of raising bias and erroneous conclusions. Historical data may come from different resources, including clinical trials, clinical practice, health record systems, insurance claims systems, etc. Ghadessi et al. (2020) present a comprehensive review of the data resources and the pros and cons. At the planning stage of clinical trials, historical data is frequently used to explore the variance of endpoints for sample size calculation, to determine the margins used in equivalence/non-inferiority clinical trials, to make the assumption of targeted product profiles, to provide information for patient selection and so on. During trial ongoing, historical data, either from internal studies or external competitive studies, assist study adaptions such as sample size re-estimation, study population enrichment, Go-No-Go criteria, etc. The use of historical data provides efficiency to revisit study design at pre-planned interim analysis or at a critical time point before study being unblinded, thus could potentially increase study success probability. In recent years, with the development of real-world data resources, historical data used to support regulatory approval has raised much more interest. One of the applications is to use disease natural histories as control in a single-arm study to support the approval in rare diseases. Such use of historical data only makes sense if sufficient information could be provided to justify traditional RCTs are inapplicable or unethical. Based on single-arm design with historical control, FDA accepted several new drugs for rare diseases. An example could be found on the website https://www.fda.gov/news-events/press-announcements/fda-approves-first-treatment-form-batten-disease for the approval of Brineura. Another use of historical data from the real-world is to support label expansion. If one product has already been approved for one indication, then subsequently it could be used off-label for some indications that do not get approved yet. Based on such historical data, new indications could be added to original label with risk-benefit evaluation.

There are a lot of literatures discussing historical data borrowing, generally speaking, the methodology can be divided into simple pooling, power priors, commensurate priors and robust mixture priors. Simple pooling approach assumes historical data coming from the same distribution as current study data come from, thus by using Bayes rule, historical posterior could be formulated as $\pi(\theta \mid D_0) \approx L(\theta \mid D_0)\pi_0(\theta)$, where $\pi_0(\theta)$ is prior distribution and $L(\theta \mid D_0)$ is historical data. Ibrahim and Chen (2000) proposed power priors, which allows to define how much historical data to borrow, $\pi(\theta \mid D_0) \propto L(\theta \mid D_0)^{\alpha_0} \pi_0(\theta)$, where α_0 indicate borrow strength. This method gives the flexibility to use historical data depending on the similarity of historical data with current observed data. One criticism of power priors is that they do not parameterise the concordance of historical data with current data, to solve this problem, Hobbs et al. (2011) proposed to add a commensurate part which is centered at the historical locations with variance σ, $\pi(\theta, \theta_0 \mid D_0, \sigma) \propto L(\theta_0 \mid D_0)\pi(\theta \mid \theta_0, \sigma)\pi_0(\theta_0)$. If σ is larger, this method will reduce the borrowing of historical data, however if σ is small, it will increase the borrowing of historical data. Neuenschwander et al. (2010) proposed Meta-Analytic-Predictive (MAP) framework based on a normal random effects distribution with the assumption of exchangeability. Schmidli et al. (2014) further extended MAP method by approximating MAP priors using mixture distributions consisting of two or three components of standard priors, which leads to good approximations and straightforward posterior calculations. To reflect prior data conflict, they proposed robust MAP prior by adding an extra weakly-informative mixture component.

All the above methods, except the simple pooling method, require a tuning parameter which defines the amount of borrowing. This tuning parameter is important when we decide to use historical data because it reflects the confidence we have in the similarity of historical data to our current study. The chosen this parameter need the collaboration between clinical physician and statistical experts. Another challenge when using historical data borrowing is the drift of data, especially for the scenario when historical data was observed a long time before the current study was conducted. Drift will impact study power and inflate Type I error. One of the solutions is to use a longitudinal model to estimate how treatment effect has evolved over the time (Berry et al. 1999)

7.3.3 Platform Trial Design and Master Protocol

Platform trial design is far away from traditional Randomized Control Trials (RCTs), and the latter one has been regarded as gold-standard in the past decades to generate solid evidence to support the assessment of risk and benefit for a new therapeutic agent. However traditional RCTs was lacking efficiency considering the need to compare multiple interventions in a single trial and sometimes the need to compare treatment effects across different populations with distinct mutations. Stemming from the weakness of traditional RCTs, platform trial design has been proposed to minimize the gap between clinical practice and traditional RCTs. Platform trials can study multiple interventions in a single therapeutic area in a perpetual manner, with interventions allowed to enter or leave the platform on the basis of a decision algorithm. To support the flexibility of platform trials, they are always conducted under master protocol, which is defined as a protocol designed with multiple substudies, which may have different objectives and involves coordinated efforts to evaluate one or more investigational drugs in one or more disease subtypes within the overall trial structure (US Food and Drug Administration (FDA) 2018f). Besides the flexibility to study multiple interventions simultaneously through a perpetual platform, platform trials also have the advantage to well compatible with trial adaptions, including but not limited to Bayesian inference models which are well suited for iterative updating by cooperating various sources of information, response-adaptive randomization which gradually assign patients to the interventions that perform most favorably, and decision making criteria used to trigger the addition or termination of a treatment arm. Considering its tremendous benefits, several platform trials have been proposed and launched, such as I-SPY 2 (Barker et al. 2009), REMAP-CAP (https://www.remapcap.org/), GBM AGILE (Alexander et al. 2018), INSIGhT (Alexander et al. 2019). In Section 7.5.1, we will give a detailed introduction to I-SPY 2.

To facilitate the standard of platform trial designs in terms of the definitions, common design features, trial oversight, results reporting and case sharing, Adaptive Platform Trials Coalition was assembled. In the review paper they wrote in 2019 (Adaptive Platform Trials Coalition 2019), platform trial design was grouped into five broad areas. In the following section, we will debrief the five broad areas and point out the challenges within each area.

7.3.3.1 Patient Selection and Enrichment Strategies

Patients enrolled in platform trials usually have common characteristics, e.g., under the same disease with different subtypes, harbor the same mutation or biomarkers. To treat individuals precisely, it is recommended to use enrichment strategy to enroll appropriate patients and assign the most effective treatment to selected sub-populations according to biomarker expression. FDA has released a guidance that tried to help industry develop enrichment strategies in clinical development (US Food and Drug Administration (FDA) 2019c). In this guidance, not only the commonly used enrichment strategies with fruitful case studies were summarized, but also it points out some challenges that we need to pay attention to. The most important one is the sensitivity and specificity of screening measurement used for patient selection. With the poor performance of measurement methods, the effect of enrichment will be diluted.

7.3.3.2 Organization of Study Arms

Since platform trials allow multiple interventions to be explored simultaneously, usually multiple arms will be incorporated with a single experimental therapy assigned to each arm and a common control arm designed to facilitate the comparisons between new investigational agents and standard of care. Considering the dependence among multiple arms and relatively small sample size within each arm, statistical model that is able to borrow information across multiple arms is demanded. Bayesian Hierarchical Model (BHM) firstly proposed by Thall et al. (2003) could be used to fit this purpose. However, this model will lack power and inflate Type I error when treatment effect across multiple arms is heterogeneous. To solve this problem, Jiang et al. (2020) proposed Optimal Bayesian Hierarchical Model (OBHM) to trade-off power and Type I error through a utility function and maximize this utility function by considering homogeneous or heterogeneous treatment effects.

7.3.3.3 Within-Trial Learning and Adaptions

Response-Adaptive Randomization (RAR) is always combined with adaptive enrichment design, based on which, randomization probability could be updated with accruing within-study data in a continuous learning process. RAR intend to protect the patient from exposure to non-effective agents. Since randomization probability needs to be updated once the efficacy endpoint from the previous patients has been collecting, it is recommended to use a short-term efficacy endpoint to save enrollment time, and the predictive of short-term efficacy endpoint to long-term efficacy endpoint (OS) need to be demonstrated. However, it is unavoidable that sometimes long-term efficacy endpoint is the only option. Xu and Yin (2013) proposed a two-stage adaptive randomization method with an optimal allocation scheme to tackle the common problem caused by delayed efficacy response.

7.3.3.4 Integration of Patient Selection, Study Arms and Adaptations

Integrating information from multiple interventions, multiple subtypes and multiple combinations is a challenge in platform design. Learning from the existing platform designs, the majority of them use Bayesian method as an overarching model to incorporate all information. Before fitting the Bayesian model, we need to carefully consider which is the interaction term, intervention-by-subtypes, or intervention-by-intervention-by-subtype.

7.3.3.5 Miscellaneous Features

Conducting platform trials usually require comprehensive statistical experience. Much attention should be paid to, but not limited to, multiple comparisons, the inflations of Type I error, drift in standard of care for prolonged platform period, interim analysis, simulations to demonstrate well controlled study operational characteristics, handling of missing data and so no.

7.3.4 Confirmatory Adaptive Design for Trials with Time-to-Event Endpoints

Confirmatory adaptive design refers to prospectively planned modifications to future course of an ongoing trial on the basis of comparative (i.e., unblinded) or non-comparative (i.e., blinded) analysis of accumulating data, ensuring statistical validity in the conclusion. For adaptions based on comparative analysis, statistical methods to withstand type I error inflation and estimation bias, and operational steps to ensure appropriate trial conduct are critical to regulatory agencies (US Food and Drug Administration (FDA) 2018g, National Medical Products Administration (NMPA) 2021). The common confirmatory adaptions based on comparative analysis include group sequential designs, unblinded sample size re-estimation, and two-stage adaptive design, e.g., in a seamless Phase II/III framework with treatment selection and/or population enrichment. There could be combined implementation of different types. For example, the TAPPAS trial as discussed in the Section 7.5.2 incorporated both unblinded sample size re-estimation and adaptive population enrichment. Bhatt and Mehta (2016) have comprehensively reviewed different types of confirmatory adaptive designs, discussing general benefits and limitations and presenting case studies. In this review, we focus on discussing the general challenges of confirmatory adaptive designs based on comparative analysis for cancer trials with TTE endpoints.

7.3.4.1 Challenges Due to Non-Proportional Hazards (NPH)

For adaptive designs, the information at an interim analysis which is defined by a number of events must be useful for predicting the results that would achieve at the latter analyses if the trial were to continue. Meanwhile, as discussed in Section 7.2.2, the prediction can be controversial in the presence of NPH. Especially, in the presence of delayed treatment effect, a "trial within a trial" design (Choueiri et al. 2015) that analyze the endpoint within first enrolled batch of patients to ensure enough data maturity (i.e., number of events over number of patients is not so small) for interim analysis could be useful.

7.3.4.2 Use of Surrogate Endpoint for Defining Interim Decision Rules

Adaptive trial usually requires interim decisions to be made on outcome information from a reasonable number of participants and within a relatively quick period (compared to the planned length of the trial) to allow for modification of the trial designs (e.g., for treatment selection and population enrichment). Due to this reason, for clinical trials with OS as primary endpoint, surrogate endpoints are usually used for interim decision rules. Poor surrogacy between the endpoints can impact the efficiency and increase error rates of the modification decision.

7.3.4.3 Nature of Event-Driven Trial Due to Censoring

The number of events, rather than the number of sample size is the primary driver of power and analysis timing for an event-driven trial. This property especially complicates design for a two-stage adaptive trial with adaptions to treatment or population following interim analysis. For a two-stage adaptive trial, the statistical validity of making adaptive changes upon comparative interim analysis rests with the independence between data used for interim analysis and the data generated after adaptive change(s). Also, the common utilization of P-value combination methodology requires the complete independence of the P-values of the two stages. For TTE endpoints like OS, some patients who are administratively censored in the interim analysis dataset might have the event by the time of final analysis. Therefore, these patients may contribute to both the stage 1 and stage 2 log-rank test statistic and break the independence. To tackle the issue, Jenkins et al. (2011) proposed the solution of "patient-wising" staging to define test statistics (illustrated in Figure 7.4). In the proposed approach, p-values for comparisons of OS based on log-rank tests are produced separately for those patients recruited to stage 1 and those recruited to stage 2. In particular, the additional follow-up of stage 1 patients during stage 2 contributes to stage 1 p-values. Also, the extent of total follow-up of stage 1 patients for OS final analysis is pre-specified and, hence, not affected by their results of the interim analysis. This approach ensures complete independence of P-values from the two stages, and thus enable combination to produce a statistically valid final analysis.

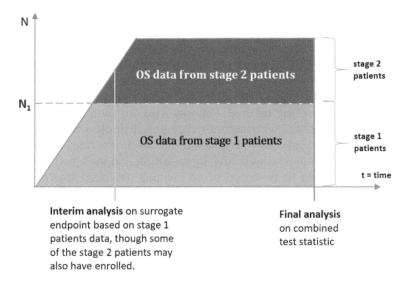

Interim analysis on surrogate
endpoint based on stage 1
patients data, though some
of the stage 2 patients may
also have enrolled.

Final analysis
on combined
test statistic

FIGURE 7.4
"Patient-wising" option for the combination of stage 1 and stage 2 time-to-event data (e.g., OS is the primary endpoint) to protect statistical validity in a two-stage adaptive trial.

7.3.5 Treatment Switching

Treatment switching commonly occurs in drug development, especially for oncology, which allows patients originally randomized to control group switch to administrate experimental treatment at some point during trial follow-up. In oncology, this time point could be disease progression. It is well acknowledged that treatment switching may bring some benefits to trial either from an ethical perspective or a practical perspective. Such as, from an ethical perspective, it is not ethical to keep patients in control arm beyond disease progression if experimental treatment shows promising treatment effects and no other non-palliative treatments available for progressed patients. From a practical perspective, allowing treatment switching can attract patients to join the study as they know they have the potential to receive new treatment, which ultimately boosts enrollment. With so many benefits, is it possible to design all trials with treatment switching allowed? Definitely, the answer is no. If treatment switching was allowed only after disease progression, the assessment and comparison of PFS will not be impacted because the event (death or disease progression) had already been observed before switching to a new therapy. However, in many occasions, PFS alone lacks evidence to support full regulatory approval. OS as the golden standard will always be expected to show promising trends or statistical significance in some cases to support drug approval. In addition, the estimation of OS is a key for reimbursement by Health Technology Assessment (HTA) agencies.

Based on Intend-To-Treat (ITT) population, the true survival benefit of comparing purely experimental treatment versus purely control group will be underestimated if control group patients switch to experimental drugs and benefit from it. The magnitude of survival benefits will be distorted with subsequent use of experimental treatment for switched patients from control arm. To reflect true treatment benefit of survival, we would like to estimate the benefit that would have been observed had treatment switching not been allowed. This request facilitates the methodology research which can adjust survival benefits from switched treatment. Simple methods, including excluding patients who are switched or censoring those patients at the timing of switching, will lead to substantial bias because switching usually is related to patient's prognosis and thus are not recommended. Many complex methods are proposed to handle treatment switching and we will introduce some of the methods in the following.

Inverse Probability of Censoring Weights (IPCW) (Robins and Finkelstein 2000) is an extension of a simple censoring method. Patients who are switched will be censored at the time of switch, and patients who are not switched will apply a weight, in which larger weights will be assigned to patients who have similar baseline factors and time-dependent prognostic factors to patients who switched. By weighing non-switched patients, a pseudo population was established to be based on to estimate adjusted treatment effect. This method relies on the assumption of 'no unmeasured confounders', without which, selection bias and informative censoring can not be avoided. However, this assumption really depends on comprehensive data collection, which is difficult to be guaranteed. When applied to real cases, it is recommended to collect confounders as many as possible and use the confounders to build weights.

Rank Preserving Structural Failure Time Model (RPSFTM) (Robins and Tsiatis 1991) is based on the randomized control structure, so it is reasonable to adjust treatment for a well-designed randomized control study. This method will construct counterfactual survival time as if the patients never take experimental treatment, which is calculated by multiplying acceleration factor with the time patients spend on experimental treatment. For patients in experimental arm and patients in control arm who switched to take experimental treatment, counterfactual survival time can be constructed in above way, and for patients who remain on control arm, counterfactual survival time is actually the observed survival time. Since no treatment difference was expected for treatment arm and control arm in terms of counterfactual survival time, the acceleration factor can be estimated as the one with maximum p-value from the log-rank test comparing counterfactual survival time between treatment group and control group through G-estimation. RPSFT method depends on the assumption of 'common treatment effect', which means the relative treatment effect is equal for all patients no matter when the treatment is received. In oncology, this assumption is challenging, as it is common to see the treatment effect for patients in the front-line treatment setting tends to be larger than for the patients heavily treated.

Two-stage method (Latimer et al. 2017) was designed according to the switching commonly observed in oncology studies, where switch can happen only after disease progression or other disease-related time points. In two-stage method, specific disease-related time point that trigger treatment switching, e.g. disease progression, was required, which is called second baseline. Survival time beyond this second baseline was compared for patients who switched from control arm and for patients who did not switch from control arm by fitting an Accelerated Failure Time (AFT) model. The acceleration factor estimated from AFT model can be used to derive counterfactual survival time for patients who switched. Two-stage method also depends on the assumption of 'no unmeasured confounders' at second baseline. In real practice, a lot of laboratory tests and safety monitor could happen before treatment switching to ensure the patient is tolerable for experimental drug, which will provide as many confounder measurements as possible. When estimating acceleration factor, both baseline factors that could affect post second baseline survival time and were not balanced between switchers and non-switchers are recommended to be included in AFT model.

Besides the above three methods, many other approaches are available to adjust for treatment switching. Latimer et al. (2020) proposed improved two-stage method when there are time-dependent confounders between the time of disease-related event and the time of switching, which could not be handled by simple two-stage method. Luo et al. (2016) proposed an approach that can be used to adjust treatment effect caused by treatment switching from both directions, which means, not only patients from control arm can switch to take treatment therapy, but also patients from treatment arm can take the therapy from control arm. Zhang et al. (2014) proposed a Bayesian gamma frailty model which is more appropriate for the scenario that the patient immediately switch to experimental treatment once he/she experiences an event. As a sum, there are many methods can be reached to handle treatment switching, and each method has its own assumptions and application conditions. Cautious thinking before taking these methods was recommended, as only appropriate method could provide 'true' treatment effect that we are looking for.

7.4 Regulatory Guidance

This section collectively reviewed challenges and corresponding statistical considerations in cancer clinical trials. The regulatory guidance related to each topic are reviewed in corresponding sub-sections. In general, regulatory authorities are in supportive attitude to clinical development innovations, and lots of guidance were released to support drug development with Agency's latest thinking and recommendations during decades. For the hot topics and challenges we mentioned above, including but not limited to adaptive design, enrichment design, master protocol, surrogate endpoint, and Bayesian methods in design, regulatory guidance is a good reference to find the answer. Almost all the guidance will emphasize the importance of early interaction with regulatory authorities. Especially for some complex design, there definitely exist a knowledge gap between regulators and sponsors, therefore, an efficient and comprehensive interaction allow both sides to exchange idea and ultimately facilitate development progress.

7.5 Case Studies

7.5.1 The I-SPY2 Study: An Oncology Platform Trial

I-SPY 2 (investigation of serial studies to predict your therapeutic response with imaging and molecular analysis 2, NCT01042379) is an open-label phase II trial aiming to evaluate the efficacy and safety of experimental drugs combined with standard chemotherapy compared with standard chemotherapy alone for women diagnosed with local metastatic breast cancer before surgical resection. It is by far the longest-running platform trial that has established a new benchmark for early phase study in the area of neoadjuvant setting for women with locally advanced breast cancer. This platform is a collaborative effort among pharmaceutical companies, academic investigators, and health authorities.

Over the past decades, the research of breast cancer has achieved significant progress, especially for patients with disease stage I and II due to the improved adjuvant therapy. However, for locally advanced breast cancer patients, the long-term benefit from adjuvant therapy still remains limited. To further improve survival for locally advanced patients, neoadjuvant therapy that was used prior to surgical resection has become standard of care. Another challenge of breast cancer is patient heterogeneity, where patient could have different molecular characteristics, and drugs designed to target molecular subtypes of cancer may increase the chances of good responses. So, the development of target therapy directing to specific molecular pathways was encouraged for patients with breast cancer. Motivated by the challenges, I-SPY 2 was proposed aiming to bring a new treatment to patients with breast cancer at an earlier, more treatable stage of disease in a rapid, bio-marker-focused and innovative clinical development process.

The overall trial design for I-SPY 2 was provided in Figure 7.5. Generally speaking, I-SPY 2 platform will be used to compare multiple investigational therapies with a common control in subgroups of breast cancer with ten distinct biomarker signatures. The platform was initiated by randomizing patients adaptively to investigational therapies or standard of care on the basis of molecular characteristics. Then Bayesian method will be used to predict the probability of being more effective than standard therapy. If the probability is high, this investigational therapy will graduate from the platform to move for further evaluation in following Phase III studies. Otherwise, investigational therapy will be dropped if a low predictive probability was observed. As platform design, multiple investigational therapies could be under assessment simultaneously, and new investigational drugs were allowed to enter the platform at any time during trial ongoing.

I-SPY 2 integrated several innovative elements. Due to content limit, this section will focus on adaptive randomization, Bayesian decision framework and master protocol, which attract a lot of attention currently in early phase clinical development. To benefit more patients to potential promising investigational therapy, adaptive randomization was used to increase the likelihood of assignment to a given therapy if accrued information from previous patients demonstrates this assignment is more efficacious than control. Unlike

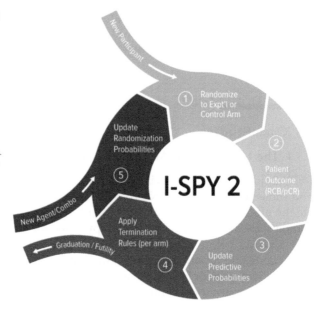

At consent, a new participant's breast cancer is classified into one of 10 molecular subtypes. Then, for each participant in the trial:

1) I-SPY 2's adaptive randomization engine assigns a participant to a study arm; it gives greater weight to arms that have been successful in the participant's tumor subtype.

2) The endpoint is assessed at time of surgery. Primary endpoint is RCB 0 or pathologic complete response meaning the tumor has disappeared completely.

3) Based on the participant's tumor subtype, outcome (i.e. MRI volume, pCR) and treatment received, the predictive probabilities of the agent in the various subtypes are updated in real time.

4) If predictive probabilities for an experimental agent reach a pre-determined level of efficacy in one or more molecular subtypes, it is declared a success ("graduates"). Alternatively, it may be stopped for futility after reaching a maximum number of participants. At any point new agents can enter the trial through a protocol amendment.

5) The participant's serial MRI measures, RCB scores and tumor subtype are used to update the prior probabilities of the randomization engine -- over time this refines the targeting of subsequent participants.

FIGURE 7.5
Trial design of I-SPY2.

traditional randomization methods, the balance of baseline characteristics may be broken in adaptive randomization, so it may trigger more discussion on how to estimate treatment effect without bias. One goal of I-SPY 2 platform is speeding up the process of drug development, accordingly, only the investigational drug that performs well were deserved to be further explored, and the drug lack of preliminary efficacy signal could be terminated earlier to save time and budget. Stem from this idea, Bayesian method was used to establish go/nogo criteria by predicting success probability of each investigational drug dynamically once there is new efficacy data available. Bayesian methods are often well suited to oncology settings in which inference and decisions benefit from adaptation based on accruing information (Harrington and Parmigiani 2016) and health authorities encourage the use of Bayesian method through recent guidance releases. The last, but not the least innovative point is master protocol, which gives plenty of flexibility in clinical development. Because of master protocol, sub-studies were carried out under the same framework by sharing key design components and operational aspects, which further increase the efficiency of drug development compared to several single trials conducted separately.

As presented in I-SPY 2 website, till 2021, up to 22 investigational drugs have been explored in this platform, among which, seven drugs have graduated from this platform and move forward to the next stage of development. Benefit from platform design, up to five agents were able to be evaluated in parallel. On the basis of trial results from I-SPY 2, pivotal Phase III design with registration purpose has been proposed for graduated agents, and active regular's contact with US FDA was planned for an accelerated approval (Park et al. 2016).

7.5.2 The TAPPAS Trial: An Adaptive Phase III Trial

7.5.2.1 Study Background

The TAPPAS trial (ClinicalTrials.gov identifier: NCT02979899) is a Phase III trial of TRC105 (cartuximab) in combination with pazopanib versus pazopanib alone in advanced Angiosarcoma (AS), an ultra-orphan oncology disease and aggressive form of soft tissue sarcoma. The approved standard of care pazopanib for treating AS is of modest benefit with median Progression-Free Survival (PFS) ranging from 3.0 to 6.6 months (Mehta et al. 2019). In a single-arm Phase I/II study of TRC105 in combination with pazopanib in soft tissue sarcoma (ClinicalTrials.gov Identifier: NCT01975519), the combination showed durable complete response and median PFS of 7.8 months in the AS cohort of 22 patients at the time of designing TAPPAS study (Mehta et al. 2019). In addition, further subgroup analysis indicates the benefit in patients with cutaneous lesions appeared to be superior to that of patients with non-cutaneous disease. The promising results from this Phase I/II study encourages further development of the combination regimen, thus the setup of TAPPAS trial. Meanwhile, the limit size of the early phase data brings uncertainty of treatment effect size and concerns for possible differences in treatment effect on the cutaneous and non-cutaneous AS subgroups.

7.5.2.2 Overview of Study Design

In TAPPAS trial, patients will be stratified by AS type (cutaneous vs non-cutaneous) and the number of lines of prior systemic therapy for AS (zero versus one or two) and randomized in a 1:1 ratio to TRC105 in combination with pazopanib (treatment arm) vs pazopanib alone (control arm). A PFS hazard ratio of 0.55, corresponds to an improvement of median PFS from 4 months to 7.27 months, is considered to be clinically relevant. Based on the use of log-rank test at the 2-sided alpha of 0.05 level of significance, 95 PFS events will provide 83% power. Considering the rarity of the disease, 190 patients were planned to be enrolled to complete the trial within three years in the absence of adaption.

Due to the uncertainty of the treatment effect, and possible heterogeneity among the cutaneous and non-cutaneous subgroups, an adaptive two-stage design was employed in TAPPAS trial with allowing for potential sample size re-estimation and population enrichment. The adaptive design called for enrolling the 190 patients into two cohorts, with 120 adult patients in Cohort 1, and 70 adult patients in Cohort 2. In the design schema (Figure 7.6 as blow), cohort 1 will be enrolled first and an interim analysis will be performed after observing 40 events or 30 days after enrolling 120 patients in cohort 1. Based

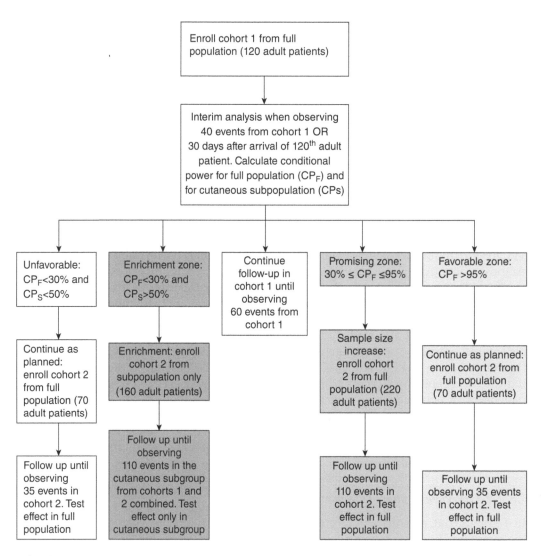

FIGURE 7.6
Schematic representation of adaptive trial design in TAPPAS trial, as originated from figure 7.3 of TAPPAS study protocol (ClinicalTrials.gov identifier: NCT02979899).

on the conditional power for full population (CP_F) and for the cutaneous subgroup (CP_S), the interim analysis results could result in different following decisions:

1. no change to the study design and sample size when data fall in favorable zone or unfavorable zone,
2. no change to the study design but an increase in the sample size when data is in promising zone,
3. or termination of enrollment of the non-cutaneous subtype and adjustment of the sample size of the cutaneous subtype when data is in enrichment zone.

An Independent Data Monitoring Committee (IDMC) was employed to review the interim results and made corresponding recommendation. In addition to the above decisions, the IDMC might also recommend termination of the trial for futility by exercising its judgment based on the totality of the data at interim time if TRC105 arm showed doing worse than the control arm.

7.5.2.3 Statistical Methodology for Preserving Type 1 Error

The statistical validity of making adaptive changes to an ongoing trial based on comparative interim analysis requires keeping the dataset that was utilized for the interim analysis independent of the data that will result from the adaptive change. The TAPPAS trial is an event-driven trial, and in such trials, patients who are censored administratively at interim analysis might subsequently experience a PFS event before final analysis. If one were to avail the treatment assignment sensitive data of these patients, the study level type-1 error could be inflated due to manipulating patients' disposition. Considering the challenges, the TAPPAS trial utilizes the Jenkins, Stone et al. (2011) suggested approach of "patient wise" staging. The approach suggested the split of the patients and PFS events between the two cohorts and suggested pre-specify the timing of the interim analysis and final analysis. The TAPPAS trial first enroll 120 patients to cohort 1 and will be followed until 40 events in the cohort for interim analysis and until 60 PFS events in the cohort for final analysis. Following decision made after interim analysis, 70 (in the absence of adaption) up to 220 patients would be enrolled in cohort 2 and cohort 2 patients will be followed till 35 PFS events (in the absence of adaption) up to 110 PFS events for final analysis. The inverse normal method will be applied to combine the p-values from the two cohorts for the final analysis.

More technical details, including definitions of conditional power, the closed testing approach to control Type-I-error considering multiplicity due to selecting either the full population or the cutaneous subgroup following the interim analysis, and combination of two cohorts data under different scenarios can be found in the supplementary material of Mehta CR et al. 2019.

7.5.2.4 Statistical Simulation on Trial Operating Characteristics

Trial operational characteristics are evaluated by statistical simulation and are summarized in Table 7.3. For the same average total sample size and PFS events, the fixed design has higher "total power" than the adaptive design when the sub-groups have similar hazard ratios (short as HRs), and this is because the adaptive design faces the statistical penalty from closed hypothesis testing procedure. However, the adaptive design has higher

TABLE 7.3

Operating Characteristics of Adaptive and Fixed Sample Designs of TAPPAS Study Based on 10,000 Simulations

HR for Cutanous/ Non-Cutaneous		Zone	Prob of Zone	Power		Average Study Duration (Months)		Average PFS Events		Average Sample Size (Number of Patients)	
				Adaptive Enrichmnt	Fixed Sampl Design	Adaptive Enrichmnt	Fixed Sampl Design	Adaptive Enrichment	Fixed Sample Design	Adaptive Enrichmnt	Fixed Sample Design
0.55	0.55	Enrch	5%	81%		56		140		277	
		Unfav	14%	32%		40		95		190	
		Prom	38%	94%		52		170		339	
		Fav	42%	92%		40		95		190	
		Total	100%	84%	92%	45	40	126	126	252	252
0.55	0.65	Enrch	9%	80%		56		139		275	
		Unfav	19%	24%		39		95		190	
		Prom	40%	89%		50		170		338	
		Fav	32%	88%		39		95		190	
		Total	100%	76%	83%	45	40	129	129	257	257
0.55	0.75	Enrch	14%	81%		57		139		275	
		Unfav	22%	18%		38		95		190	
		Prom	40%	84%		50		170		338	
		Fav	24%	86%		38		95		190	
		Total	100%	70%	71%	45	40	131	131	261	261
0.55	0.85	Enrch	19%	79%		57		138		274	
		Unfav	24%	15%		37		95		190	
		Prom	38%	79%		49		170		336	
		Fav	19%	80%		38		95		190	
		Total	100%	64%	58%	45	40	131	131	261	261
0.55	01.0	Enrch	27%	80%		57		138		272	
		Unfav	29%	10%		37		95		190	
		Prom	33%	76%		49		170		335	
		Fav	12%	75%		36		95		190	
		Total	100%	58%	40%	46	39	131	131	260	260

Source:　Table 1 of Mehta et.al., 2019

power than the fixed design when the HRs become disparate (e.g., HR of 0.55 for cutaneous subgroup and 0.85 for non-cutaneous subgroup), and this is because that the adaptive design allows for learning and sub-sequent improvement in sample size or change in population so that generates higher power when data falls into "promising zone" or "enrichment zone". This is the real benefit of adaptive design. Across all scenarios, the adaptive design has longer trial duration than the fixed design and this is because of the splitting of study into two cohorts and the awaiting time of the data maturity in cohort 2 which is enrolled after the interim analysis.

7.5.2.5 Study Results

In April 2019, the TAPPAS study was terminated following the planned interim analysis for trend of worse efficacy than control arm. Based on 123 patients in cohort 1, the median PFS in TRC105 treatment arm is 4.2 months (95% CI: 2.8–8.3 months) as compared to the median PFS of 4.3 months (95% CI: 2.9 to NA) in the control arm. The results reverse the findings from the Ph1/2 study. The application of adaptive design in TAPPAS study for learning and sub-sequent adaption helps mitigate the potential risks of large investment at trial set-up.

References

Aalen, O. O. and S. Johansen (1978). "An Empirical Transition Matrix for Non-Homogeneous Markov Chains Based on Censored Observations." Scandinavian Journal of Statistics **5**: 141–150.

Aaronson, N. K., et al. (1993). "The European Organization for Research and Treatment of Cancer QLQ-C30: a quality-of-life instrument for use in international clinical trials in oncology." J Natl Cancer Inst **85**(5): 365–376.

Adaptive Platform Trials Coalition (2019). "Adaptive platform trials: definition, design, conduct and reporting considerations." Nat Rev Drug Discov **18**(10): 797–807.

Albertsen, P. C., et al. (1998). "Competing Risk Analysis of Men Aged 55 to 74 Years at Diagnosis Managed Conservatively for Clinically Localized Prostate Cancer." JAMA **280**(11): 975–980.

Alexander, B. M., et al. (2018). "Adaptive Global Innovative Learning Environment for Glioblastoma: GBM AGILE." Clin Cancer Res **24**(4): 737–743.

Alexander, B. M., et al. (2019). "Individualized Screening Trial of Innovative Glioblastoma Therapy (INSIGhT): A Bayesian Adaptive Platform Trial to Develop Precision Medicines for Patients With Glioblastoma." JCO Precis Oncol **3**.

Barker, A. D., et al. (2009). "I-SPY 2: an adaptive breast cancer trial design in the setting of neoadjuvant chemotherapy." Clin Pharmacol Ther **86**(1): 97–100.

Bellera, C. A., et al. (2015). "Guidelines for time-to-event end point definitions in sarcomas and gastrointestinal stromal tumors (GIST) trials: results of the DATECAN initiative (Definition for the Assessment of Time-to-event Endpoints in CANcer trials)†." Annals of Oncology **26**(5): 865–872.

Bellera, C. A., et al. (2013). "Protocol of the Definition for the Assessment of Time-to-event Endpoints in CANcer trials (DATECAN) project: formal consensus method for the development of guidelines for standardised time-to-event endpoints' definitions in cancer clinical trials." Eur J Cancer **49**(4): 769–781.

Berry, S. D., et al. (2010). "Competing risk of death: an important consideration in studies of older adults." J Am Geriatr Soc **58**(4): 783–787.

Berry, S. M., et al. (1999). "Bridging Different Eras in Sports." Journal of the American Statistical Association **94**(447): 661–676.

Bhatt, D. L. and C. Mehta (2016). "Adaptive Designs for Clinical Trials." New England Journal of Medicine **375**(1): 65–74.

Blumenthal, G. M., et al. (2017). "Oncology Drug Approvals: Evaluating Endpoints and Evidence in an Era of Breakthrough Therapies." Oncologist **22**(7): 762–767.

Bonnetain, F., et al. (2014). "Guidelines for Time-to-Event Endpoint Definitions in trials for Pancreatic Cancer. Results of the DATECAN initiative (Definition for the Assessment of Time-to-event End-points in CANcer trials)." European Journal of Cancer **50**(17): 2983–2993.

Branchoux, S., et al. (2019). "Immune-Checkpoint Inhibitors and Candidate Surrogate Endpoints for Overall Survival across Tumor types: A Systematic Literature Review." Crit Rev Oncol Hematol **137**: 35–42.

Buyse, M., et al. (2000). "The Validation of Surrogate Endpoints in Meta-Analyses of Randomized Experiments." Biostatistics **1**(1): 49–67.

Cella, D. F., et al. (1993). "The Functional Assessment of Cancer Therapy scale: development and validation of the general measure." J Clin Oncol **11**(3): 570–579.

Centers for Disease Control and Prevention (CDC), et al. (2020). "Annual Report to the Nation on the Status of Cancer."

Chen, T.-T. (2013). "Statistical Issues and Challenges in Immuno-Oncology." Journal for Immuno-Therapy of Cancer **1**(1): 18.

Cheson, B. D., et al. (2016). "Refinement of the Lugano Classification lymphoma response criteria in the era of immunomodulatory therapy." Blood **128**(21): 2489–2496.

Cheson, B. D., et al. (2014). "Recommendations for Initial Evaluation, Staging, and Response Assessment of Hodgkin and Non-Hodgkin Lymphoma: The Lugano Classification." Journal of Clinical Oncology **32**(27): 3059–3067.

Choueiri, T. K., et al. (2015). "Cabozantinib versus Everolimus in Advanced Renal-Cell Carcinoma." New England Journal of Medicine **373**(19): 1814–1823.

Daniels, M. J. and M. D. Hughes (1997). "Meta-analysis for the evaluation of potential surrogate markers." Statistics in Medicine **16**(17): 1965–1982.

de Glas, N. A., et al. (2016). "Performing Survival Analyses in the Presence of Competing Risks: A Clinical Example in Older Breast Cancer Patients." J Natl Cancer Inst **108**(5).

De Gruttola, V. G., et al. (2001). "Considerations in the Evaluation of Surrogate Endpoints in Clinical Trials: Summary of a National Institutes of Health Workshop." Controlled Clinical Trials **22**(5): 485–502.

Degtyarev, E., et al. (2019). "Estimands and the Patient Journey: Addressing the Right Question in Oncology Clinical Trials." JCO Precision Oncology: 1–10.

Duke and FDA (2018). "Public workshop: Oncology clinical trials in the presence of non-proportional hazards."

Eisenhauer, E. A., et al. (2009). "New Response Evaluation Criteria in Solid Tumors: Revised RECIST Guideline (version 1.1)." Eur J Cancer **45**(2): 228–247.

European Medicines Agency (EMA) (2014). "The role of the Pathological Complete Response as an Endpoint in Neoadjuvant Breast Cancer Studies." Committee for Medicinal Products for Human Use (CHMP), London, United Kingdom.

European Medicines Agency (EMA) (2018). "Guideline on the use of minimal residual disease as a clinical endpoint in multiple myeloma studies." Committee for Medicinal Products for Human Use (CHMP), London, United Kingdom.

Ferris, R. L., et al. (2016). "Nivolumab for Recurrent Squamous-Cell Carcinoma of the Head and Neck." N Engl J Med **375**(19): 1856–1867.

Fine, G. D. (2007). "Consequences of Delayed Treatment Effects on Analysis of Time-to-Event Endpoints." Drug Information Journal **41**(4): 535–539.

Fine, J. P. and R. J. Gray (1999). "A Proportional Hazards Model for the Subdistribution of a Competing Risk." Journal of the American Statistical Association **94**(446): 496–509.

Fleming, T. and D. Harrington (1991). Counting Processes and Survival Analysis.

Fleming, T. R. and J. H. Powers (2012). "Biomarkers and Surrogate Endpoints in Clinical Trials." Stat Med **31**(25): 2973–2984.

Ford, R., et al. (2009). "Lessons Learned from Independent Central Review." European Journal of Cancer **45**(2): 268–274.

Gail, M. H., et al. (2000). "On Meta-analytic Assessment of Surrogate Outcomes." Biostatistics **1**(3): 231–246.

Ghadessi, M., et al. (2020). "A Roadmap to using Historical Controls in Clinical Trials – by Drug Information Association Adaptive Design Scientific Working Group (DIA-ADSWG)." Orphanet Journal of Rare Diseases **15**(1): 69.

Gourgou-Bourgade, S., et al. (2015). "Guidelines for Time-to-event Endpoint Definitions in Breast Cancer Trials: Results of the DATECAN Initiative (Definition for the Assessment of Time-to-event Endpoints in CANcer trials)†." Ann Oncol **26**(5): 873–879.

Harrington, D. and G. Parmigiani (2016). "I-SPY 2 — A Glimpse of the Future of Phase 2 Drug Development?" New England Journal of Medicine **375**(1): 7–9.

Hobbs, B. P., et al. (2011). "Hierarchical Commensurate and Power Prior Models for Adaptive Incorporation of Historical Information in Clinical Trials." Biometrics **67**(3): 1047–1056.

Hoering, A., et al. (2017). "Endpoints and Statistical Considerations in Immuno-Oncology Trials: Impact on Multiple Myeloma." Future Oncol **13**(13): 1181–1193.

Hoering, A., et al. (2011). "Seamless Phase I-II Trial Design for Assessing Toxicity and Efficacy for Targeted Agents." Clin Cancer Res **17**(4): 640–646.

Hoering, A., et al. (2013). "Early Phase Trial Design for Assessing Several Dose Levels for Toxicity and Efficacy for Targeted Agents." Clinical Trials **10**(3): 422–429.

Hunsberger, S., et al. (2005). "Dose Escalation Trial Designs based on a Molecularly Targeted Endpoint." Stat Med **24**(14): 2171–2181.

Ibrahim, J. and M.-H. Chen (2000). "Power Prior Distributions for Regression Models." Statistical Science **15**.

Iqvia (2019). "Global Oncology Trends 2019."

Jenkins, M., et al. (2011). "An Adaptive Seamless Phase II/III Design for Oncology Trials with Subpopulation Selection using Correlated Survival Endpoints." Pharm Stat **10**(4): 347–356.

Jenkins, M., et al. (2011). "An Adaptive Seamless Phase II/III Design for Oncology Trials with Subpopulation Selection using Correlated Survival Endpoints†." Pharmaceutical Statistics **10**(4): 347–356.

Jiang, L., et al. (2020). "Optimal Bayesian Hierarchical Model to Accelerate the Development of Tissue-Agnostic Drugs and Basket Trials." arXiv:2012.0237.

Karrison, T. (1987). "Restricted Mean Life with Adjustment for Covariates." Journal of the American Statistical Association **82**(400): 1169–1176.

Karrison, T. G. (2016). "Versatile Tests for Comparing Survival Curves Based on Weighted Log-rank Statistics." The Stata Journal **16**(3): 678–690.

Kemp, R. and V. Prasad (2017). "Surrogate Endpoints in Oncology: When are they Acceptable for Regulatory and Clinical Decisions, and are they Currently Overused?" BMC Med **15**(1): 134.

Koller, M. T., et al. (2012). "Competing Risks and the Clinical Community: Irrelevance or Ignorance?" Stat Med **31**(11–12): 1089–1097.

Korn, E. L. and B. Freidlin (2018). "Interim Futility Monitoring Assessing Immune Therapies With a Potentially Delayed Treatment Effect." J Clin Oncol **36**(23): 2444–2449.

Lachin, J. M. and M. A. Foulkes (1986). "Evaluation of Sample Size and Power for Analyses of Survival with Allowance for Nonuniform Patient Entry, Losses to Follow-up, Noncompliance, and Stratification." Biometrics **42**(3): 507–519.

Lakatos, E. (1988). "Sample Sizes Based on the Log-rank Statistic in Complex Clinical Trials." Biometrics **44**(1): 229–241.

Latimer, N. R., et al. (2017). "Adjusting for Treatment Switching in Randomised Controlled Trials - A Simulation Study and a Simplified Two-Stage Method." Stat Methods Med Res **26**(2): 724–751.

Latimer, N. R., et al. (2020). "Improved Two-stage Estimation to adjust for Treatment Switching in Randomised Trials: G-estimation to Address time-Dependent Confounding." Stat Methods Med Res **29**(10): 2900–2918.

Lee, S.-H. (2007). "On the Versatility of the Combination of the Weighted Log-rank Statistics." Computational Statistics & Data Analysis 51(12): 6557–6564.

Li, J., et al. (2019). "Reply to Z. McCaw and L-J. Wei." J Clin Oncol 37(12): 1034.

Lin, R. S., et al. (2020). "Alternative Analysis Methods for Time to Event Endpoints Under Nonproportional Hazards: A Comparative Analysis." Statistics in Biopharmaceutical Research 12(2): 187–198.

Lipscomb, J., et al. (2007). "Patient-Reported Outcomes Assessment in Cancer Trials: Taking Stock, Moving Forward." J Clin Oncol 25(32): 5133–5140.

Luo, X., et al. (2016). "A Proposed Approach for Analyzing Post-Study Therapy Effect in Survival Analysis." Journal of Biopharmaceutical Statistics 26(4): 790–800.

Mehta, C. R., et al. (2019). "An Adaptive Population Enrichment Phase III trial of TRC105 and Ppazopanib versus Pazopanib alone in Patients with Advanced Angiosarcoma (TAPPAS trial)." Ann Oncol 30(1): 103–108.

Miller, K., et al. (2007). "Paclitaxel plus Bevacizumab versus Paclitaxel Alone for Metastatic Breast Cancer." New England Journal of Medicine 357(26): 2666–2676.

Mok, T. S., et al. (2009). "Gefitinib or Carboplatin–Paclitaxel in Pulmonary Adenocarcinoma." New England Journal of Medicine 361(10): 947–957.

Mok, T. S. K., et al. (2019). "Pembrolizumab versus Chemotherapy for Previously Untreated, PD-L1-expressing, Locally Advanced or Metastatic Non-small-cell Lung Cancer (KEYNOTE-042): A Randomised, Open-label, Controlled, Phase 3 Trial." The Lancet 393(10183): 1819–1830.

National Medical Products Administration (NMPA) (2020). "Techinical Guidance for Imaging Endpoint Process Standards for Oncology Clinical Trials."

National Medical Products Administration (NMPA) (2021). "Guidelines for adaptive design of drug clinical trials."

Neuenschwander, B., et al. (2008). "Critical Aspects of the Bayesian Approach to Phase I Cancer Trials." Statistics in Medicine 27(13): 2420–2439.

Neuenschwander, B., et al. (2010). "Summarizing Historical Information on Controls in Clinical Trials." Clinical Trials 7(1): 5–18.

O'Quigley, J., et al. (1990). "Continual Reassessment Method: A Practical Design for Phase 1 Clinical Trials in Cancer." Biometrics 46(1): 33–48.

Overcash, J., et al. (2001). "Validity and Reliability of the FACT-G Scale for Use in the Older Person With Cancer." American Journal of Clinical Oncology 24(6): 591–596.

Panageas, K. S., et al. (2007). "When you look Matters: The Effect of Assessment Schedule on Progression-free Survival." J Natl Cancer Inst 99(6): 428–432.

Park, J. W., et al. (2016). "Adaptive Randomization of Neratinib in Early Breast Cancer." N Engl J Med 375(1): 11–22.

Patrick, D. L., et al. (2011). "Content Validity–establishing and Reporting the Evidence in Newly Developed Patient-Reported Outcomes (PRO) Instruments for Medical Product Evaluation: ISPOR PRO Good Research Practices Task Force Report: Part 1–Eliciting Concepts for a new PRO Instrument." Value Health 14(8): 967–977.

Pocock, S. J. (1977). "Group Sequential Methods in the Design and Analysis of Clinical Trials." Biometrika 64(2): 191–199.

Prentice, R. L. (1989). "Surrogate Endpoints in Clinical Trials: Definition and Operational Criteria." Stat Med 8(4): 431–440.

Putter, H., et al. (2007). "Tutorial in Biostatistics: Competing Risks and Multi-state Models." Stat Med 26(11): 2389–2430.

Ranganathan, P. and C. S. Pramesh (2012). "Censoring in Survival Analysis: Potential for Bias." Perspect Clin Res 3(1): 40.

Robins, J. M. and D. M. Finkelstein (2000). "Correcting for Noncompliance and Dependent Censoring in an AIDS Clinical Trial with Inverse Probability of Censoring Weighted (IPCW) Log-rank Tests." Biometrics 56(3): 779–788.

Robins, J. M. and A. A. Tsiatis (1991). "Correcting for Non-compliance in Randomized Trials using Rank Preserving Structural Failure Time Models." Communications in Statistics - Theory and Methods 20(8): 2609–2631.

Roychoudhury, S., et al. (2019). "Robust Design and Analysis of Clinical Trials With Non-proportional Hazards: A Straw Man Guidance from a Cross-pharma Working Group." arXiv: Applications.

Royston, P. and M. K. Parmar (2011). "The Use of Restricted Mean Survival Time to Estimate the Treatment Effect in Randomized Clinical Trials when the Proportional Hazards Assumption is in Doubt." Stat Med **30**(19): 2409–2421.

Rufibach, K. (2019). "Treatment Effect Quantification for Time-to-event Endpoints–Estimands, Analysis Strategies, and Beyond." Pharmaceutical Statistics **18**(2): 145–165.

Schmidli, H., et al. (2014). "Robust Meta-analytic-predictive priors in Clinical Trials with Historical Control Information." Biometrics **70**(4): 1023–1032.

Seymour, L., et al. (2017). "iRECIST: Guidelines for Response Criteria for use in Trials Testing Immunotherapeutics." The Lancet Oncology **18**(3): e143–e152.

Shen, W., et al. (2015). "Cancer-specific Mortality and Competing Mortality in Patients with Head and Neck Squamous Cell Carcinoma: A Competing Risk Analysis." Ann Surg Oncol **22**(1): 264–271.

Storer, B. E. (1989). "Design and Analysis of Phase I clinical trials." Biometrics **45** 3: 925–937.

Templeton, A. J., et al. (2020). "Informative Censoring - A Neglected Cause of Bias in Oncology Trials." Nat Rev Clin Oncol **17**(6): 327–328.

Thall, P. F., et al. (2003). "Hierarchical Bayesian Approaches to Phase II trials in Diseases with Multiple Subtypes." Stat Med **22**(5): 763–780.

Therasse, P., et al. (2000). "New Guidelines to Evaluate the Response to Treatment in Solid Tumors." JNCI: Journal of the National Cancer Institute **92**(3): 205–216.

Tian, L., et al. (2018). "Efficiency of Two Sample Tests via the Restricted Mean Survival Time for Analyzing Event Time Observations." Biometrics **74**(2): 694–702.

Turnbull, B. W. (1976). "The Empirical Distribution Function with Arbitrarily Grouped, Censored and Truncated Data." Journal of the Royal Statistical Society: Series B (Methodological) **38**(3): 290–295.

Turner, R. R., et al. (2007). "Patient-reported Outcomes: Instrument Development and Selection Issues." Value Health **10 Suppl 2**: S86–93.

Uno, H., et al. (2014). "Moving Beyond the Hazard Ratio in Quantifying the Between-group Difference in Survival Analysis." J Clin Oncol **32**(22): 2380–2385.

US Food and Drug Administration (FDA) (2014). "Guidance for Industry - Pathological Complete Response in Neoadjuvant Treatment of High-Risk Early-Stage Breast Cancer: Use as an Endpoint to Support Accelerated Approval." Center for Drug Evaluation and Research (CDER).

US Food and Drug Administration (FDA) (2015a). "Clinical Trial Endpoints for the Approval of NonSmall Cell Lung Cancer Drugs and Biologics." Center for Drug Evaluation and Research (CDER).

US Food and Drug Administration (FDA) (2015b). "Guidance for Industry - Clinical Trial Endpoints for the Approval of Non-Small Cell Lung Cancer Drugs and Biologics." Center for Drug Evaluation and Research (CDER).

US Food and Drug Administration (FDA) (2018). "Adaptive Designs for Clinical Trials of Drugs and Biologics Guidance for Industry." Center for Drug Evaluation and Research (CDER).

US Food and Drug Administration (FDA) (2018). "Master Protocols: Efficient Clinical Trial Design Strategies to Expedite Development of Oncology Drugs and Biologics Guidance for Industry." Center for Drug Evaluation and Research (CDER).

US Food and Drug Administration (FDA) (2018a). "Surrogate Endpoint Resources for Drug and Biologic Development." Center for Drug Evaluation and Research (CDER).

US Food and Drug Administration (FDA) (2018b). "Guidance for Industry - Clinical Trial Endpoints for the Approval of Cancer Drugs and Biologics." Center for Drug Evaluation and Research (CDER).

US Food and Drug Administration (FDA) (2018c). "Guidance for Industry - Nonmetastatic, Castration-Resistant Prostate Cancer: Considerations for Metastasis-Free Survival Endpoint in Clinical Trials." Center for Drug Evaluation and Research (CDER).

US Food and Drug Administration (FDA) (2018d). "Clinical Trial Endpoints for the Approval of Cancer Drugs and Biologics Guidance for Industry." Center for Drug Evaluation and Research (CDER).

US Food and Drug Administration (FDA) (2018f). "Clinical Trial Imaging Endpoint Process Standards Guidance for Industry." Center for Drug Evaluation and Research (CDER).

US Food and Drug Administration (FDA) (2019). "Enrichment Strategies for Clinical Trials to Support Determination of Effectiveness of Human Drugs and Biological Products Guidance for Industry." Center for Drug Evaluation and Research (CDER).

US Food and Drug Administration (FDA) (2019a). "Guidance for Industry - Demonstrating Substantial Evidence of Effectiveness for Human Drug and Biological Products Guidance for Industry." Center for Drug Evaluation and Research (CDER).

US Food and Drug Administration (FDA) (2019b). "Guidance for Industry - Advanced Prostate Cancer: Developing Gonadotropin Releasing Hormone Analogues." Center for Drug Evaluation and Research (CDER).

US Food and Drug Administration (FDA) (2020a). "Table of Surrogate Endpoints That Were the Basis of Drug Approval or Licensure." Center for Drug Evaluation and Research (CDER).

US Food and Drug Administration (FDA) (2020b). "Guidance for Industry - Pathological Complete Response in Neoadjuvant Treatment of High-Risk Early-Stage Breast Cancer: Use as an Endpoint to Support Accelerated Approval." Center for Drug Evaluation and Research (CDER).

Wages, N. A. and C. Tait (2015). "Seamless Phase I/II Adaptive Design for Oncology Trials of Molecularly Targeted Agents." J Biopharm Stat 25(5): 903–920.

Wang, L., et al. (2019). "A Simulation-free Group Sequential Design with Max-combo Tests in the Presence of Non-proportional Hazards." arXiv: Methodology.

Weir, C. J. and R. J. Walley (2006). "Statistical Evaluation of Biomarkers as Surrogate Endpoints: A Literature Review." Stat Med 25(2): 183–203.

Wilson, M. K., et al. (2015). "Outcomes and Endpoints in Trials of Cancer Treatment: The Past, Present, and Future." The Lancet Oncology 16(1): e32–e42.

Xu, J. and G. Yin (2013). "Two-stage Adaptive Randomization for Delayed Response in Clinical Trials." Journal of the Royal Statistical Society: Series C (Applied Statistics) 63.

Yang, S. and R. Prentice (2010). "Improved Logrank-Type Tests for Survival Data Using Adaptive Weights." Biometrics 66(1): 30–38.

Zang, Y. and J. J. Lee (2014). "Adaptive Clinical Trial Designs in Oncology." Chin Clin Oncol 3(4).

Zhang, W., et al. (2006). "An Adaptive Dose-finding Design Incorporating Both Toxicity and Efficacy." Stat Med 25(14): 2365–2383.

Zhang, Y., et al. (2014). "Bayesian Gamma Frailty Models for Survival Data with Semi-Competing Risks and Treatment Switching." Lifetime Data Anal 20(1): 76–105.

8

Statistical Methods for Assessment of Biosimilars

Yafei Zhang[1], Vivian Gu[1], Xiuyu Julie Cong[2], and Shein-Chung Chow[3]

[1]PPC China, Shanghai, China

[2]Everest Medicines, Shanghai, China

[3]Duke University School of Medicine, Durham, NC, USA

CONTENTS

DOI: 10.1201/9781003107323-8

8.1 Introduction

Biosimilars are Similar Biological Drug Products (SBDP), which are the *generic versions* of biological products. The SBDP are *not* generic drug products, which are drug products with *identical* active ingredient(s) as the innovative drug product. Thus, the concept for development of SBDP, which are made of living cells, is very different from that of the generic drug products for small molecule drug products. The SBDP is usually referred to as biosimilars by European Medicines Agency (EMA) of European Union (EU), Follow-on Biologics (FOB) by the United States FDA, and Subsequent Entered Biologics (SEB) by the Public Health Agency (PHA) of Canada. In 2009, the United States Congress passed the BPCI Act (as part of the *Affordable Care* Act), which has given FDA the authority to approve biosimilar drug products. The up-to-date regulatory guidance is listed in table 8.1.

8.1.1 Definition and Basic Principles

As indicated in the BPCI Act, a biosimilar product is defined as a product that is *highly similar* to the reference product notwithstanding minor differences in clinically inactive components and there are no clinically meaningful differences in terms of safety, purity and potency. Based on this definition, we would interpret that a biological medicine is biosimilar to a reference biological medicine if it is highly similar to the reference in *safety*, *purity* and *potency*, where purity may be related to some important *quality* attributes at critical stages of a manufacturing process and potency has something to do with the *stability* and *efficacy* of the biosimilar product. However, little or no discussion regarding how similar is considered highly similar in the BPCI Act.

The BPCI Act seems to suggest that a biosimilar product should be highly similar to the reference drug product in all spectrums of good drug characteristics such as identity, strength (potency), quality, purity, safety and stability as described in the US Pharmacopeia and National Formulary (see, e.g., USP/NF, 2000). In practice, however, it is almost impossible to demonstrate that a biosimilar product is highly similar to the reference product in all aspects of good drug characteristics in a *single* study. Thus, to ensure a biosimilar product is highly similar to the reference product in terms of these good drug characteristics, different biosimilar studies may be required. For example, if safety and efficacy is a concern, then a clinical trial must be conducted to demonstrate that there are no clinically meaningful differences in terms of safety and efficacy between a biosimilar product and the innovator biological product. On the other hand, to ensure highly similar in important quality attributes at critical stages of a manufacturing process, assay development/validation, process control/validation, and product specification of the reference product is necessarily established. In addition, comparability studies need to be conducted for testing comparability in manufacturing process (raw materials, in-use materials, and end-product) between biosimilars and the reference product. This is extremely important because biosimilar products are known to be sensitive to a small change or variation in environmental factors such as light and temperature during the manufacturing process. In some cases, if a surrogate endpoint such as PK, PD, or genomic marker is predictive of the primary efficacy/safety clinical endpoint, then a PK/PD or genomic study may be used to assess biosimilarity between biosimilar and the reference product.

8.1.2 Regulatory Requirement

8.1.2.1 World Health Organization (WHO)

As an increasingly wide range of Similar Biotherapeutic Products (SBPs) are under development or are already licensed in many countries, WHO formally recognized the need for the guidance for their evaluation and overall regulation in 2007. "Guidelines on Evaluation of SBPs" was developed and adopted by the 60th meeting of the WHO Expert Committee on Biological Standardization in 2009. The intention of the guidelines is to provide globally acceptable principles for licensing biotherapeutic products that are claimed to be similar to the reference products that have been licensed based on a full licensing dossier (WHO, 2009). The scope of the guidelines includes well-established and well-characterized biotherapeutic products that have been marketed for a suitable period of time with a proven quality, efficacy and safety, such as recombinant DNA-derived therapeutic proteins.

8.1.2.2 European Union (EU)

The European Union (EU) has pioneered in developing a regulatory system for biosimilar products. The European Medicines Agency (EMA) began formal consideration of scientific issues presented by biosimilar products at least as early as January 2001, when an ad hoc working group discussed the comparability of medicinal products containing biotechnology-derived proteins as active substances. In 2003, the European Commission amended the provisions of EU secondary legislation governing requirements for marketing authorization applications for medicinal products to establish a new category of applications for "similar biological medicinal products" (EMA, 2003). In 2005, the EMA issued a general guideline on similar biological medicinal products, in order to introduce the concept of similar biological medicinal products, to outline the basic principles to be applied and to provide applicants with a 'user guide', showing where to find relevant scientific information (EMA, 2005a–f, 2006, 2009, 2010, 2011). Since then, 13 biosimilar products have been approved by EMA under the pathway. Two of them are somatropins, five are epoetins, and six are filgrastims.

8.1.2.3 US Food and Drug Administration

On 23 March 23 2010, the BPCI *Act* (as part of the Affordable Care Act) was written into law, which has given the FDA the authority to approve similar biological drug products. Following the passage of the BPCI Act, in order to obtain input on specific issues and challenges associated with the implementation of the BPCI Act, the US FDA conducted a two-day public hearing on *Approval Pathway for Biosimilar and Interchangeability Biological Products* held on 2–3 November 2010 at the FDA in Silver Spring, Maryland, USA. Several scientific factors were raised and discussed at the public hearing. These scientific factors include criteria for assessing biosimilarity, study design and analysis methods for assessment of biosimilarity, and tests for comparability in quality attributes of manufacturing process and/or immunogenicity (see, e.g., Chow and Liu, 2010). These issues primarily focus on the assessment of biosimilarity. The issue of interchangeability in terms of the concepts of alternating and switching was also mentioned and discussed. The discussions of these scientific factors have led to the development of regulatory guidance. On 9 February 2012, the US FDA circulated three draft guidance on the demonstration of biosimilarity for comments. These three draft guidance include (i) *Scientific Considerations in Demonstrating Biosimilarity to a Reference Product*, (ii) *Quality Considerations in Demonstrating Biosimilarity to a Reference Protein Product*, (iii) *Biosimilars: Questions and Answers Regarding Implementation of the BPCI Act of 2009* (FDA, 2012a–c). Subsequently, another FDA Public Hearing on the discussion of these draft guidance was held at the FDA on 11 May 2012. These three guidance were finalized in 2015.

As indicated in the guidance on scientific consideration, FDA recommends a stepwise approach for obtaining the totality-of-the-evidence for demonstrating biosimilarity between a proposed biosimilar (test) product and an innovative biological (reference) product. The stepwise approach starts with analytical studies for structural and functional characterization of critical quality attributes and followed by the assessment of PK/PD similarity and the demonstration of clinical similarity including immunogenicity and safety/efficacy evaluation. For analytical similarity assessment, the FDA recommended equivalence test for Critical Quality Attributes (CQAs) that are relevant to clinical outcomes with high criticality or risk ranking (FDA, 2017). When performing the equivalence test, FDA recommended an Equivalence Acceptance Criterion (EAC), i.e., a similarity margin of $1.5\sigma_R$ be used for demonstrating that the test product is highly similar to the reference product. Although this equivalence test is considered the most rigorous test, it has been criticized for being not efficient and not flexible (Shutter, 2017; Lee etc., 2019). For PK/PD similarity, two products are said to be highly similar if the 90% confidence interval of Geometric Mean Ratio (GMR) of PK responses such as AUC (area under the blood or plasma concentration-time curve) or C_{max} (peak concentration) falls entirely within biosimilarity limits of 0.80 to 1.25.

Similar to requirements of the WHO and EMA, a number of factors are considered important by the FDA when assessing applications for biosimilars, including the robustness of the manufacturing process, the demonstrated structural similarity, the extent to which mechanism of action was understood, the existence of valid, mechanistically related pharmacodynamics assays, comparative pharmacokinetics and immunogenicity, and the amount of clinical data and experience available with the original products. FDA is now seeking public comment on the guidance within 60 days of the notice of publication in the

Federal Register. Even though the guidance does not provide clear standards for assessing biosimilar products, they are the first step towards removing the uncertainties surrounding the biosimilar approval pathway in the United States.

8.1.2.4 Canada (Health Canada)

Health Canada, the federal regulatory authority that evaluates the safety, efficacy, and quality of drugs available in Canada also recognize that with the expiration of patents for biologic drugs, manufacturers may be interested in pursuing subsequent entry versions of these biologic drugs, which is called Subsequent Entry Biologics (SEB) in Canada. In 2010, Health Canada issued the "Guidance for Sponsors: Information and Submission Requirements for SEBs" (HC,2010), whose objective is to provide guidance on how to satisfy the data and regulatory requirements under the Food and Drugs Act and Regulations for the authorization of SEBs in Canada.

The concept of an SEB applies to all biologic drug products, however, there are additional criteria to determine whether the product will be eligible to be authorized as SEBs: (i) a suitable reference biologic drug exists that was originally authorized based on a complete data package, and has significant safety and efficacy data accumulated; (ii) the product can be well characterized by state-of-the-art analytical methods; (iii) the SEB can be judged similar to the reference biologic drug by meeting an appropriate set of pre-determined criteria. With regard to the similarity of products, Health Canada requires the manufacturer to evaluate the following factors: (i) relevant physicochemical and biological characterization data; (ii) analysis of the relevant samples from the appropriate stages of the manufacturing process; (iii) stability data and impurities data; (iv) data obtained from multiple batches of the SEB and reference to understand the ranges in variability; (v) non-clinical and clinical data and safety studies. In addition, Health Canada also has stringent postmarket requirements including the adverse drug reaction report, periodic safety update reports, suspension or revocation of NOC (notice of compliance). The guidance of Canada shares similar concepts and principles as indicated in the WHO's guidelines, since it is clearly mentioned in the guidance that Health Canada has the intention to harmonize as much as possible with other competent regulators and international organizations.

8.1.2.5 Asian Pacific Region (Japan and Korea)

Japanese Ministry of Health, Labor and Welfare (MHLW) have also been confronted with the new challenge of regulating biosimilar/follow-on biologic products (MHLW, 2009). Based on the similarity concept outlined by the EMA, Japan has published a guideline for quality, safety and efficacy of biosimilar products in 2009. The scope of the guideline includes recombinant plasma proteins, recombinant vaccines, PEGylated recombinant proteins and non-recombinant proteins that are highly purified and characterized. Unlike EU, polyglucans such as low-molecular weight heparin has been excluded from the guideline. Another class of product excluded is synthetic peptides, since the desired synthetic peptides can be easily defined by structural analyses and can be defined as generic drugs. Same as the requirements by the EU, the original biologic should be already approved in Japan. However, there are some differences in the requirements of stability test and toxicology studies for impurities in biosimilar between EU and Japan. A comparison of the stability of a biosimilar with the reference innovator products as a strategy for the development of biosimilar is not always necessary in Japan. In addition, it is not required to evaluate the safety of impurities in the biosimilar product through non-clinical studies without comparison to the original product. According to this guideline, two follow-on biologics, "Somatropin" and "Epoetin alfa BS" have been recently approved in Japan.

In Korea, *Pharmaceutical Affairs Act* is the high-level regulation to license all medicines including biologic products. The South Korea's Ministry of Food and Drug Safety (MFDS) notifications serve as a lower-level regulation. Biological products and biosimilars are subject to the "Notification of the regulation on review and authorization of biological products". The MFDS takes an active participation in promoting a public dialogue on the biosimilar issues. In 2008 and 2009, the MFDS held two public meetings and co-sponsored a workshop to gather input on scientific and technical issues. The regulatory framework of biosimilar products in Korea is a three-tiered system: (i) Pharmaceutical Affairs Act; (ii) notification of the regulation on review and authorization of biological products; (iii) guideline on evaluation of biosimilar products (KFDA, 2009; Suh and Park, 2011). As Korean guideline for biosimilar products was developed along with that of the WHO's (WHO,2009), most of the requirements are similar except for that of the clinical evaluation to demonstrate similarity. The MFDS requires that equivalent rather than non-inferior efficacy should be shown in order to open the possibility of extrapolation of efficacy data to other indications of the reference product. Equivalence margins need to be pre-defined and justified, and should be established within the range which is judged not to be clinically different from reference products in clinical regards.

8.1.2.6 Global Harmonization

According to the regulatory requirements of different regions described in the previous section, there seems to be no significant difference in the general concept and basic principles in these guidelines. There are five well recognized principles with regard to the assessment of biosimilar products: (i) generic approach is not appropriate for biosimilars; (ii) biosimilar products should be similar to the reference in terms of quality, safety, efficacy; (iii) a step-wise comparability approach is required that indicates the similarity of

TABLE 8.1

List of Up-to-Date Regulatory Guidance

Year (Version)	Title of the Guidance
2014 (Draft)	Reference Product Exclusivity for Biological Products filed Section 351(a) of the PHS Act
2015 (Draft)	Biosimlars: Additional Questions and Answers Regarding Implementation of the Biologics Price Competition and Innovation Act of 2009
2015 (Final)	Scientific Considerations in Demonstrating Biosimilarity to a Reference Product
2015 (Final)	Quality Considerations in Demonstrating Biosimilarity to a Reference Product
2015 (Final)	Biosimilars: Questions and Answers Regarding Implementation of the Biologics Price Competition and Innovation Act of 2009
2015 (Final)	Formal Meetings between the FDA and Biosimilar Biological Product Sponsors or Applicants
2016 (Draft)	Labeling for Biosimilar Products
2016 (Final)	Clinical Pharmacology Data to Support a Demonstration of Biosimilarity to a Reference Product
2017 (Draft)	Considerations in Demonstrating Interchangeability With a Reference Product
2017 (Final)	Nonproprietary Naming of Biological Products
2017 (Draft)	Statistical Approaches to Evaluate Analytical Similarity

the SBP to RBP in terms of quality is a prerequisite for reduction of non-clinical and clinical data submitted; (iv) the assessment of biosimilar is based on a case-by-case approach for different classes of products; (v) the importance of pharmacovigilance is stressed.

However, differences have been noted in the scope of the guidelines, the choice of the reference product, and the data required for product approval. The concept of a "similar biological medicinal product" in the EU is applicable to a broad spectrum of products ranging from biotechnology-derived therapeutic proteins to vaccines, blood-derived products, monoclonal antibodies, gene and cell-therapy, etc. However, the scopes of other organizations or countries are limited to recombinant protein drug products. Concerning the choice of the reference product, the EU and Japan require that the reference product should be previously licensed in their own jurisdiction, while other countries do not have this requirement. More details can be found in Wang and Chow (2012).

8.1.3 Current Issues

8.1.3.1 Interchangeability

As indicated in the Subsection (b)(3) amended to the Public Health Act Subsection 351(k)(3), the term *interchangeable* or *interchangeability* in reference to a biological product that is shown to meet the standards described in subsection (k)(4), means that the biological product may be substituted for the reference product without the intervention of the health care provider who prescribed the reference product. Along this line, in what follows, definition and basic concepts of interchangeability (in terms of switching and alternating) are given. The Subsection (a)(2) amends the Public Health Act Subsection 351(k)(3) states that a biological product is considered to be interchangeable with the reference product if (i) the biological product is biosimilar to the reference product; and (ii) it can be expected to produce the same clinical result in *any given patient*. In addition, for a biological product that is administered more than once to an individual, the risk in terms of safety or diminished efficacy of alternating or switching between the use of the biological product and the reference product is not greater than the risk of using the reference product without such alternation or switch.

Thus, there is a clear distinction between biosimilarity and interchangeability. In other words, biosimilarity does not imply interchangeability which is much more stringent. Intuitively, if a test product is judged to be interchangeable with the reference product, then it may be substituted, even alternated, without a possible intervention, or even notification, of the health care provider. However, the interchangeability is expected to produce the *same* clinical result in *any given patient*, which can be interpreted as that the same clinical result can be expected in *every single patient*. In reality, conceivably, lawsuits may be filed if adverse effects are recorded in a patient after switching from one product to another.

It should be noted that when FDA declares the biosimilarity of two drug products, it may not be assumed that they are interchangeable. Therefore, labels ought to state whether for a follow-on biologic which is biosimilar to a reference product, interchangeability has or has not been established. However, payers and physicians may, in some cases, switch products even if interchangeability has not been established.

8.1.3.2 Extrapolation

For biosimilar product development, the sponsors often select one or two indications and seek approval of all indications of the innovative biological product. For a given indication and a Critical Quality Attribute (CQA), the validity of extrapolation depends upon whether there is a well-established relationship (linear or non-linear) between the CQA and PK/PD and clinical outcomes. Under a well-established relationship, a notable difference in Tier 1 CQAs, which leads to a clinically meaningful difference in clinical outcomes may vary from one indication to another even they have similar PK profile or mechanism of action (MOA). Thus, extrapolation across indications without collecting any clinical data is a great concern. In this case, statistical evaluation of extrapolation from one indication to another is recommended.

8.2 Statistical Considerations

8.2.1 Study Design

As indicated in the *Federal Register* [Vol. 42, No. 5, Section 320.26(b) and Section 320.27(b), 1977], a bioavailability study (single-dose or multi-dose) should be crossover in design, unless a parallel or other design is more appropriate for valid scientific reasons. Thus, in practice, a standard two-sequence, two-period (or 2×2) crossover design is often considered for a bioavailability or bioequivalence study. Denote by T and R the test product and the reference product, respectively. Thus, a 2×2 crossover design can be expressed as (TR, RT), where TR is the first sequence of treatments and RT denotes the second sequence of treatments. Under the (TR, RT) design, qualified subjects who are randomly assigned to sequence 1 (TR) will receive the test product (T) first and then cross-over to receive the reference product (R) after a sufficient length of wash-out period. Similarly, subjects who are randomly assigned to sequence 2 (RT) will receive the reference product (R) first and then cross-over to receive the test product (T) after a sufficient length of wash-out period.

One of the limitations of the standard 2×2 crossover design is that it does not provide independent estimates of intra-subject variabilities since each subject receives the same treatment only once. In the interest of assessing intra-subject variabilities, the following alternative crossover designs for comparing two drug products are often considered:

Design 1: Balaam's design – e.g., (TT, RR, RT, TR);

Design 2: Two-sequence, three-period dual design – e.g., (TRR, RTT);

Design 3: Four-period design with two sequences – e.g., (TRRT, RTTR);

Design 4: Four-period design with four sequences – e.g., (TTRR, RRTT, TRTR, RTTR).

The above study designs are also referred to as higher-order crossover designs. A higher-order crossover design is defined as a design with the number of sequences or the number of periods greater than the number of treatments to be compared.

For comparing more than two drug products, a Williams' design is often considered. For example, for comparing three drug products, a six-sequence, three-period (6×3) Williams' design is usually considered, while a 4×4 Williams' design is employed for comparing four drug products. Williams' design is a variance stabilizing design. More information regarding the construction and good design characteristics of Williams' designs can be found in Chow and Liu (2008).

8.2.2 Statistical Methods

8.2.2.1 Two One-Sided Tests (TOST) Procedure

Under a valid study design, biosimilarity can then be assessed by means of an equivalence test under the following interval hypotheses:

$$H_0: \mu_T - \mu_R \leq \theta_L \quad \text{or} \quad \mu_T - \mu_R \geq \theta_U \quad \text{vs.} \quad H_a: \theta_L < \mu_T - \mu_R < \theta_U, \tag{8.1}$$

where (θ_L, θ_U) are pre-specified equivalence limits (margins) and μ_T and μ_R are the population means of a biological (test) product and an innovator biological (reference) product, respectively. That is, biosimilarity is assessed in terms of the *absolute* difference between the two population means. Alternatively, biosimilarity can be assessed in terms of the *relative* difference (i.e., ratio) between the population means.

The concept of interval hypotheses (8.1) is to show average biosimilarity by rejecting the null hypothesis of average bio-dis-similarity. In most biosimilar studies, δ_L and δ_U are often chosen to be $-\theta_L = \theta_U = 20\%$ of the reference mean (μ_R). When the natural logarithmic transformation of the data is considered, the hypotheses corresponding to hypotheses (8.1) can be stated as

$$H'_0: \mu_T / \mu_R \leq \delta_L \quad \text{or} \quad \mu_T / \mu_R \geq \delta_U \quad \text{vs.} \quad H'_a: \delta_L < \mu_T / \mu_R < \delta_U \tag{8.2}$$

where $\delta_L = \exp(\theta_L)$ and $\delta_U = \exp(\theta_U)$. Note that FDA recommends that $(\delta_L, \delta_U) = (80\%, 125\%)$ for assessing average bioequivalence.

Note that the test for hypotheses in (8.2) formulated on the log-scale is equivalent to testing for hypotheses (8.1) on the raw scale. The interval hypotheses (8.1) can be decomposed into two sets of one-sided hypotheses

$$H_{01}: \mu_T - \mu_R \leq \theta_L \quad \text{vs.} \quad H_{a1}: \mu_T - \mu_R > \theta_L$$

and

$$H_{02}: \mu_T - \mu_R \geq \theta_U \quad \text{vs.} \quad H_{a2}: \mu_T - \mu_R < \theta_U. \tag{8.3}$$

The first set of hypotheses is to verify that the average biosimilarity of the test product is not too low, whereas the second set of hypotheses is to verify that the average biosimilarity of the test product is not too high. A relatively low (or high) average biosimilarity may refer to the concern of efficacy (or safety) of the test product. If one concludes that $\theta_L < \mu_T - \mu_R$ (i.e., reject H_{01}) and $\mu_T - \mu_R < \theta_U$ (i.e., reject H_{02}), then it has been concluded that

$$\theta_L < \mu_T - \mu_R < \theta_U.$$

Thus, μ_T and μ_R are equivalent. The rejection of H_{01} and H_{02}, which leads to the conclusion of average bioequivalence, is equivalent to rejecting H_0 in (8.1). Under hypotheses (8.1), Schuirmann (1987) introduced the Two One-Sided Tests (TOST) procedure for assessing average biosimilarity between drug products. The proposed TOST procedure suggests the conclusion of similarity of μ_T and μ_R at the α level of significance if, and only if, H_{01} and

H_{02} in (8.3) are rejected at a pre-determined α level of significance. Under the normally assumptions, the two sets of one-sided hypotheses can be tested with ordinary one-sided t tests. We conclude that of μ_T and μ_R are biosimilar if

$$T_L = \frac{(\bar{Y}_T - \bar{Y}_R) - \theta_L}{\hat{\sigma}_d \sqrt{\dfrac{1}{n_1} + \dfrac{1}{n_2}}} > t(\alpha, n_1 + n_2 - 2)$$

and

$$T_U = \frac{(\bar{Y}_T - \bar{Y}_R) - \theta_U}{\hat{\sigma}_d \sqrt{\dfrac{1}{n_1} + \dfrac{1}{n_2}}} < -t(\alpha, n_1 + n_2 - 2). \tag{8.4}$$

Note that the two one-sided t tests procedure is operationally equivalent to the classic (shortest) confidence interval approach; that is, both the classic confidence interval approach and Schuirmann's two one-sided tests procedure will lead to the same conclusion on bioequivalence. Under a parallel group design, Schuirmann's two one-sided tests procedure can be similarly derived with a slightly modification from a pair-t test statistic to a two-sample t test statistic.

8.2.2.2 Confidence Interval Approach

Confidence interval approach is usually performed after log-transformation of the data. Let $\bar{Y}_T$ and $\bar{Y}_R$ be the respective least squares means for the test and reference formulations, which can be obtained from the sequence-by-period means. The classic (or shortest) $(1 - 2\alpha) \times 100\%$ confidence interval can then be obtained based on the following t statistic:

$$T = \frac{(\bar{Y}_T - \bar{Y}_R) - (\mu_T - \mu_R)}{\hat{\sigma}_d \sqrt{\dfrac{1}{n_1} + \dfrac{1}{n_2}}}, \tag{8.5}$$

where n_1 and n_2 are the numbers of subjects in sequences 1 and 2, respectively, and $\hat{\sigma}_d$ is an estimate of the variance of the period differences for each subject within each sequence, which are defined as follows

$$d_{ik} = \frac{1}{2}(Y_{i2k} - Y_{i1k}), \quad i = 1, 2, \ldots, n_k; \quad k = 1, 2.$$

Thus, $V(d_{ik}) = \sigma_d^2 = \sigma_e^2 / 2$. Under normality assumptions, T follows a central student t distribution with degrees of freedom $n_1 + n_2 - 2$. Thus, the classic $(1 - 2\alpha) \times 100\%$ confidence interval for $\mu_T - \mu_R$ can be obtained as follows:

$$L_1 = \left(\bar{Y}_T - \bar{Y}_R\right) - t\left(\alpha, n_1 + n_2 - 2\right)\hat{\sigma}_d \sqrt{\frac{1}{n_1} + \frac{1}{n_2}},$$

$$U_1 = \left(\bar{Y}_T - \bar{Y}_R\right) - t\left(\alpha, n_1 + n_2 - 2\right)\hat{\sigma}_d \sqrt{\frac{1}{n_1} + \frac{1}{n_2}}. \tag{8.6}$$

The above a $(1 - 2\alpha) \times 100\%$ confidence interval for $\log(\mu_T) - \log(\mu_R) = \log(\mu_T/\mu_R)$ can be converted into a $(1 - 2\alpha) \times 100\%$ confidence interval for μ_T/μ_R by taking an anti-log transformation. Biosimilarity is concluded if the obtained $(1 - 2\alpha) \times 100\%$ confidence interval falls entirely within the biosimilarity limits of 0.8 to 1.25.

8.2.2.3 Remarks

In practice, it should be noted that in some cases, TOST for testing interval hypotheses is not operationally equivalent to the $(1 - 2\alpha) \times 100\%$ CI approach. Although hypotheses testing procedure for evaluation of the safety and efficacy of drug products is currently recommended by the FDA, CI approach is often mis-used for evaluation of the safety and efficacy of the drug products regardless the framework of hypotheses testing (see, e.g., Chow and Zheng, 2019). The concept of hypotheses testing procedure (e.g., point hypotheses testing for equality and interval hypotheses testing for equivalence) and CI approach are very different. For example, hypotheses testing procedure focuses on the control of type-II error (i.e., power), while the CI approach is based on type-I error. In practice, it is desirable to have a high probability that the constructed CI is totally within the equivalence (e.g., bioequivalence or biosimilarity) limits. This probability is not the power under the framework of hypotheses testing.

8.2.3 Sample Size Considerations

Let Y_{ijk} be the response of the ith subject in the kth sequence at the jth period. Then the following model without consideration of unequal carryover effects can be used to describe a standard two-sequence, two-period crossover design:

$$Y_{ijk} = \mu + S_{ik} + P_j + T_{(j,k)} + e_{ijk},$$ (8.7)

where i(subject) $= 1, 2, \ldots, n_k$, j(period), k(sequence) $= 1, 2$. In model (8.7), μ is the overall mean, S_{ik} is the random effect of the ith subject in the kth sequence, P_j is the fixed effect of the jth period, $T_{(j,k)}$ is the direct fixed effect of the treatment administered at period j in sequence k, namely

$$T_{(j,k)} = \begin{cases} \text{Placebo} & \text{if } k = j. \\ \text{Test Drug} & \text{if } k \neq j, k = 1, 2, j = 1, 2, \end{cases}$$

and e_{ijk} is the within-subject random error in observing Y_{ijk}. For model (8.7) it is assumed that $\{S_{ik}\}$ are independently and identically distributed with mean 0 and variance σ_S^2 and that $\{e_{ijk}\}$ are independently distributed with mean 0 and variance σ^2. $\{S_{ik}\}$ and $\{e_{ijk}\}$ are assumed to be mutually independent.

8.2.3.1 Test for Equality

Let us test the following hypotheses:

$$H_0: \mu_T = \mu_P \quad \text{vs.} \quad H_a: \mu_T \neq \mu_P$$ (8.8)

Under model (8.7), we can consider period differences for each subject within each sequence which are defined as

$$d_{ik} = \frac{1}{2}(Y_{i2k} - Y_{i1k}),$$

where $i = 1, \ldots, n_k; k = 1, 2$. Then a test for hypotheses (8.8) can be obtained based on a two-sample t statistic as follows:

$$T_d = \frac{\bar{Y}_T - \bar{Y}_P}{\hat{\sigma}_d \sqrt{(1/n_1) + (1/n_2)}},$$

where

$$\bar{Y}_T = \frac{1}{2}\left(\bar{Y}_{.21} + \bar{Y}_{.12}\right)$$

$$\bar{Y}_P = \frac{1}{2}\left(\bar{Y}_{.11} + \bar{Y}_{.22}\right)$$

$$\hat{\sigma}_d^2 = \frac{1}{n_1 + n_2 - 2}\sum_{k=1}^{2}\sum_{i=1}^{n_k}\left(d_{ik} - \bar{d}_{.k}\right)^2,$$

and

$$\bar{Y}_{.jk} = \frac{1}{n_k}\sum_{i=1}^{n_k}Y_{ijk},$$

$$\bar{d}_{.k} = \frac{1}{n_k}\sum_{i=1}^{n_k}d_{ijk}.$$

Under the null hypothesis (8.8), T_d follows a t distribution with $n_1 + n_2 - 2$ degrees of freedom. We can reject the null hypothesis of (8.8) if

$$|T_d| > t(\alpha/2, n_1 + n_2 - 2).$$

Under the alternative hypothesis that $\mu_T = \mu_P + \Delta$, the power of the test T_d can be similarly evaluated. In the interest of balance, we assume that $n_1 = n_2 = n$; that is, each sequence will be allocated the same number of subjects at random. As a result, the sample size per sequence for testing the hypotheses of equality (11.7.2) can be determined by the formula

$$n \geq \frac{2\sigma_d^2\left[t(\alpha/2, 2n-2) + t(\beta, 2n-2)\right]^2}{\Delta^2}, \tag{8.9}$$

where σ_d^2 can be estimated from previous studies and A is the clinically meaningful difference which we want to detect. If we need to have a power of 80% for detection of a difference of at least 20% of the unknown placebo mean, then (8.9) can be simplified as

$$n \geq \left[t(\alpha/2, 2n-2) + t(\beta, 2n-2) \right]^2 \left[\frac{CV}{20} \right]^2, \tag{8.10}$$

where

$$CV = \frac{\sqrt{2}\sigma_d}{\mu_P} \times 100\%$$

Since $(2n-2)$ in (8.9) and (8.10) are unknown, a numerical iterative procedure is required to solve for n.

8.2.3.2 Interval Hypotheses for Similarity

As pointed out by Chow and Liu (2000), the power approach for sample size determination based on the hypothesis of equality (8.8) is not statistically valid in assessing *similarity* between treatments. For the assessment of similarity between treatments under the standard two-sequence, two-period crossover design, it is suggested that the following interval hypotheses be tested:

$$H_0: \mu_T - \mu_P \leq \theta_L \quad \text{or} \quad \mu_T - \mu_P \geq \theta_L \quad \text{vs.} \quad H_a: \theta_L < \mu_T - \mu_P < \theta_U. \tag{8.11}$$

where θ_L and θ_U are some clinically meaningful limits for equivalence. The concept of interval hypotheses is to show equivalence by rejecting the null hypothesis of dis-similarity. The above hypotheses can be decomposed into two sets of one-sided hypotheses:

$$H_{01}: \mu_T - \mu_P \leq \theta_L \quad \text{vs.} \quad H_{a1}: \mu_T - \mu_P > \theta_L.$$

and

$$H_{02}: \mu_T - \mu_P \geq \theta_U \quad \text{vs.} \quad H_{a2}: \mu_T - \mu_P < \theta_U.$$

Under model (8.1), Schuirmann (1987) proposes two one-sided test procedures for the above two one-sided hypotheses. We can reject the null hypothesis of dis-similarity if

$$T_L = \frac{\bar{Y}_T - \bar{Y}_P - \theta_L}{\hat{\sigma}_d \sqrt{(1/n_1) + (1/n_2)}} > t(\alpha, n_1 + n_2 - 2)$$

and

$$T_U = \frac{\bar{Y}_T - \bar{Y}_P - \theta_U}{\hat{\sigma}_d \sqrt{(1/n_1) + (1/n_2)}} < -t(\alpha, n_1 + n_2 - 2)$$

Let $\theta = \mu_T - \mu_P$ and $\phi_S(\theta)$ be the power of Schuirmann's two one-sided tests at θ. Assuming that $n_1 = n_2 = n$, the power at $\theta = 0$ is given by

$$1 - \beta = \phi_S(0)$$

$$= P\left\{\frac{-\Delta}{\hat{\sigma}_d\sqrt{2/n}} + t(\alpha, 2n-2) < \frac{Y}{\hat{\sigma}_d\sqrt{2/n}} < \frac{\Delta}{\hat{\sigma}_d\sqrt{2/n}} - t(\alpha, 2n-2)\right\} \qquad (8.12)$$

where $Y = \bar{Y}_T - \bar{Y}_P$. Since a central t distribution is symmetric about 0, the lower and upper endpoints of (8.12) are also symmetric about 0:

$$\frac{-\Delta}{\hat{\sigma}_d\sqrt{2/n}} + t(\alpha, 2n-2) = -\left\{\frac{\Delta}{\hat{\sigma}_d\sqrt{2/n}} - t(\alpha, 2n-2)\right\}$$

Therefore, $\phi_S(0) \geq 1 - \beta$ implies that

$$\left|\frac{\Delta}{\hat{\sigma}_d\sqrt{2/n}} - t(\alpha, 2n-2)\right| \geq t(\beta/2, 2n-2)$$

or that

$$n(\theta = 0) \geq 2\left[t(\alpha, 2n-2) + t(\beta/2, 2n-2)\right]^2 \left[\frac{\hat{\sigma}_d}{\Delta}\right]^2 \qquad (8.13)$$

If we must have an 80% power for detection of a 20% difference of placebo mean, then (8.13) becomes

$$n(\theta = 0) \geq \left[t(\alpha, 2n-2) + t(\beta/2, 2n-2)\right]^2 \left[\frac{CV}{20}\right]^2, \qquad (8.14)$$

We will now consider the case where $\theta \neq 0$. Since the power curves of Schuirmann's two one-sided test procedures are symmetric about zero (Phillips, 1990), we will only consider the case where $0 < \theta = \theta_0 < \Delta$. In this case, the statistic

$$\frac{Y - \theta_0}{\hat{\sigma}_d\sqrt{2/n}}$$

has a central t distribution with $2n - 2$ degrees of freedom. The power of Schuirmann's two one-sided test procedures can be evaluated at θ_0, which is given by

$$1 - \beta = \phi_S(\theta_0)$$

$$= P\left\{\frac{-\Delta - \theta_0}{\hat{\sigma}_d\sqrt{2/n}} - t(\alpha, 2n-2) < \frac{Y - \theta_0}{\hat{\sigma}_d\sqrt{2/n}} < \frac{\Delta - \theta_0}{\hat{\sigma}_d\sqrt{2/n}} - t(\alpha, 2n-2)\right\} \qquad (8.15)$$

Note that unlike the case where $\theta = 0$, the lower and upper endpoints of (8.15) are not symmetric about 0. Therefore, as indicated by Chow and Liu (2000), if we choose

$$\frac{\Delta - \theta_0}{\hat{\sigma}_d\sqrt{2/n}} - t(\alpha, 2n-2) = t(\beta/2, 2n-2)$$

then the resultant sample size may be too large to be of practical interest, and the power may be more than we need. As an alternative, Chow and Liu (2000) consider the inequality for obtaining an approximate formula for n

$$\phi_S\left(\theta_0\right) \le P\left\{\frac{Y-\theta_0}{\hat{\sigma}_d\sqrt{2/n}} < \frac{\Delta-\theta_0}{\hat{\sigma}_d\sqrt{2/n}} - t(\alpha, 2n-2)\right\}.$$

As a result, $\phi_S(\theta_0) \ge 1-\beta$ gives

$$\frac{\Delta-\theta_0}{\hat{\sigma}_d\sqrt{2/n}} - t(\alpha, 2n-2) = t(\beta, 2n-2)$$

or

$$n(\theta_0) \ge 2\left[t(\alpha, 2n-2) + t(\beta, 2n-2)\right]^2\left[\frac{\hat{\sigma}_d}{\Delta-\theta_0}\right]^2 \qquad (8.16)$$

Similarly, if we must have an 80% power for detection of a 20% difference of placebo mean, then (8.16) becomes

$$n(\theta_0) \ge \left[t(\alpha, 2n-2) + t(\beta, 2n-2)\right]^2\left[\frac{CV}{20-\theta_0'}\right]^2 \qquad (8.17)$$

where

$$\theta_0' = 100 \times \frac{\theta_0'}{\mu_P}$$

8.2.3.3 Higher-Order Crossover Designs

For a given higher-order crossover design, the sample size is similarly determined based on either the point hypotheses for equality or the interval hypotheses for equivalence under model (8.1). Let us consider the sample size determined by the interval hypotheses (8.11). Let $n_i = n$ be the number of subjects in sequence i of a higher-order crossover design, and let F_v denote the cumulative distribution function of the t distribution with v degrees of freedom. Then it can be verified that the power of Schuirmann's two one-sided tests at the a level of significance for the mth design is given by

$$\phi_m\left(\theta\right) = F_{V_m}\left(\frac{\Delta-\theta}{CV\sqrt{b_m/n}} - t(\alpha, v_m)\right) - F_{V_m}\left(t(\alpha, v_m) - \frac{\Delta+\theta}{CV\sqrt{b_m/n}}\right)$$

Hence the formula of n required to achieve a $1-\beta$ power at the α level of significance for the mth design when $\theta = 0$ is given by

$$n \ge b_m\left[t(\alpha, v_m) + t(\beta/2, v_m)\right]^2\left[\frac{CV}{\Delta}\right]^2, \qquad (8.18)$$

and if $\theta = \theta_0 > 0$, the approximate formula for n is given

$$n(\theta_0) \geq b_m \left[t(\alpha, v_m) + t(\beta, v_m)\right]^2 \left[\frac{CV}{\Delta - \theta}\right]^2, \tag{8.19}$$

for $m = 1$ (Balaam design), 2 (two-sequence dual design), 3 (four-period design with two sequences), and 4 (four-period design with four sequences), where

$$v_1 = 4n - 3, \quad v_2 = 4n - 4, \quad v_3 = 6n - 5, \quad v_4 = 12n - 5;$$

$$b_1 = 2, \quad b_2 = \frac{3}{4}, \quad b_3 = \frac{11}{20}, \quad b_4 = \frac{1}{4}.$$

8.3 Analytical Similarity

FDA recommends that a stepwise approach be considered for providing the totality-of-the-evidence to demonstrating biosimilarity of a proposed biosimilar product as compared to a reference product (FDA, 2015a). The stepwise approach starts with analytical studies for structural and functional characterization. Analytical similarity assessment is referred to as the comparisons of functional and structural characterizations between a proposed biosimilar product and a reference product in terms of CQAs that are relevant to clinical outcomes. FDA suggests that the sponsors identify CQAs that are relevant to clinical outcomes and classify them into three tiers depending on the criticality or risk ranking (e.g., most, mild to moderate, and least) relevant to clinical outcomes. At the same time, FDA also recommends some statistical approaches for the assessment of analytical similarity for CQAs from different tiers. FDA recommends an equivalence test for CQAs from Tier 1, quality range approach for CQAs from Tier 2, and descriptive raw data and graphical presentation for CQAs from Tier 3 (see, e.g., Chow, 2014).

8.3.1 Equivalence Test

For CQAs in Tier 1, FDA recommends that an equivalency test be performed for the assessment of analytical similarity. As indicated by the FDA, a potential approach could be a similar approach to bioequivalence testing for generic drug products (FDA, 2003; Chow, 2015). In other words, for a given critical attribute, we may test for equivalence by the following interval (null) hypothesis:

$$H_0: \mu_T - \mu_R \leq -\delta \quad \text{or} \quad \mu_T - \mu_R \geq \delta, \tag{8.20}$$

where $\delta > 0$ is the equivalence limit (or similarity margin), and μ_T and μ_R are the mean responses of the test (the proposed biosimilar) product and the reference product lots, respectively. Analytical equivalence (similarity) is concluded if the null hypothesis of non-equivalence (*dis*-similarity) is rejected. Note that Yu (2004) defined inequivalence as when the confidence interval falls entirely outside the equivalence limits. Similarly to the confidence interval approach for bioequivalence testing under the raw data model, analytical similarity would be accepted for a quality attribute if the $(1 - 2\alpha)100\%$ two-sided confidence interval of the mean difference is within $(-\delta, \delta)$.

Under the null hypothesis (8.20), FDA indicates that the equivalence limit (similarity margin), δ, would be a function of the variability of the reference product, denoted by σ_R. It should be noted that each lot contributes one test value for each attribute being assessed. Thus, σ_R is the population standard deviation of the lot values of the reference product.

Suppose there are k lots of a Reference Product (RP) and n lots of a Test Product (TP) available for analytical similarity assessment, where $k > n$. For a given CQA, Tier 1 equivalence test can be summarized in the following steps:

Step 1. Matching number of RP lots to TP lots – Since $k > n$, there are more reference lots than test lots. The first step is then to match the number of RP lots to TP lots for a head-to-head comparison. To *match* RP lots to TP lots, FDA suggests *randomly* selecting n lots out of the k RP lots. If the n lots are not randomly selected from the k RP lots, justification needs to be provided to prevent from *selection bias*.

Step 2. Use the remaining independent RP lots for estimating σ_R – After the matching, the remaining $k - n$ lots are then used to *estimate* σ_R in order to set up the equivalency acceptance criterion (EAC). It should be noted that if $k - n \leq 2$, it is suggested that all RP lots should be used to estimate σ_R.

Step 3. Calculate the equivalency acceptance criterion (EAC): EAC = 1.5 × $\hat{\sigma}_R$ – Based on the estimate of σ_R, denoted by $\hat{\sigma}_R$, FDA recommends EAC be set as $1.5 \times \hat{\sigma}_R$, where $c = 1.5$ is considered a regulatory standard.

Step 4. Based on c (regulatory standard), $\hat{\sigma}_R$, and $\Delta = \mu_T - \mu_R$, an appropriate sample size can be chosen for the analytical similarity assessment – As an example, suppose that there are 21 RP lots and 7 TP lots. We first randomly select 7 out of the 21 RP lots to match the 7 TP lots. Suppose that based on the remaining 14 lots, an estimate of σ_R is given by $\hat{\sigma}_R = 1.039$. Also, suppose that the true difference between the biosimilar product and the reference product is proportional to σ_R, say $\Delta = \sigma_R/8$. Then, the following table with various sample sizes (the number of TP lots available and the corresponding test size and statistical power for detecting the difference of $\sigma_R/8$ is helpful for the assessment of analytical assessment.

To assist the sponsor in performing Tier 1 equivalence test, recently, FDA circulated a draft guidance on analytical similarity assessment in September 2017, which was subsequently withdrawn and replaced with a guidance on comparability analytical assessment (FDA, 2019). In the 2019 draft guidance, FDA recommends that a minimum of ten lots should be used when performing analytical similarity assessment.

8.3.2 Quality Range (QR) Method

A Quality Range (QR) is established based on the values obtained from the reference product for a specific quality attribute. It is derived from $(\hat{\mu}_R - k\hat{\sigma}_R, \hat{\mu}_R + k\hat{\sigma}_R)$, where $\hat{\mu}_R$ and $\hat{\sigma}_R$ are the sample mean and sample standard deviation estimated from the reference product lot values. The k is the multiplicative factor that determines the width of the range. In practice, $k = 3$ is frequently used in the pharmaceutical industry for comparative analytical assessment. When sufficient percentage (e.g., 90%) of CQA measures of a proposed biosimilar product falls within the QR, it is considered to be highly similar to the reference product. If any less than 90% of proposed biosimilar product values are within the QR, it is considered not similar for the CQA. The QR method is often used under assumptions that the population mean values and variances of the test product and the reference product do not significantly differ $\mu_T \approx \mu_R$ and $\sigma_T \approx \sigma_R$, however, using the QR method can be misleading in situations where the true mean responses and variabilities are different. In such circumstances, the QR method can misclassify the non-similar proposed product as similar to the reference.

8.3.3 Challenging Issues and Recent Development

8.3.3.1 Flexible Equivalence Test

Lee, Oh, and Chow (2019) studied equivalence test with flexible margin. For analytical similarity assessment of a given critical quality attribute between a proposed biosimilar (test) product and an innovative (reference) biological product, FDA recommended an equivalence test with an Equivalence Acceptance Criterion (EAC), a margin of 1.5 σ_R (standard deviation of the reference product) be performed. This EAC, however, has been criticized due to its inflexibility (Shutter, 2017). An estimate of σ_R can be considered as any values from a 95% confidence interval of σ_R, $(\hat{\sigma}_L, \hat{\sigma}_U)$ let f be a flexible index such as $\hat{\sigma}_R^* = f \times \hat{\sigma}_R$. then the flexible margin becomes $\delta = 1.5 \times \hat{\sigma}_R^* = 1.5 f \times \hat{\sigma}_R$. One idea is to select f achieving the maximum power for testing the following interval hypotheses for equivalence or similarity, H_0: $|\varepsilon| \geq \delta$ versus H_a: $|\varepsilon| < \delta$, where $\varepsilon = \mu_T - \mu_R$ and $\delta = 1.5 f \hat{\sigma}_R$. For $n = 6,7,8,9$, and 10, the optimal choice of f maximizing power for $\varepsilon = 0$ and $\varepsilon = 1/8 \ \sigma_R$, respectively. More details can be found in Lee, Oh, and Chow (2019).

8.3.3.2 Modified QR (mQR) Method

Son et al. (2020) indicated that the QR method for analytical similarity evaluation as it stands is not statistically valid and hence not acceptable based on the following reasons: (i) the QR method is designed for quality assessment of the proposed biosimilar product rather than analytical similarity evaluation between the proposed biosimilar product and the US-licensed (reference) product; (ii) the QR method is unable to control the risk of approving products not deemed biosimilar; (iii) the EMA discourages the use of the QR method for evaluation of analytical similarity; (iv) the QR method is not statistically valid in general; (v) the QR method alone cannot replace "equivalence test (for CQA with high risk ranking) with QR method (for CQA with lower risk ranking)" for evaluation of analytical similarity.

To overcome the limitations and potential risk of the QR method for analytical similarity evaluation, alternative methods based on modified versions of the QR method proposed by Son et al. (2020) are suggested. Such approaches are referred to as the modified QR (mQR) methods. Since the FDA recommends QR method, Son et al. (2020) suggested using the Modified QR (mQR) methods that take into account (i) the difference (or shift) between μ_T and μ_R and (ii) the relative difference between σ_T and σ_R in the process of constructing a QR.

8.4 PK/PD Similarity

8.4.1 Fundamental Biosimilarity Assumption

Bioequivalence assessment for approval of generic drug products is often done under the following Fundamental Bioequivalence Assumption:

If two drug products are shown to be bioequivalent, it is assumed that they will reach the same therapeutic effect or they are therapeutically equivalent and hence can be used interchangeably.

Under the Fundamental Bioequivalence Assumption, one of the controversial issues is that bioequivalence may not necessarily imply therapeutic equivalence and therapeutic equivalence does not guarantee bioequivalence either. The assessment of average bioequivalence for generic approval has been criticized that it is based on legal/political deliberations rather than scientific considerations. In the past several decades, many sponsors/researchers have made an attempt to challenge this assumption with no success. In practice, the verification of the Fundamental Bioequivalence Assumption is often difficult, if not impossible, without the conduct of clinical trials. In practice, there are following four possible scenarios:

  i. Drug absorption profiles are similar and they are therapeutic equivalent;
  ii. Drug absorption profiles are not similar but they are therapeutic equivalent;
  iii. Drug absorption profiles are similar but they are not therapeutic equivalent;
  iv. Drug absorption profiles are not similar and they are not therapeutic equivalent.

The Fundamental Bioequivalence Assumption is nothing but scenario (i). Scenario (i) works if the drug absorption (in terms of the rate and extent of absorption) is predictive of clinical outcome. In this case, PK responses such as AUC (area under the blood or plasma concentration-time curve for measurement of the extent of drug absorption) and C_{max} (maximum concentration for measurement of the rate of drug absorption) serve as surrogate endpoints for clinical endpoints for assessment of efficacy and safety of the test product under investigation. Scenario (ii) is the case where generic companies use to argue for generic approval of their drug products especially when their products fail to meet regulatory requirements for bioequivalence. In this case, it is doubtful that there is a relationship between PK responses and clinical endpoints. The innovator companies usually argue with the regulatory agency against generic approval with scenario (iii). However, more studies are necessarily conducted in order to verify scenario (iii). There are no arguments with respect to scenario (iv).

In practice, the Fundamental Bioequivalence Assumption is applied to all drug products across therapeutic areas without convincing scientific justification. In the past several decades, however, no significant safety incidences were reported for the generic drug products approved under the Fundamental Bioequivalence Assumption. One of the convincing explanations is that the Fundamental Bioequivalence Assumption is for drug products with *identical* active ingredient(s). Whether the Fundamental Bioequivalence Assumption is applicable to drug products with similar but different active ingredient(s) as in the case of follow-on products becomes an interesting but controversial question.

Current methods for the assessment of bioequivalence for drug products with identical active ingredients are *not* applicable to biosimilar products due to fundamental differences as described in the previous chapter. The assessment of biosimilarity between biosimilar products and the innovative biological product in terms of surrogate endpoints (e.g., pharmacokinetic parameters and/or pharmacodynamics responses) or biomarkers (e.g., genomic markers) requires the establishment of the Fundamental Biosimilarity Assumption in order to bridge the surrogate endpoints and/or biomarker data to clinical safety and efficacy.

8.4.2 Complete n-of-1 Trial Design

In recent years, the n-of-1 trial design has become a very population design for evaluation of the difference in treatment effect within the same individual when n treatments are administered at different dosing periods. Thus, n-of-1 trial design is in fact a crossover design. Following similar ideas of switching designs with single switch and/or multiple switches, Chow et al. (2017) proposed the use of so-called complete n-of-1 trial design for assessment of relative risk between switching/alternation and without switching/alternation.

The construction of a complete n-of-1 trial design depending upon m, the number of switches. For example, if $m = 1$ (single switch), the complete n-of-1 trial design will consist of $m + 1 = 2$ periods. At each dosing period, there are two choices (i.e., either R or T). Thus, there are a total of $2^{m+1} = 2^2 = 4$ sequences (i.e., combination of R and T). This results in a 4×2 Balaam design, i.e., (RR, TT, RT, TR). When $m = 2$ (two switches), the complete n-of-1 trial design will consist of $m + 1 = 3$ periods. At each dosing period, there are two choices (i.e., either R or T). Thus, there are a total of $2^{m+1} = 2^3 = 8$ sequences. This results in an 8×3 crossover design. Similarly, where there are three switches (i.e., $m = 3$), the complete n-of-1 trial design will consist of $m + 1 = 4$ periods. At each dosing period, there are two choices (i.e., either R or T). Thus, there are a total of $2^{m+1} = 2^4 = 16$ sequences (i.e., combinations of R and T). This results in a 16×4 crossover design.

The switching designs with single switch, i.e., (RT, RR), with two switches, i.e., (RTR, RRR), and three switches, i.e., (RTRT, RRRR) are partial designs of the n-of-1 trial designs with single switch (two periods), two switches (three periods), and three switches (four periods), respectively.

8.4.3 PK/PD Bridging Studies

For assessing biosimilar products, however, there may be multiple references, e.g., an EU approved reference product and a US licensed reference product of the same innovative product. Suppose that a sponsor is interested in developing a proposed biosimilar product in US, while there is an EU-approved reference product. In this case, the sponsor often conducts a PK/PD biosimilar bridging study not only to evaluate PK/PD similarity between the proposed biosimilar product and the reference (i.e., US-licensed reference) product, but also to establish a bridge to justify the use of relevant comparative data such as clinical data generated using EU-approved as the comparator in support of a demonstration of biosimilarity between the proposed biosimilar (test) product and the reference product for regulatory approval.

When conducting a PK/PD biosimilar bridging study comparing a proposed biosimilar product (BP) and multiple (two) references such as an EU-approved reference product (EU) and a US-licensed reference product (US), one of the major concerns is that the two reference products (EU and US) are not biosimilar. In practice, reference products could be different due to the following reasons: (i) different batches from the same manufacturing process, (ii) different sites (locations) of the same manufacturer, (iii) different countries such as EU and US. In this case, it is of particular interest to determine which product should be used as the reference product for assessing biosimilarity of BP.

To address this issue, Kang and Chow (2013) proposed the use of a 3-arm parallel-group design and suggested that after the conduct of the study, data can be analyzed by comparing the test product with either the average of EU and US or the max(EU, US). The observed difference between EU and US could be used to (i) verify the criteria for biosimilarity, and (ii) serve as reference standard for future studies. However, a controversial issue has been raised: what if we fail to meet the biosimilarity criteria when comparing with EU (say) but meet the criterion when comparing with US or vice versa.

The United States FDA, on the other hand, suggests pairwise comparisons should be performed. FDA's recommendation three comparisons, namely, (i) BP vs US, (ii) BP vs EU, and (iii) US vs EU. As indicated by the ODAC (held on 13 July 2017), FDA's recommended method of pairwise comparison suffers from the following limitations: (i) pairwise comparison does not use the same reference product in the comparison (i.e., these comparisons use different similarity margins), and (ii) pairwise comparison does not utilize all data collected from the test and two reference groups. In addition, pairwise comparison may not be able to detect the following possible relationship (pattern) among BP, US, and EU under the three-arm parallel-group design: (i) US > BP > EU, (ii) US > EU > BP, (iii) BP > US > EU, (iv) BP > EU > US, (v) EU > BP > US, and (vi) EU > US > BP.

To overcome the problem of pairwise comparison, Zheng et al. (2017) proposed a simultaneous confidence approach based on the fiducial inference theory as an alternative to the method of pairwise comparison for similarity assessment of the three arms (i.e., one test group and two reference groups).

8.5 Clinical Similarity

8.5.1 Selection of Similarity Margin

8.5.1.1 FDA's Recommendations

For the selection of similarity margin, the 2010 and 2016 FDA guidance are commonly considered. The 2010 and 2016 FDA guidance recommends two non-inferiority margins, namely M_1 and M_2 should be considered. The 2010 and 2016 FDA guidance indicated that M_1 is based on (i) the treatment effect estimated from the historical experience with the active control drug, (ii) assessment of the likelihood that the current effect of the active control is similar to the past effect (the constancy assumption), and (iii) assessment of the quality of the non-inferiority trial, particularly looking for defects that could reduce a difference between the active control and the new drug. Thus, M_1 is defined as the entire effect of the active control assumed to be present in the non-inferiority study

$$M_1 = C - P. \tag{8.21}$$

On the other hand, FDA indicates that it M_2 is selected based on a clinical judgment which is never be greater than M_1 even if for active control drugs with small effects. It should be noted that a clinical judgment might argue that a larger difference is not clinically important. Ruling out that a difference between the active control and test treatment that is larger than M_1 is a critical finding that supports the conclusion of effectiveness. Thus, M_2 can be obtained as

$$M_2 = (1 - \delta_0) M_1 = (1 - \delta_0)(C - P), \tag{8.22}$$

where

$$\delta_0 = 1 - r = 1 - \frac{T - P}{C - P} = \frac{C - T}{C - P}$$

is referred to as the ratio of the effect of the active control agent as compared to the test treatment and the effect of the active control agent as compared to the placebo. Thus, δ_0 becomes smaller if the difference between C and T decreases, i.e., T is close to C (the retention rate of T is close to 1). In this case, the FDA suggests a wider margin for the non-inferiority testing.

8.5.1.2 Chow and Shao's Method

By the 2010 and 2016 FDA draft guidance, there are essentially two different approaches to analysis of the non-inferiority study: one is the fixed margin method (or the two confidence interval method) and the other one is the synthesis method. In the fixed margin method, the margin M_1 is based on estimates of the effect of the active comparator in previously conducted studies, making any needed adjustment for changes in trial circumstances. The non-inferiority margin is then pre-specified and it is usually chosen as a margin smaller than M_1 (i.e., M_2). The synthesis method combines (or synthesizes) the estimate of treatment effect relative to the control from the non-inferiority trial with the estimate of the control effect from a meta-analysis of historical trials. This method treats both sources of data as if they came from the same randomized trial to project what the placebo effect would have been having the placebo been present in the non-inferiority trial.

Following the idea of the ICH E10 (2000) that the selected margin should not be greater than the smallest effect size that the active control has, Chow and Shao (2006) introduced another parameter δ which is a superiority margin if the placebo ($\delta > 0$) and assumed that the non-inferiority margin M is proportional to δ, i.e., $M = \lambda\delta$ then, Under the worst scenario, i.e., T-C achieves its lower bound $-M$, then the largest possible M is given by $M = C - P - \delta$, which leads to

$$M = \frac{\lambda}{1+\lambda}(C-P),$$

where

$$\lambda = \frac{r}{1-r}.$$

It can be seen that if $0 < r \leq 1$, then $0 < \lambda \leq 1/2$.

To account for the variability of $C - P$, Chow and Shao suggested the non-inferiority margins, M_1 and M_2 be modified as follows, respectively,

$$M_3 = M_1 - (z_{1-\alpha} + z_\beta)SE_{C-T} = C - P - (z_{1-\alpha} + z_\beta)SE_{C-T}, \qquad (8.23)$$

where SE_{C-T} is the standard error of $\hat{C} - \hat{T}$ and $z_a = \Phi^{-1}(a)$ assuming that

$$SE_{C-P} \approx SE_{T-P} \approx SE_{C-T}.$$

Similarly, M_2 can be modified as follows

$$M_4 = rM_3 = r\left\{C - P - (z_{1-\alpha} + z_\beta)SE_{C-T}\right\} \qquad (8.24)$$

$$= \frac{\lambda}{1+\lambda} \left\{ C - P - \left(z_{1-\alpha} + z_\beta \right) SE_{C-T} \right\},$$

$$= \left(1 - \frac{1}{1+\lambda} \right) M_3,$$

where δ_0 is chosen to be $\frac{1}{1+\lambda}$ as suggested by Chow and Shao (2006).

8.5.2 Post-Approval Non-Medical Switch

Post-approval non-medical switch is referred to as the switch from the reference product (more expensive) to an approved biosimilar product (less expensive) based on factors unrelated to clinical/medical considerations. Typical approaches for the assessment of non-medical switch include (i) observational studies and (ii) limited clinical studies. However, there are concerns regarding (i) validity, quality and integrity of the data collected, and (ii) scientific validity of design and analysis of studies conducted for assessment of safety and efficacy of non-medical switch (see also Chow, 2018).

In recent years, several observational studies and a national clinical study (e.g., NOR-SWITCH) were conducted to evaluate the risk of non-medical switch from a reference product to an approved biosimilar product (Glintborg, 2016). The conclusions from these studies, however, are biased and hence may be somewhat misleading due to some scientific and/or statistical deficiencies in design and analysis of the data collected. Chow (2018) recommended some valid study designs and appropriate statistical methods for a more accurate and reliable assessment of potential risk of medical/non-medical switch between a proposed biosimilar product and a reference product. The results can be easily extended for evaluation of the potential risk of medical/non-medical switch among multiple biosimilar products and a reference product.

8.6 Case Studies

8.6.1 Avastin Biosimilar Regulatory Submission

Amgen submitted a Biologics License Application (BLA# 761028) under section 351(k) of the PHS Act for ABP215, a proposed biosimilar to US-licensed Avastin (bevacizumab) of Genentech. Genentech's Avastin (BLA# 125085) was initially licensed by FDA on 26 February 2004. Amgen's submission was discussed and voted approved by the Oncologic Drugs Advisory Committee (ODAC) meeting held within FDA in Silver Spring on 13 July 2017.

In this section, the case of Amgen's Avastin biosimilar regulatory submission is studied by focusing on similarity assessment of data collected from the analytical studies. In what follows, Amgen's strategy for biosimilar submission is outlined followed by the introduction of the mechanism of action of the US-licensed reference product, analytical data generation, results of analytical similarity assessment, and FDA's assessment of analytical data.

8.6.1.1 Amgen's Strategy for Biosimilar Submission

Amgen adopted strategy for biosimilar submission with multiple references (i.e., US-licensed Avastin and EU-approved bevacizumab). Thus the application consists of the following:

1. Extensive analytical data intended to support (i) a demonstration that ABP215 and US-licensed Avastin are highly similar; (ii) a demonstration that ABP215 can be manufactured in a well-controlled and consistent manner that is sufficient to meet appropriate quality standards; and (iii) a justification of the relevance of the comparative data generated using EU-approved bevacizumab to support a demonstration of biosimilarity of ABP215 to US-licensed Avastin;

2. A single-dose PK study providing a three-way comparison of ABP215, US-licensed Avastin, and EU-approved bevacizumab intended to (i) support PK similarity of ABP215 and US-licensed Avastin and (ii) provide the PK portion of the scientific bridge to support the relevance of the comparative data generated using EU-approved bevacizumab to support a demonstration of the biosimilarity of ABP215 to US-licensed Avastin;

3. A comparative clinical study (Study 20120265) between ABP215 and EU-approved bevacizumab in patients with advanced/metastatic non-small cell lung cancer (NSCLC) to support the demonstration of no clinically meaningful differences in terms of response, safety, purity, and potency between ABP215 and US-licensed Avastin. This was a randomized, double-blind, parallel group study conducted in 642 patients with previously untreated NSCLC who were randomized (1:1) to receive carboplatin and paclitaxel with ABP215 or EU-approved bevacizumab (15 mg/kg dose every 3 weeks for up to 6 cycles). The primary endpoint of Study 20120265 was the risk ratio of the overall response rate (ORR). The study met its primary endpoint, as the risk ratio of ORR fell within the pre specified margin. In addition to meeting the primary endpoint, the study showed that cardinal anti-VEGF effects (e.g., hypertension) were similar between arms;

4. A scientific justification for extrapolation of data to support biosimilarity in each of the additional indications for which Amgen is seeking licensure.

Note that ABP215 was developed as 100 mg per 4 mL and 400 mg per 16 mL single-use vials to reflect the same strength and presentations approved for US-licensed Avastin. Proposed dosing and administration labeling instructions are the same as those approved for US-licensed Avastin. Amgen is seeking licensure of ABP215 for indications for which US-licensed Avastin is approved (Table 8.2).

8.6.1.2 Extensive Analytical Data Generated

In the regulatory submission of ABP215 (BLA# 761028), extensive analytical data regarding structural and functional characterization were generated. Critical quality attributes (CQAs) that are related to bevacizumab structure mechanism of action. These CQAs were classified into three tiers according to their criticality or risk ranking relevant to clinical outcomes and tested on some selected reference and test (ABP 215) lots using tired approach as recommended by the FDA.

These CQAs were tested on 19 lots of ABP215, 27 lots of US-licensed Avastin, and 29 lots of EU-approved bevacizumab. Tier 1 CQAs, Tier 2 CQAs, and Tier 3 CQAs were evaluated using equivalence test, quality range approach, and graphical comparison, respectively

TABLE 8.2

Approved Indications for Avastin

No. Indication
1. Metastatic colorectal cancer, with intravenous 5-fluorouracil–based chemotherapy for first- or second-line treatment
2. Metastatic colorectal cancer, with fluoropyrimidine-irinotecan- or fluoropyrimidine oxaliplatin-based chemotherapy for second-line treatment in patients who have progressed on a first-line Avastin-containing regimen
3. Non-squamous non-small cell lung cancer, with carboplatin and paclitaxel for first line treatment of unresectable, locally advanced, recurrent or metastaticdisease
4. Glioblastoma, as a single agent for adult patients with progressive disease following prior therapy
5. Metastatic renal cell carcinoma with interferon alfa
6. Cervical cancer, in combination with paclitaxel and cisplatin or paclitaxel and topotecan in persistent, recurrent, or metastatic disease

TABLE 8.3

Product Lots Used Data Analysis

Product	Number of Lots	CQA Assessment	Statistical Analysis
ABP 215 DP	19	Tier 1	Equivalence test
ABP 215 DS	13*		
US-licensed Avastin	27	Tier 2	Quality range
EU-approved bevacizumab	29	Tier 3	Graphical comparison

DP = drug product
DS = drug substance
*13 independent DS lots were used to derive 19 DP lots

(Table 8.3). Note that Tier 1 CQAs such as assays that assessed the primary mechanism of action were tested based on the endpoints of (i) % relative potency as assessed by proliferation inhibition bioassay, and (ii) VEGF-A binding by Enzyme-Linked Immunosorbent Assay (ELISA).

8.6.1.3 Analytical Similarity Assessment

As it can be seen from Table 8.4, a total of 19 ABP215, 27 US-licensed Avastin, and 29 EU-approved bevacizumab lots were used in the analytical similarity assessment. However, not all lots were used. Amgen indicated that the number of lots used to evaluate each quality attribute was determined based on their assessment of the variability of the analytical

TABLE 8.4

Equivalence Testing Results for the VEGF-A Binding by ELISA

Comparison	#of Lots	Mean Difference,%	90% Confidence Interval	Equivalence Margin,%	Equivalent
ABP215 vs. US	(13, 14)	0.63	(–2.93, 4.18)	(–9.79, +9.79)	Yes
ABP215 vs. EU	(13, 14)	4.85	(1.23, 8.45)	(–9.57, +9.57)	Yes
EU vs. US	(13, 14)	–4.22	(–8.47, 0.03)	(–9.79, +9.79)	Yes

method and availability of US-licensed Avastin and EU-approved bevacizumab. Both the 100 mg/vial and 400 mg/vial strengths were used in the analytical similarity assessment.

Pairwise comparisons of ABP215 to EU-approved bevacizumab and EU-approved bevacizumab to US-licensed Avastin were performed for the purpose of establishing the analytical portion of the scientific bridge necessary to support the use of the data derived from the clinical studies that used the EU-approved bevacizumab as the comparator. The results are summarized in Table 8.4. The results show that the 90% confidence interval for the mean difference in VEGFA binding by ELISA between ABP215 and US-licensed Avastin is (–2.93%, 4.18%) which falls entirely within the equivalence margin of (–9.79%, 9.79%). This result supports a demonstration that ABP215 is highly similar to US-licensed Avastin. On the other hand, the 90% confidence interval for the mean difference in VEGFA binding by ELISA between ABP215 and EU-approved bevacizumab is (1.24%, 8.45%) which is also within the equivalence limit of (–9.79%, 9.79%). The result supports analytical portion of the scientific bridge to justify the relevance of EU-approved bevacizumab data from the comparative clinical study.

However, several quality attribute differences were noted. These notable differences include differences in glycosylation content (galactosylation and high mannose), FcgRIlla (158) binding, and product related species (aggregates, fragments, and charge variants). Actions were taken to address these notable differences. For example, for glycosylation and Fcγ RIlla (158V) binding differences, *in vitro* cell based ADCC and CDC activities were assessed and were not detected for all three products. In addition, clinical pharmacokinetic data further addressed the residual uncertainty and showed that differences between the three products were unlikely to have clinical impact. For differences in charge variants, Amgen was able to isolate and characterize acidic and basic peaks and identify the same types of product variants in each peak for all three products, albeit in different amounts. In addition, the carboxypeptidase treatment of ABP215 also resulted in similar basic peak levels as US-licensed Avastin and EU-approved bevacizumab. Similar potency was demonstrated for all three products. As a result, the totality-of-the-evidence provided supports a conclusion that ABP215 is highly similar to US-licensed Avastin notwithstanding minor differences in clinical inactive components.

8.6.1.4 FDA's Assessment

The FDA performed confirmatory statistical analyses of the submitted data. As indicated by the FDA, the sponsor employed numerous analytical methods that compared the primary and higher order structures, product-related variants such as aggregate levels and charge variants, process-related components such as host cell DNA, and biological functions to support a demonstration that ABP215 is highly similar to US-licensed Avastin. In addition, the sponsor supported the analytical portion of the scientific bridge to justify the relevance of data obtained from the use of EU-approved bevacizumab as the comparator product in clinical studies.

The analytical data submitted supports a demonstration that ABP215 is highly similar to US-licensed Avastin. All three products demonstrated similar binding affinities to VEGFA and similar potency, which are product quality attributes associated with the mechanism of action for ABP215 and US-licensed Avastin. Lastly, the higher order structure determinations showed the presence of similar secondary and tertiary structures and further support the binding and potency results. The impurity profiles also demonstrated that ABP215 has acceptably low levels of impurities that are similar to US-licensed Avastin.

Some quality attributes were found to be slightly different between products but unlikely to have a clinical impact and do not preclude a demonstration that ABP215 is highly similar to US-licensed Avastin. For example, the differences in charge variants for ABP215 were due to lower levels of the product variants in US-licensed Avastin and are likely due to the age difference between ABP215 and US-licensed Avastin at the time of the analytical similarity assessment. Furthermore, the differences in the glycan species were shown to not affect PK in clinical studies and no effector functions were observed *in vitro* that could be impacted by differences in the level of glycoforms.

The analytical similarity data comparing ABP215, EU-approved bevacizumab and US-licensed Avastin supported the relevance of clinical data derived from using EU-approved bevacizumab as the comparator to support a demonstration of biosimilarity of ABP215 to US-licensed Avastin.

8.6.1.5 Remarks

The Applicant used a non-US-licensed comparator (EU-approved bevacizumab) in the comparative clinical study intended to support a demonstration of no clinically meaningful differences from US-licensed Avastin. Accordingly, the Applicant provided scientific justification for the relevance of that data by establishing an adequate scientific bridge between EU-approved bevacizumab, US-licensed Avastin, and ABP215. Review of an extensive battery of test results provided by the Applicant confirmed the adequacy of the scientific bridge and hence the relevance of comparative clinical data obtained with EU-approved bevacizumab to support a demonstration of biosimilarity to US-licensed Avastin. This battery of tests included both analytical studies and a comparative PK study in humans.

In considering the totality of the evidence, the data submitted by the Applicant support a demonstration that ABP215 is highly similar to US-licensed Avastin, not withstanding minor differences in clinically inactive components, and support a demonstration that there are no clinically meaningful differences between ABP215 and US-licensed Avastin in terms of the safety, purity, and potency of the product.

The Applicant has also provided an extensive data package to address the scientific considerations for extrapolation of data to support biosimilarity to other conditions of use and potential licensure of ABP215 for each of the indications for which US-licensed Avastin is currently licensed and for which the Applicant is eligible for licensure.

8.6.2 Herceptin Biosimilar

Mylan submitted a Biologics License Application (BLA# 761074) under section 351(k) of the PHS Act for MYL-1401O, a proposed biosimilar to US-licensed Herceptin of Genentech. Genentech's Herceptin (BLA# 103792) was initially licensed by FDA on 25 September 1998. Mylan's submission was discussed and voted approval by the Oncologic Drugs Advisory Committee (ODAC) meeting held within FDA in Silver Spring on 13 July 2017.

In this section, the case of Mylan's Herceptin biosimilar regulatory submission is studied by focusing on similarity assessment of data collected from the analytical studies. In what follows, Mylan's strategy for biosimilar submission is outlined followed by introduction to pathophysiology of HER2 and mechanism of action of trastuzumab, analytical data generation, results of analytical similarity assessment, and FDA's assessment of analytical data.

8.6.2.1 Mylan's Strategy for Biosimilar Submission

Mylan adopted strategy for biosimilar submission with multiple references (i.e., US-Herceptin and EU-Herceptin). Thus the application consists of:

1. Extensive analytical data intended to support (i) a demonstration that MYL-1401O and US-Herceptin are highly similar; (ii) a demonstration that MYL-1401O can be manufactured in a well-controlled and consistent that is sufficient to meet appropriate quality standards; and (iii) a justification of the relevance of the comparative data generated using EU-Herceptin to support a demonstration of biosimilarity of MYL-1401O to US-Herceptin;

2. A single-dose (PK) study providing a three-way comparison of MYL-1401O, US-Herceptin, and EU-Herceptin intended to (i) support PK similarity of MYL-1401O and US-Herceptin, and (ii) provide the PK portion of the scientific bridge to support the relevance of the comparative data generated using EU-Herceptin to support a demonstration of the biosimilarity of MYL-1401O to US-Herceptin;

3. A comparative clinical study between MYL-1401O and EU-Herceptin in patients with untreated metastatic HER2 positive breast cancer to support the demonstration of no clinically meaningful differences in terms of safety, purity, and potency between MYL-1401O and US-Herceptin. This was a randomized, double-blind, parallel group study conducted in 493 patients with previously untreated breast cancer who were randomized (1:1) to receive MYL-1401O or EU-Herceptin (loading dose 8 mg/kg in cycle 1 followed by maintenance dose 6 mg/kg three week cycles up to eight cycles; if stable disease after eight cycles, can continue combination treatment at investigator's discretion). The primary endpoint of MYL-Her 3001 study was the risk ratio of the overall response rate (ORR). The study met its primary endpoint, as the risk ratio of ORR fell within the pre-specified margin of (0.81, 1.24);

4. A scientific justification for extrapolation of data to support biosimilarity in each of the additional indications for which Mylan is seeking licensure.

Trastuzumab is a humanized IgG1κ monoclonal antibody directed against an epitope on the extracellular juxta membrane domain of HER2. Multiple mechanisms of action have been proposed for trastuzumab, including inhibition of HER2 receptor dimerization, increased destruction of the endocytic portion of the HER2 receptor, inhibition of extracellular domain shedding, and activation of cell-mediated immune defenses such as ADCC activity. Trastuzumab has not been shown to inhibit the dimerization of HER2 with the other isoforms; therefore, signaling through the other three receptor isoforms is maintained in the presence of the antibody. Studies have supported a mechanism by which trastuzumab is bound to the HER2 receptor and taken up by the target cell through endocytosis and subsequently degrades the receptor leading to a downregulation of downstream survival signaling, cell cycle arrest and apoptosis. Trastuzumab has also been shown to block the cleavage/shedding of the HER2 receptor extracellular domain thereby preventing the formation of the activated truncated p95, which has been correlated with a poor prognosis based on the detection of the released extracellular domain of HER2 in the serum of metastatic breast cancer patients. In addition, the initiation of ADCC activity plays a role in the mechanism of action of trastuzumab; it appears that Natural Killer (NK) cells are important mediators of ADCC activity in the context of trastuzumab-treated breast cancer. Receptor-ligand binding between trastuzumab and HER2 lead to the recruitment of immune cells

TABLE 8.5

Approved Indications for US-Herceptin

No. Indication

1. Adjuvant breast cancer
   a. As part of a treatment regimen consisting of doxorubicin, cyclophosphamide, and either paclitaxel or docetaxel
   b. With docetaxel and carboplatin
   c. As a single agent following multi-modality anthracycline based therapy

2. Metastatic breast cancer (MBC)
   a. In combination with paclitaxel for first-line treatment of HER2-overexpressing metastatic breast cancer
   b. As a single agent for treatment of HER2-overexpressing breast cancer in patients who have received one or more chemotherapy regimens for metastatic disease

3. Metastatic gastric cancer
   a. In combination with cisplatin and capecitabine or 5-fluorouracil, for the treatment of patients with HER2 overexpressing metastatic gastric or gastroesophageal junction adenocarcinoma who have not received prior treatment for metastatic disease

(e.g., NK cells, macrophages, neutrophils) that express FcγRIIIa or certain other Fc receptors. The effector cell Fc receptor binds to the Fc region of the antibody, triggering release of cytokines and recruitment of more immune cells. These immune cells release proteases that effectively lyse the HER2 expressing target cell, resulting in cell death. Trastuzumab has also been demonstrated to inhibit angiogenesis and proliferation by reducing the expression of pro-angiogenic proteins, such as Vascular Endothelial Growth Factor (VEGF) and the transforming growth factor beta (TGF-β) in a mouse model.

Note that MYL-1401O is produced using a mammalian cell line expanded in bioreactor cultures followed by a drug substance purification process that includes various steps designed to isolate and purify the protein product. The MYL-1401O drug product was developed as a multi-dose vial containing 420 mg of lyophilized powder, to reflect the same strength, presentation and route of administration as US-Herceptin (420 mg).

Mylan is seeking licensure of MYL-1401O for the indications for which US-Herceptin is approved (Table 8.5). The purpose of the Oncologic Drugs Advisory Committee (ODAC) meeting is to discuss whether the totality-of-the-evidence presented support licensure of MYL-1401O as a biosimilar to US-Herceptin. Based on the information provided, the ODAC is to determine whether MYL-1401O meet the following criteria that (i) MYL-1401O is highly similar to US-Herceptin, notwithstanding minor differences in clinically inactive components, (ii) there are no clinically meaningful differences between MYL-1401O and US-Herceptin.

8.6.2.2 Analytical Similarity Assessment

The analytical similarity assessment was performed to demonstrate that MYL-1401O and US Herceptin are highly similar, notwithstanding minor differences in clinically inactive components, and to establish the analytical portion of the scientific bridge among MYL-1401O, US-Herceptin, and EU-Herceptin to justify the relevance of the comparative clinical and nonclinical data generated using EU-Herceptin. The similarity assessments were based on pairwise comparisons of the analytical data generated by the Applicant or their contract laboratory using several lots of each product. The FDA performed confirmatory statistical analyses of the data submitted, which included results from an assessment of up to 16 lots of MYL-1401O, 28 lots of US-Herceptin, and 38 lots of EU-Herceptin. All lots of each product were not included in every assessment; the number of lots analyzed in each assay was determined by the Applicant based on the availability of test material at the time of analysis, orthogonal analytical techniques, variability of the analytical method, method qualification, and use of a common internal reference material.

The expiration dates of the US-Herceptin and EU-Herceptin lots included in the similarity assessment spanned approximately six years (2013 to 2019), and the MYL-1401O lots used for analysis were manufactured between 2011 and 2015.

The analytical similarity exercise included a comprehensive range of methods, which included orthogonal methods for the assessment of critical quality attributes. A number of assays were designed to specifically assess the potential mechanisms of action of trastuzumab, including Fc-mediated functions. All methods were validated or qualified prior to the time of testing and were demonstrated to be suitable for the intended use.

8.6.2.3 *FDA's Assessment of Analytical Data*

The MYL-1401O drug product was evaluated and compared to US-Herceptin and EU-Herceptin using a battery of biochemical, biophysical, and functional assays, including assays that addressed each major potential mechanism of action. The analytical data submitted to support the conclusion that MYL-1401O is highly similar to US-Herceptin. The amino acid sequences of MYL-1401O and US-Herceptin are identical. A comparison of the secondary and tertiary structures and the impurity profiles of MYL-1401O and US-Herceptin support the conclusion that the two products are highly similar. HER2 binding, inhibition of proliferation, and ADCC activity, which reflect the presumed primary mechanisms of action of US-Herceptin, were determined to be equivalent.

Some tests indicate that subtle shifts in glycosylation (sialic acid, high mannose, and NG-HC) exist and are likely an intrinsic property of the MYL-1401O product due to the manufacturing process. High mannose and sialic acid containing glycans can impact PK, while NG-HC is associated with loss of effector function through reduced FcγRIIIa binding and reduced ADCC activity. However, FcγRIIIa binding was similar among products and ADCC activity was equivalent among products. The residual uncertainties related to the increases in total mannose forms and sialic acid and decreases in NG-HC were addressed by the ADCC similarity and by the PK similarity between MYL-1401O and US-Herceptin as discussed in the section on Clinical Pharmacology below. Additional subtle differences in size and charge related variants were detected; however, these variants generally remain within the quality range criteria. Further, the data submitted by the Applicant support the conclusion that MYL-1401O and US Herceptin can function through the same mechanisms of action for the indications for which Herceptin is currently approved, to the extent that the mechanisms of action are known or can reasonably be determined. Thus, based on the extensive comparison of the functional, physicochemical, protein and higher order structure attributes, MYL-1401O is highly similar to US-Herceptin, notwithstanding minor differences in clinically inactive components.

In addition, the three pairwise comparisons of MYL-1401O, US-Herceptin and EU-Herceptin establish the analytical component of the scientific bridge among the three products to justify the relevance of comparative data generated from clinical and nonclinical studies that used EU-Herceptin to support a demonstration of biosimilarity of MYL-1401O to US-Herceptin.

8.6.3 Remarks

In both case studies, there are notable differences in some CQAs in Tier 1. The sponsors provided scientific rationales and/or justifications indicating that the notable differences have little or no impact on clinical outcomes based on known MOA. The scientific rationales/ justifications were accepted by the ODAC panel with some reservation because no data were collected to support the relationship between the analytical similarity and clinical similarity. In other words, it is not clear whether a notable change in CQAs is translated to a clinically meaningful difference in clinical outcome. Thus, in practice, the relationship between Tier 1 CQAs (which are considered most relevant to clinical outcomes) and clinical outcomes should be studied whenever possible.

In both biosimilar regulatory submissions, pairwise comparisons among the proposed biosimilar product, US-licensed product, and EU-approved product were performed to support (i) a demonstration that the proposed biosimilar product and the US-licensed reference product are highly similar, and (ii) a justification of the bridging of the relevance of the comparative data generated using EU-approved reference to support a demonstration of biosimilarity of the proposed biosimilar product to the US-licensed reference product under the following primary assumptions:

i. Analytical similarity assessment is predictive of PK/PD similarity in terms of drug absorption);

ii. PK/PD similarity is predictive of clinical similarity (in terms of safety and efficacy);

iii. Analytical similarity assessment is predictive of clinical similarity.

These primary assumptions, however, are difficult (if not impossible) to be verified. Thus, analytical similarity assessment using pairwise comparisons among the proposed biosimilar, US-licensed product, and EU-approved product is critical. However, at the ODAC meeting for evaluation of Avastin and Herceptin held on 13 July, the ODAC panel indicated that pairwise comparisons suffer from the disadvantages of (i) each comparison was made based on the data collected from the two products to be compared and hence did not fully utilize all of the data collected, (ii) the three comparisons used different products as reference product. For example, when comparing the proposed product with US-licensed product and when comparing EU-approved product with the US-licensed product, the US-licensed product was used as the reference product. On the other hand, when comparing the proposed biosimilar product with the EU-approved product, the EU-approved product is used as the reference product. Thus, the ODAC panel suggested a simultaneous confidence interval approach, which fully utilizes all data collected from the three products and the same reference product (i.e., US-licensed product), be considered for providing a more accurate and reliable comparison among the proposed biosimilar product, US-licensed product and EU-approved product.

8.7 Concluding Remarks

For assessment of biosimilar products, the official method recommended by the FDA is the TOST for testing interval hypotheses (each one-sided test is performed at the 5% level of significance). TOST is a size-α test and is operationally equivalent to the 90% CI approach (Chow and Shao, 2002). Thus, for convenience's sake, many practitioners *wrongly* use a

90% confidence interval approach for similarity evaluation because TOST is not generally equivalent to the 90% CI approach, e.g., for the study endpoint of binary responses.

For analytical similarity assessment, EU EMA considers raw data model based on absolute difference, i.e., $\mu_T - \mu_R$ while US FDA uses log-transformed model (or multiplicative model) based on relative difference, i.e., μ_T / μ_R. this has created some confusion between the sponsors and regulatory agencies.

After the withdrawn of the 2017 FDA draft guidance on analytical similarity assessment, FDA is seeking efficient test procedures with flexible margins. Before such an efficient test with flexible margin is developed, it is suggested that the methods discussed at previous ODAC meetings should be used with caution. If a QR or MQR method is used for analytical similarity evaluation, it is suggested that some operating characteristics (such as false positive rate) of the QR method be provided. When the FDA recommended sample size, i.e., 6–10 lots per product is used, scientific justification should be provided whenever possible.

Regulatory guidance are necessarily developed for addressing the issues of reference product changes over time and extrapolation across indications.

As indicated earlier, we claim that a test drug product is bioequivalent to a reference (innovative) drug product if the 90% confidence interval for the ratio of means of the primary PK parameter is totally within the bioequivalence limits of (80%, 125%). This one size-fits-all criterion only focuses on average bioavailability and ignores heterogeneity of variability. Thus, it is not scientifically/statistically justifiable for assessment of biosimilarity of follow-on biologics. In practice, it is then suggested that appropriate criteria, which can take the heterogeneity of variability into consideration be developed since biosimilars are known to be variable and sensitive to small variations in environmental conditions (Chow and Liu, 2010; Chow et al., 2014, Hsieh et al., 2010).

At the FDA public hearing, questions that are commonly asked are *"How similar is considered similar?"* and *"How the degree of similarity should be measured and translated to clinical outcomes (e.g., safety and efficacy)?"* These questions are closely related to drug interchangeability of biosimilars or follow-on biologics which have been shown to be biosimilar to the innovative product (Roger, 2006; Roger and Mikhail, 2007).

For assessment of bioequivalence for chemical drug products, a crossover design is often considered, except for drug products with relatively long half-lives. Since most biosimilar products have relatively long half-lives, it is suggested that a parallel group design should be considered. However, parallel group design does not provide independent estimates of variance components such as inter- and intra-subject variabilities and variability due to subject-by-product interaction. Thus, it is a major challenge for assessing biosimilars under parallel group designs.

Although EMA of EU has published several product-specific guidance based on the concept papers (e.g., EMEA 2003a-b, 2005a-g), it has been criticized that there are no objective *standards* for assessment of biosimilars because it depends upon the nature of the products. Product-specific standards seem to suggest that a *flexible* biosimilarity criterion should be considered and the flexible criterion should be adjusted for variability and/or the therapeutic index of the innovative (or reference) product.

As described above, there are many uncertainties for assessment of biosimilarity and interchangeability of biosimilars. As a result, it is a major challenge to both clinical scientists and biostatisticians to develop valid and robust clinical/statistical methodologies for assessment of biosimilarity and interchangeability under the uncertainties. In addition, how to address the issues of quality and comparability in manufacturing process is another challenge to both the pharmaceutical scientists and biostatisticians. The proposed general approach using the bioequivalence/biosimilarity index (derived based on the concept of reproducibility probability) may be useful. However, further research on the statistical properties of the proposed bioequivalence/biosimilarity index is required.

References

Chow, S. C. (2014). On assessment of analytical similarity in biosimilar studies. Drug Designing: Open Access, 3(3), 1–4.

Chow, S. C. (2015). Challenging issues in assessing analytical similarity in biosimilar studies. Biosimilars.

Chow, S. C. (2018). Analytical similarity assessment in biosimilar product development. CRC Press.

Chow, S. C. and Liu, J. P. (2008). Design and analysis of bioavailability and bioequivalence studies, third edition. CRC Press.

Chow, S. C. and Liu, J. P. (2010). Statistical assessment of biosimilar products. Journal of Biopharmaceutical Statistics, 20(1), 10–30.

Chow, S. C. and Liu, J. P. (2000). Preface. Bioequilavence measures. Statistics in Medicine, 20, 2719.

Chow, S. C., Endrenyi, L., Lachenbruch, P. A., and Mentré, F. (2014). Scientific factors and current issues in biosimilar studies. Journal of Biopharmaceutical Statistics, 24(6), 1138–1153.

Chow, S. C. and Zheng, J. (2019). The use of 95% CI or 90% CI for drug product development – a controversial issue? Journal of Biopharmaceutical Statistics, 29, 834–844.

Chow, S. C. and Shao, J. (2002). A note on statistical methods for assessing therapeutic equivalence. Controlled Clinical Trials. 23, 515–20.

Chow, S. C. and Liu, J. P. (2010). Statistical assessment of biosimilar products. Journal of Biopharmaceutical Statistics, 20(1), 10–30.

Chow, S. C. and Jun, S. (2006). On non-inferiority margin and statistical tests in active control trials. Statistics in Medicine, 25(7), 1101–1113.

Chow, S.C., Song, F., and Can, C. (2017) On hybrid parallel–crossover designs for assessing drug interchangeability of biosimilar products, Journal of Biopharmaceutical Statistics, 27(2), 265–271.

EMA (2003). Commission Directive 2003/63/EC of 25 June 2003 amending Directive 2001/83/EC of the European Parliament and of the Council on the Community code relating to medicinal products for human use. Official Journal of the European Union L 159/46.

EMA (2005a). Guideline on Similar Biological Medicinal Products. The European Medicines Agency Evaluation of Medicines for Human Use. EMEA/CHMP/437/04, London, United Kingdom.

EMA (2005c). Draft Annex Guideline on Similar Biological Medicinal Products Containing Biotechnology-derived Proteins as Drug Substance – Non Clinical and Clinical Issues – Guidance on Biosimilar Medicinal Products containing Recombinant Erythropoietins. EMEA/CHMP/94526/05, London, United Kingdom.

EMA (2005d). Draft Annex Guideline on Similar Biological Medicinal Products Containing Biotechnology-derived Proteins as Drug Substance – Non Clinical and Clinical Issues – Guidance on Biosimilar Medicinal Products containing Recombinant Granulocyte-Colony Stimulating Factor. EMEA/CHMP/31329/05, London, United Kingdom.

EMA (2005e). Draft Annex Guideline on Similar Biological Medicinal Products Containing Biotechnology-derived Proteins as Drug Substance – Non-Clinical and Clinical Issues – Guidance on Biosimilar Medicinal Products containing Somatropin. EMEA/CHMP/94528/05, London, United Kingdom.

EMA (2005f). Draft Annex Guideline on Similar Biological Medicinal Products Containing Biotechnology-derived Proteins as Drug Substance – Non Clinical and Clinical Issues – Guidance on Biosimilar Medicinal Products containing Recombinant Human Insulin. EMEA/CHMP/32775/05, London, United Kingdom.

EMA (2006). Guideline on similar biological medicinal products containing biotechnology-derived proteins as active substance: non-clinical and clinical issues. EMEA/CHMP/BMWP/42832, London, United Kingdom.

EMA (2009). Guideline on non-clinical and clinical development of similar biological medicinal products containing low-molecular-weight-heparins. EMEA/CHMP/BMWP/118264/07, London, United Kingdom.

EMA (2010). Draft guideline on similar biological medicinal products containing monoclonal antibodies. EMA/CHMP/BMWP/403543/2010, London, United Kingdom.

EMA (2011). Concept paper on the revision of the guideline on similar biological medicinal product. EMA/CHMP/BMWP/572643, London, United Kingdom.

EMA. (2005b). Guideline on Similar Biological Medicinal Products Containing Biotechnology-derived Proteins as Active Substance: Quality Issues. EMEA/CHMP/BWP/49348, London, United Kingdom.

FDA (2012a). Draft Guidance for Industry from FDA: Scientific Considerations in Demonstrating Biosimilarity to a Reference Product. Center for Drug Evaluation and Research (CDER) and Center for Biologics Evaluation and Research (CBER), the United States Food and Drug Administration, Silver Spring, Maryland.

FDA (2012b). Draft Guidance for Industry from FDA: S Quality Considerations in Demonstrating Biosimilarity to a Reference Protein Product. Center for Drug Evaluation and Research (CDER) and Center for Biologics Evaluation and Research (CBER), the United States Food and Drug Administration, Silver Spring, Maryland.

FDA (2012c). Draft Guidance for Industry from FDA: Biosimilars: Questions and Answers Regarding Implementation of the Biologics Price Competition and Innovation (BPCI) Act of 2009. Center for Drug Evaluation and Research (CDER) and Center for Biologics Evaluation and Research (CBER), the United States Food and Drug Administration, Silver Spring, Maryland.

FDA (2015). Guidance for Industry – Scientific Considerations in Demonstrating Biosimilarity to a Reference Product. Center for Drug Evaluation and Research (CDER) and Center for Biologics Evaluation and Research (CBER), the United States Food and Drug Administration, Silver Spring, Maryland.

FDA (2017). Guidance for Industry – Statistical Approaches to Evaluate Analytical Similarity. Center for Drug Evaluation and Research (CDER) and Center for Biologics Evaluation and Research (CBER), the United States Food and Drug Administration, Silver Spring, Maryland, September 2017.

FDA (2019). Guidance for Industry – Development of Therapeutic Protein Biosimilars: Comparative Analytical Assessment and Other Quality-Related Considerations. Center for Drug Evaluation and Research (CDER) and Center for Biologics Evaluation and Research, the United States Food and Drug Administrations, Silver Spring, Maryland.

FDA (2003). Guidance on bioavailability and bioequivalence studies for orally administrated drug products – general considerations, center for drug evaluation and research, the United States Food and Drug Administration, Rockville, Maryland, USA.

Glintborg, B. et al. (2016). Thu0123non-medical switch from originator to biosimilar infliximab among patients with inflammatory rheumatic disease – impact on s-infliximab and antidrug-antibodies. results from the national danish rheumatologic biobank and the danbio registry. Annals of the Rheumatic Diseases, 75(Suppl 2), 224.2–224.

HC (2010). Authority of the Minister of Health. Guidance for sponsors: information and submission requirements for subsequent entry biologics (SEBs).

Hsieh, T. C., Nicolay, B. N., Frolov, M. V., and Moon, N. S. (2010). Tuberous sclerosis complex 1 regulates de2f1 expression during development and cooperates with rbf1 to control proliferation and survival. Plos Genetics, 6(8), e1001071.

Kang, S. H., and Chow, S. C. (2013). Statistical assessment of biosimilarity based on relative distance between follow-on biologics. Statistics in Medicine 32(3), 382–92. https://doi.org/10.1002/sim.5582.

KFDA (2009). Korean guidelines on the evaluation of similar biotherapeutic products (SBPs). Seoul, Korea,

Lee, S. J., Oh, M., and Chow, S. C. (2019). Equivalence test with flexible margin in analytical similarity assessment. Enliven: Biosimilars and Bioavailability, 3(2), 5–11.

Li, J. and Chow. S. C. (2015). Confidence region approach for assessing bioequivalence and biosimilarity accounting for heterogeneity of variability. Journal of Probability and Statistics 2015.

MHLW (2009). Guidelines for the quality, safety and efficacy Assurance of follow-on biologics. Japan, 2009.

Roger S. D. (2006). Biosimilars: how similar or dissimilar are they? Nephrology (Carlton). 11(4), 341–346.

Roger, S. D. and Mikhail, A. (2007). Biosimilars: opportunity or cause for concern. Journal of Pharmacy and Pharmaceutical Sciences, 10(3), 405–410.

Schuirmann D. J. (1987). A comparison of the two one-sided tests procedure and the power approach for assessing the equivalence of average bioavailability. Journal of Pharmacokinetics and Pharmacodynamics, 15(6), 657–680.

Shutter, S. (2017). Biosimilar sponsors seek statistical flexibility when reference product change. FDA Pink Sheet.

Son, S., Oh, M., Choo, M., Chow, S. C., and Lee, S. J. (2020). Some thoughts on the QR method for analytical similarity evaluation, Journal of Biopharmaceutical Statistics, (1), 1–16.

Suh, S.K. and Park, Y. (2011). Regulatory guideline for biosimilar products in Korea. Biologicals, 39, 336–338.

Thatcher, N. et al. (2019). Efficacy & safety of biosimilar abp 215 compared with bevacizumab in patients with advanced non-small cell lung cancer (Maple): a randomized, double-blind, phase 3 study. Clinical Cancer Research, 25(10), 3193.

Wang, J. and Chow, S.C. (2012). On regulatory approval pathway of biosimilar products. Pharmaceuticals, 5, 353–368.

WHO (2009). Guidelines on evaluation of similar biotherapeutic products (SBPs). WHO, Geneva, Switzerland.

Yu L. X. (2004). Bioinequivalence: concept and definition. Presented at Advisory Committee for Pharmaceutical Science of the Food and Drug Administration. Rockville, Maryland.

Zheng, J., Chow, S. C., and Yuan, M. (2017). On assessing bioequivalence and interchangeability between generics based on indirect comparisons. Statistics in Medicine. 36(10), 100.

9

Statistical Methods for Assessment of Complex Generic Drugs

Yongpei Yu

Peking University Clinical Research Institute, Beijing, China

CONTENTS

DOI: 10.1201/9781003107323-9

9.1 Introduction: Complex Generic Products

Generic drugs are drug products that contain the same Active Pharmaceutical Drug Ingredient (API) as an already marketed brand-name drug. A generic drug should be identical with its brand-name version in dosage form, safety, strength, route of administration, quality, performance characteristics and intended use. In many countries, generic drugs are approved through an Abbreviated New Drug Application (ANDA). In other words, generic drug applications are generally not required to demonstrate safety and effectiveness of the generic product through animal and clinical studies like innovative drugs. Instead, a generic drug application should demonstrate that the generic drug would follow a similar behavior in human body as its brand-name counterparts. Bioequivalence (BE) is a primary evidence for the approval of generic drugs. In the US Food and Drug Administration (FDA) guidance, BE is defined as "the absence of a significant difference in the rate and extent to which the active ingredient or active moiety in pharmaceutical equivalents or pharmaceutical alternatives becomes available at the site of drug action when administered at the same molar dose under similar conditions in an appropriately designed study" (US FDA, 2020a).

In a typical BE study, Pharmacokinetic (PK) parameters such as Area Under Blood/ Plasma Concentration-Time Curve (AUC) and maximum concentration (C_{max}) are used as primary endpoints for comparing drug absorption profiles between the generic drug and the brand-name counterparts. For each volunteer, blood samples should be collected at scheduled times, and thus the concentration-time profile is obtained. The PK parameters of each volunteer can be estimated using Noncompartmental Analysis (NCA). Then the geometric means and corresponding Confidence Interval (CI) can be calculated based on log-transformed PK parameters (Chen, 2014). According to the current guidance of the FDA as well as most other regulated authorities, generic drugs could be claimed to be BE to the brand-name counterparts if the 90% confidence interval of geometric means of primary PK parameter lies within the BE criteria of (0.80,1.25). This procedure is commonly referred to as one-size-fits-all approach and can be used for BE assessment of most systemically acting drugs (Chow, 2014).

However, the one-size-fits-all approach may not be adequate for all cases. For example, the development of locally acting ophthalmic drugs, the systemic exposure of drugs may not represent their therapeutic effect (Kanfer & Shargel, 2007). Thus, the one-size-fits-all approach, focusing on comparison of PK parameters, may not be an optimal solution for demonstration of therapeutic equivalence. For the development of those generic drugs with challenging issues, BE methodologies should be established based on the complexities of different products. As stated in the Generic Drug User Fee Amendments (GDUFA) commitment letter (GDUFA, 2016), complex scenarios can be classified into five categories: complex active ingredients, complex formulations, complex dosage forms, complex routes of delivery, and complex drug-device combinations.

Complex active ingredients mainly include polymeric compounds, peptides, and complex mixtures of APIs. The first step in assessment of this kind of drug is the demonstration of API sameness between generic and innovative drugs. This is often a challenging issue, as the measures and criteria of API sameness vary with the characteristics of the drugs. BE would then be assessed after the API sameness is demonstrated (US FDA, 2014b, 2016b).

The second category is complex formulations/dosage forms, such as liposomes, suspensions, and emulsions. Complexities of formulations/dosage forms usually come from inactive ingredients. According to the FDA guidances, a generic drug for parenteral use should contain the same inactive ingredients, referred to as "Q1", and in the same concentration, referred to as "Q2", with the innovative drug. The demonstration of Q1/Q2 sameness should be prior to the BE assessment. Moreover, since the manufacturing condition and characteristics of inactive ingredients may affect the drug release profile, *in vitro* studies for drug release or/and other characteristics such as liposome size distribution may be necessary as supportive evidence of in vivo BE (US FDA, 2018d; Zheng et al., 2014).

Most drugs with complex routes of delivery are locally acting drugs. For locally acting drugs, the drug concentration in system circulation may not represent the target-site exposure. In addition, the drug concentration in system circulation could be very low and even undetectable. Consequently, study design, study population, endpoints, and statistical methods for BE assessment should be considered according to the characteristics of the drug and target tissue (Braddy et al., 2015).

Drug-device combinations are used in a variety of applications, such as implantable contraception for birth control, inhalers for asthma, and auto-injectors for life-threatening allergic reactions (Saluja et al., 2014). For drug-device combinations, the drug delivery performance highly depends on the devices. Therefore, *in vitro* studies are often necessary to demonstrate the generic product is equivalence in device performance with the reference product. On the other hand, many drug-device combinations are locally acting drugs, such as oral inhalers for treating pulmonary disease and nasal sprays for nasal diseases (Choi et al., 2018). Traditional PK-based BE studies may not be adequate, and additional studies well pharmacodynamics (PD) or clinical endpoints are often required for BE assessment of drug-device combinations (US FDA, 2019c, 2020b).

In practice, a drug product could have several forms of complexity. Identifying the complexities and determining the necessary studies for BE assessment are primary challenges in the development of complex generic drugs. FDA has issued a series of Product-Specific Guidance (PSG) documents that cover a range of critical issues, including scientific concerns, required studies, study design, analytical methods and statistical methods for BE assessment of specific complex generic drugs (Lunawat & Bhat, 2020). In this chapter, we focus on statistical methods and considerations of study design in BE assessment of complex generic drugs. The remainder of this chapter is organized as follows. Section 9.2 discusses regulatory aspect of complex generic drugs. In addition, for each category of complexity, at least one representative PSGs are introduced in this section. Section 9.3 and Section 9.4 discuss statistical design and analysis of *in vivo* and *in vitro* studies in development of complex generic drugs, respectively. Several representative cases of development of complex generic drugs are illustrated in Section 9.5. Some concluding remarks are given in Section 9.6.

9.2 Regulatory Perspectives

9.2.1 Current Regulatory Framework of FDA for Complex Generic Drugs

Controlling the cost of healthcare is a major public health issue that regulatory authorities, such as US FDA, should be concern. Regulatory authorities generally don't involve price making directly but affect drug pricing through policy-making. The price of generic drugs is significantly lower than the price of brand-name drugs, approval of generic drugs could help lower drug costs by increasing competition in the biopharmaceutical market. Thus, we can see policies of different regulatory authorities are intended to make the development process of generic drugs more scientific and efficient.

In 1984, the US FDA issued the *Drug Price Competition and Patent Term Restoration Act*, which assumes that BE is an effective surrogate for safety and efficacy (Kanfer & Shargel, 2007). Based on this act, the current approval pathway of generic drugs is established. Generic drugs could be approved based on evidence of average BE in drug absorption through the conduct of bioavailability and BE studies. However, for some drugs with one or more features that make them difficult to be genericized, the traditional one-size-fits-all approach may not be adequate or appropriate. As stated in the GDUFA commitment letter (Choi et al., 2018; GDUFA, 2016), complex scenarios can be classified into five categories:

- Complex active ingredients;
- Complex formulations;
- Complex dosage forms;
- Complex routes of delivery;
- Complex drug-device combinations.

Complex drugs may have one or more of these complexities. In some cases, costly, complex brand-name drugs have lost their exclusivity but are still not subject to any generic competition. FDA has carried out a number of different policies to address insufficient competition for complex drugs.

In 2017, FDA announced the Drug Competition Action Plan (DCAP). One primary goal of this plan is to provide as much scientific and regulatory clarity as possible with respect to complex generic drugs. As the categories, indications and manufacturing process of complex drugs varies, it is difficult to develop a complete guidance to cover all possible uncertainties in development of complex generic drugs. Instead, under the framework of DCAP, FDA issued numbers of product-specific guidance documents, as well as several general guidelines for certain scientific issues, such as:

- Assessing Adhesion With Transdermal and Topical Delivery Systems (TDS) for Abbreviated New Drug Applications (Draft, October 2018),
- Assessing the Irritation and Sensitization Potential of Transdermal and Topical Delivery Systems for Abbreviated New Drug Applications (Draft, October 2018),

- General Principles for Evaluating the Abuse Deterrence of Generic Solid Oral Opioid Drug Products (Final, November 2017),
- ANDAs for Certain Highly Purified Synthetic Peptide Drug Products that Refer to Listed Drugs of rDNA Origin (Draft, October 2017),
- Comparative Analyses and Related Comparative Use Human Factors Studies for a Drug-Device Combination Product Submitted in an ANDA (Draft, January 2017).

FDA also encourages generic drug companies to communicate with FDA at each stage of generic drug development process. Generic drug companies can submit written inquiries, which is referred to as controlled correspondence, to the Office of Generic Drugs (OGD) to requests for information on a specific element of generic drug development. The scope of controlled correspondence encompasses a broad spectrum of issues in generic drug development. However, in some cases, the controlled correspondence may not be adequate for some complex inquires, such as asking for recommendations on appropriate BE study designs for a specific drug product or review of BE clinical protocols. In order to further facilitate the development of complex generic drugs, FDA permits a series of formal meetings between FDA and generic drug companies that intends to develop complex generic drugs. Such formal meetings are: (i) product develop meetings, (ii) pre-submission meetings, and (iii) mid-review-cycle meetings. These meetings will be very helpful to reduce the uncertainty in the development and regulatory review of complex generic drugs, especially for products that there are no PSGs or alternative approaches for reference. In such cases, the applicants are encouraged to propose solutions for specific scientific issues such as proposed study designs or statistical methods.

In addition to guidance documents and formal communications, FDA holds a number of public meetings as well as a public workshop on specific topics of complex generic drug development, review, and approval pathways. Moreover, FDA has conducted a series of research on regulatory science of complex generic drugs. FDA will carry out PSGs for certain products when appropriate methodologies and approval pathways are established. To date, FDA has issued more than 1650 PSGs since 2007.

9.2.2 Product-Specific Guidances (PSGs)

The PSGs are essential to reduce the uncertainty in development of complex generic drugs. Although, the features that cause the complexity of drug products to vary, the regulatory considerations for a certain category of complexity are likely to be similar. Consequently, different drugs with certain complexity may have similar approval pathways. In this section, several representative product-specific guidances for each type of complexity are briefly introduced.

9.2.2.1 Complex Active Ingredients

Drugs with complex APIs mainly include polymeric compounds, peptides, molecular complexes and complex mixtures of APIs. The complexity of these drugs mainly comes from the complex structure, impurity and may be difficult to be characterized by common analytical methods. For assessment of drugs with complex APIs, the first and foremost issue is to demonstrate the sameness of APIs. After that, BE studies would be conducted.

Glatiramer acetate is a complex mixture of synthetic polypeptides, which is a representative of drugs with complex APIs. In the PSG of glatiramer acetate, a four-stage criterion is recommended for the demonstration of API sameness (Bell et al., 2017; US FDA, 2018c): (i) equivalence of fundamental reaction scheme; (ii) equivalence of physicochemical properties including compositions; (iii) equivalence of structural signatures for polymerization and depolymerization; and (iv) equivalence of biological assay results. A biological assay can serve as a confirmatory test of equivalence and provide complementary confirmation of API sameness. As the formulation of glatiramer acetate relatively simple (parenteral solution), if the generic product is qualitatively (Q1) and quantitatively (Q2) the same in terms of API and inactive ingredients as the reference product, the requirement of *in vivo* BE study could be waived (US FDA, 2018c).

Naturally-sourced conjugated estrogens tablet is another representative instance of this category. Naturally-sourced conjugated estrogens is a complex mixture derived from pregnant mares' urine. As indicated in the PSG of naturally-sourced conjugated estrogens, the sameness of API can be established based on comparative physicochemical characterizations, and following tests should be conducted (US FDA, 2014b): (i) identification test for steroidal components; (ii) the USP quantification test for ten steroidal components; (iii) control of major non-USP steroidal components; (iv) control of additional steroidal components in the test API batches; (v) total steroidal components content test; and (vi) non-steroidal components in the test API batches. The sameness of API could be established if corresponding qualitative and quantitative criteria are met. After that, Four *in vivo* BE studies for different strengths, as well as fed and fasting state, should be conducted to establish BE between generic products and innovative products.

9.2.2.2 Complex Formulations

Complex formulations mainly encompass liposomes, suspensions and emulsions. The first and foremost issue in assessment of generic drugs with complex formulations/dosage forms is to demonstrate the sameness of inactive ingredients in terms of qualitative (Q1) and quantitative (Q2) methods. After that, *in vivo* BE studies could be conducted. In addition, since *in vitro* and *in vivo* drug release profiles are sensitive to manufacturing differences as well as characteristics of inactive ingredients, *in vitro* studies are often needed (Lee et al., 2016).

Doxorubicin hydrochloride injectable liposome is a representative of drugs with complex formulation. In the PSG of glatiramer acetate, the generic product should meet the criteria including Q1/Q2 sameness of inactive ingredients and equivalent liposome characteristics to be eligible for the bioequivalence studies. An *in vivo* BE study and an *in vitro* population BE (PBE) study for liposome size distribution are recommended to establish the BE (US FDA, 2018b).

9.2.2.3 Complex Dosage Forms

Complex dosage forms are generally products with complex release mechanisms, delivery systems, or complicated manufacturing processes, such as Long-Acting Injectables (LAIs), transdermal patches, and Metered-Dose Inhalers (MDIs). Pathways for assessment of products with complex dosage forms vary with the characteristics of the product (Kanfer & Shargel, 2007).

Risperidone depot suspension is a long-acting dosage form consisting of microspheres. Similar to the liposome drug products, the PSG of risperidone depot suspension requires the demonstration of Q1/Q2 sameness prior to BE assessment. Both *in vitro* and *in vivo* studies are required for BE assessment. The *in vitro* study is focused on drug release profiles. As risperidone depot suspension is a long-acting dosage form, the *in vivo* study would be performed in patients who are already receiving stable risperidone intramuscular treatment and at steady-state (US FDA, 2016e).

Topical delivery system is another large category of complex dosage form. For drugs with a topical delivery system, equivalence on characteristics related to dosage forms such as adhesion and dermal response should be demonstrated and included in the ANDA package (Sun et al., 2019). For instance, in the PSG document of selegiline patch, three *in vivo* studies, including a PK BE study, an adhesion study, as well as a skin irritation and sensitization study, are recommended to establish BE (US FDA, 2018e). In addition, in 2018, FDA issued two draft guidance documents, in which scientific consideration on design and analysis for adhesion and dermal response studies, respectively (US FDA, 2018f, 2018g).

9.2.2.4 Complex Routes of Delivery

Most drugs with complex routes of delivery are locally acting drugs, in which case the systemic drug exposure may not represent their therapeutic effect in the target site. For these drugs, BE studies with systemic PK endpoints can hardly yield a conclusion of therapeutic equivalence. Consequently, *in vitro* studies and *in vivo* studies with clinical endpoints, PD endpoints, as well as drug concentration in local tissues are considered in BE assessment for locally acting drugs (Braddy & Conner, 2014; Saluja et al., 2014).

In practice, clinical endpoints are used in most BE studies for locally acting drugs. Acyclovir cream, which is a topical medication for herpes infections, is a classical representative of drugs with complex routes of delivery. In guidance for acyclovir cream (US FDA, 2016a), FDA recommended two pathways to establish BE. The first option is to conduct *in vitro* studies. First, the Q1/Q2 sameness of the generic and the reference product should be demonstrated. After that, physicochemical analyses should be conducted to demonstrate that the generic product is physically and structurally similar, referred to as "Q3" with the reference product. Then an *In Vitro* Release Test (IVRT) study and an *In Vitro* Permeation Test (IVPT) study could be conducted as pivotal studies for application. The other option for establishing BE is to conduct an in vivo study with clinical endpoints. A randomized, three-arm, placebo-controlled BE study is recommended.

BE studies with clinical endpoints are relatively expensive and require large numbers of subjects. Therefore, if there exist acceptable PK or PD endpoints, these endpoints can be preferred. For instance, for topical dermatologic corticosteroid drug products, BE can be established using in vivo PD studies. The PD endpoint for dermatologic corticosteroid drug products is obtained through the McKenzie-Stoughton Vasoconstrictor Assay (VCA) approach (Smith et al., 1993). The VCA approach is based on the fact that a corticosteroid product will cause vasoconstriction of the skin microvasculature and consequently will produce a visible blanching response over time. Note that the VCA approach is limited only to dermatologic corticosteroid drug products. Mometasone furoate cream is a representative of this category. For BE assessment of mometasone furoate cream, both a pilot and pivotal vasoconstrictor study are recommended. The aim of the pilot study is to determine the appropriate dose duration for use in the subsequent pivotal BE study (US FDA, 2016c).

Ophthalmic corticosteroid drugs are another instance of BE assessment for locally acting drugs using non-clinical endpoints. Corticosteroids can be absorbed into the anterior chamber across the epithelium and corneal stroma and be eliminated by aqueous flow and by diffusion into the blood circulation. Consequently, BE of corticosteroid eye drops can be established using *in vivo* study with Aqueous Humor (AH) PK endpoints (Harigaya et al., 2018). Nepafenac ophthalmic suspension is a representative of ophthalmic corticosteroid drugs. As recommended in the PSG for Nepafenac ophthalmic suspension (US FDA, 2016d), besides of the two options of *in vitro* Q1/Q2/Q3 sameness and the *in vivo* BE study with clinical endpoint, an *in vivo* AH serial sampling (a special case of sparse sampling) PK study can be performed for BE assessment of Nepafenac ophthalmic suspension.

9.2.2.5 Complex Drug-Device Combinations

Drug-device combinations are used in a variety of applications, such as implantable contraception for birth control, inhalers for asthma and auto-injectors for life-threatening allergic reactions. Generally, drug-device combination products are consist of drug constituent part and device constituent part, where the main function of the device constituent part is drug delivery (Choi et al., 2018). The efficacy of these products depends not only on active ingredients and formulations but also on the performance of device constituent parts. Therefore, *in vitro* studies are often necessary to demonstrate the generic product is equivalence in device performance with the reference product.

Metered-Dose Inhalers (MDIs), Dry Powder Inhalers (DPIs), and nasal sprays are classical representatives of drug-device combination products. For BE assessment of these products, *in vitro* studies for evaluation of drug delivery characteristics should be conducted prior to *in vivo* PK BE study and PD BE study (or clinical endpoint BE study). In the case of albuterol sulfate aerosol, which is delivered through a metered-dose inhaler, equivalence in device characteristics including: (i) Single Actuation Content (SAC); (ii) Aerodynamic Particle Size Distribution (APSD); (iii) spray pattern; (iv) plume geometry; and (v) priming and repriming are required to be demonstrated. After that, an *in vivo* PK BE study should be conducted (Saluja et al., 2014). However, one *in vivo* PK BE study may not be adequate, as albuterol sulfate aerosol is locally acting and systemic exposure doesn't reflect therapeutic effect. Therefore, a PD study, in which PD endpoint is obtained through a bronchoprovocation test, is required to establish BE. For products that have no suitable PD endpoints, such as triamcinolone acetonide nasal spray for the treatment of allergic rhinitis, a comparative clinical endpoint BE study is generally needed (US FDA, 2020c).

9.2.2.6 Remarks

In practice, a complex generic drug may have more than one complex feature. Consequently, pathways for establishing BE can be very different for different categories of drugs. Therefore, PSGs are essential in developing complex generic drugs. For BE assessment of complex generic drugs, a variety of uncertainties, including characteristics to be evaluated, analytical methods, endpoints, study designs, BE standard and statistical methods etc. are recommended in PSGs. For a generic product that there is no PSG, the generic companies can propose methods for establishing BE or find an alternative approach in guidance for other products and then communicate with FDA through controlled correspondence or formal meetings. In addition, FDA has conducted and supported a number of researches on methodologies in development of generic drugs. Corresponding outcomes are published in terms of literature, guidance documents and public workshops.

On the other hand, in addition to the complexities listed in the GDUFA commitment letter, there are Highly Variable (HV) drugs and Narrow Therapeutic Index (NTI) drugs. Complexity of these drugs generally come from characteristics of drug substance rather than characteristics related to manufacturing process and formulation, such as impurity, excipient and particle size etc. Since the one-size-fits-all approach is not suitable for HV drugs and NTI drugs, FDA developed a Reference-Scaled Average BE (RSABE) approach for establishing BE for HV drugs and NTI drugs.

9.3 In Vivo Studies

Pathways for establishing BE vary considerably for generic drugs with different categories of complexity, and correspondingly, study design, endpoints, as well as statistical methods for BE studies could be quite different. In this section, Study design and analysis methods for *in vivo* BE studies for different application scenarios, including: (i) BE studies with clinical endpoints, (ii) vasoconstrictor BE study for topical dermatologic corticosteroids, (iii) PD BE study using the dose-scale method, (iv) AH PK BE study for topical ophthalmic corticosteroids, (v) RSABE study for NTI drugs, as well as (vi) studies for assessing adhesion, skin irritation and sensitization of TDS are introduced.

9.3.1 Bioequivalence Studies with Clinical Endpoints

Studies with clinical endpoints are not an efficient way for establishing BE as these studies are generally time-consuming and cost-intensive, but in some cases, it is the only option due to limitations in methodology. BE studies with clinical endpoints are mostly applied in studies for locally acting drugs. For simplicity, the terminology "BE studies with clinical endpoints" is referred to as "clinical BE study" in the rest of this Section.

9.3.1.1 *Study Design Considerations*

In a number of PSGs, a three-arm, placebo-controlled, parallel design is recommended for clinical BE studies. While the use of a placebo control arm in a generic drug study may have ethical challenges, as the reference products have already proved to be effective, a placebo-controlled study can provide not only evidence of BE of generic and brand-name drugs but also direct evidence of effectiveness for generic drugs. Because of these controversies, at the planning stage of a study, it should be carefully considered whether a placebo arm should be included based on the indication being treated as well as scientific necessity. To prevent a non-effective drug from being approved, BE should be concluded if the test product is clinically equivalence to the reference product, and both the test and reference product are superior to the placebo group (Peters, 2014; US FDA, 2019a).

Endpoints of clinical BE studies vary with the indication and category of product. In BE study, most endpoints are binary or continuous. For instance, in studies of triamcinolone acetonide nasal spray for treatment of seasonal allergic rhinitis, the recommended primary endpoint is the difference in the mean change in reflective total nasal symptom scores from baseline through the treatment period (US FDA, 2020c); in studies of ciclopirox cream for treatment of tinea pedis, the primary endpoint is the proportion of therapeutic cure, which is defined as both mycological cure and clinical cure (US FDA, 2011).

A Per-Protocol (PP) population and a modified Intent-to-Treat (mITT) population should be pre-defined for establishing BE. The PP population is used for equivalent analysis. Although there is not a standard definition of PP population for all products, the following criteria can be considered for reference:

i. Meet all inclusion/exclusion criteria.

ii. Well compliant with pre-specified dosing schedules.

iii. Complete the effect evaluation within the designated visit window with no protocol violations that would affect the treatment evaluation (e.g. loss to follow-up, using restricted medications during the study).

The mITT population, on the other hand, is generally defined as all randomized subjects who use at least one dose of product. The superiority tests are performed using the mITT population (Peters, 2014).

9.3.1.2 Statistical Analysis

Let θ_1 and θ_2 be the pre-specified BE limits. For binary endpoints, the hypotheses for equivalence test are given as follows:

$$H_0: \pi_T - \pi_R < \theta_1 \quad \text{or} \quad \pi_T - \pi_R > \theta_2 \quad \text{versus} \quad H_a: \theta_1 \leq \pi_T - \pi_R \leq \theta_2,$$

where π_T and π_R are the success proportion of the test group and reference group, respectively.

All statistical methods that are suitable for a non-inferiority test for proportions, such as asymptotic Wald test and Farrington-Manning (score) test, can be applied to perform the Two One-Sided Tests (TOST) for equivalence analysis(Grosser et al., 2015). BE would be established if the 90% confidence interval of $(\pi_T - \pi_R)$ lies within the interval $[\theta_1, \theta_2]$. The bioequivalence limits, θ_1 and θ_2, are different for different drugs and indications. In the case of triamcinolone acetonide nasal spray for treatment of seasonal allergic rhinitis, the BE limits are −0.20 and 0.20.

For continuous endpoints, such as the mean change in reflective total nasal symptom scores from baseline in seasonal allergic rhinitis studies, the following hypotheses are recommended in the FDA guidance:

$$H_0: \pi_T / \pi_R < \theta_1 \quad \text{or} \quad \pi_T / \pi_R > \theta_2 \quad \text{versus} \quad H_a: \theta_1 \leq \pi_T / \pi_R \leq \theta_2,$$

where π_T and π_R are the mean of the primary endpoint for the test and reference group, respectively. Unlike PK BE study, in which the study data is log-transformed and tested using the Schuirmann's TOST, log transformation is not suitable in clinical BE studies, as clinical endpoints such as change from baseline could be both positive and negative. Instead, equivalence test for clinical BE study could be performed using Fieller's method (Cox, 1990).

Assuming that the clinical endpoints of the test and reference products are mutually independent and normally distributed. Let $\hat{X}_T$ and $\hat{X}_R$ be the estimator of the treatment effect of the test and reference group, π_T and π_R, respectively. The parameter of interest is $\theta = \pi_T / \pi_R$. Using Fieller's method, a confidence interval for the parameter of interest θ is derived from the statistic:

$$T = \frac{\hat{X}_T - \theta \hat{X}_R}{\sqrt{\hat{\sigma}_T^2 + \theta^2 \hat{\sigma}_R^2 - 2\theta \hat{\sigma}_{TR}}}, \tag{9.1}$$

where $\hat{\sigma}_T^2$, $\hat{\sigma}_R^2$, and $\hat{\sigma}_{TR}$ are estimators of the variance of π_T and π_R, and the covariance of π_T and π_R, respectively. Note that in a parallel group design, the covariance σ_{TR} is zero. The statistic T has a central t distribution with $(n_1 + n_2 - 2)$ degrees of freedom. Hence, by resolving the following equation about T:

$$\left\{ \theta \mid T^2 \leq t_{\alpha, n_1 + n_2 - 2}^2 \right\}, \tag{9.2}$$

a $(1 - 2\alpha) \times 100\%$ confidence interval for θ can be obtained. The two roots of this quadratic are the lower and upper limits of the Fieller confidence interval for θ, which are given by:

$$\theta_L = \left[-B - \left(B^2 - AC \right)^{1/2} \right] / A$$

and

$$\theta_U = \left[-B + \left(B^2 - AC \right)^{1/2} \right] / A, \tag{9.3}$$

where

$$A = \hat{X}_R^2 - t_{\alpha, n_1 + n_2 - 2}^2 \hat{\sigma}_R^2,$$

$$B = t_{\alpha, n_1 + n_2 - 2}^2 \hat{\sigma}_{TR} - \hat{X}_T \hat{X}_R,$$

$$C = \hat{X}_T^2 - t_{\alpha, n_1 + n_2 - 2}^2 \hat{\sigma}_T^2. \tag{9.4}$$

If the 90% confidence interval for π_T / π_R, (θ_L, θ_U), lies within the interval $[\theta_1, \theta_2]$, the bioequivalence could be concluded. As discussed by Fieller, obtaining an interpretable confidence interval requires that $\hat{X}_T^2 / \hat{\sigma}_T^2 > t_{\alpha, n_1 + n_2 - 2}^2$ and $\hat{X}_R^2 / \hat{\sigma}_R^2 > t_{\alpha, n_1 + n_2 - 2}^2$ are both satisfied. In other words, both π_T and π_R should be statistically significant compared to 0 in order to construct a Fieller confidence interval that contains no negative values.

In addition, in some cases, baseline values and study sites are recommended to be taken into account. Therefore, a generalized linear model including treatment group, study sites, and baseline would be fitted. The Fieller's methods can also be extended to the matrix formulation of generalized linear model (Sykes, 2000). The treatment effect of each product can be expressed as a linear combination of model parameters. Hence, the parameter of interest becomes $\theta = K'\beta / L'\beta$, where K and L are $p \times 1$ vectors of constants, and respectively, $K'\hat{\beta}$ and $L'\hat{\beta}$ are least square means of test and reference products that adjusted for covariates such as sites and baseline in the model. Then the parameters A, B, and C can be obtained follow the same procedure using Fieller's method, as:

$$A = \left(L'\hat{\beta} \right)^2 - t_{\alpha, n_1 + n_2 - p - 1}^2 L' I^{-1} \left(\hat{\beta} \right) L \hat{\sigma}^2,$$

$$B = t_{\alpha, n_1 + n_2 - p - 1}^2 K' I^{-1} \left(\hat{\beta} \right) L \hat{\sigma}^2 - \left(L'\hat{\beta} \right) \left(K'\hat{\beta} \right),$$

$$C = \left(K'\hat{\beta} \right)^2 - t_{\alpha, n_1 + n_2 - p - 1}^2 K' I^{-1} \left(\hat{\beta} \right) K \hat{\sigma}^2. \tag{9.5}$$

where $I^{-1}(\hat{\beta})$ is the estimator of the information matrix. To obtain an interpretable confidence interval, both $K'\beta$ and $L'\beta$ should be statistically significantly different from zero.

9.3.1.3 Sample Size Considerations

The sample size of a clinical BE study should provide sufficient power not only for the demonstration of clinical equivalence of the test and reference products but also the superiority test comparing with placebo. For superiority tests, as well as the equivalence test for binary endpoints, the sample size can be calculated through the power function of the corresponding statistical methods. While the sample size calculation for equivalence test for continuous endpoints is relatively different.

As presented by Hauschke et al.(Hauschke et al., 1999) and Berger et al.(Berger & Hsu, 1996), a likelihood ratio test proposed by Sasabuchi (Berger, 1989), referred to as the T_1 / T_2 test, can always lead to the same decision on BE with the Fieller confidence interval. In this way, the power of the Fieller confidence interval can be analyzed using the power function of the T_1/T_2 test. The statistics of the T_1/T_2 test in a parallel clinical BE study are given by:

$$T_1 = \frac{\hat{X}_T - \theta_1 \hat{X}_R}{\sqrt{\hat{\xi}_T^2/n_1 + \theta_1^2 \hat{\xi}_R^2/n_2}} \quad \text{and} \quad T_2 = \frac{\hat{X}_T - \theta_2 \hat{X}_R}{\sqrt{\hat{\xi}_T^2/n_1 + \theta_2^2 \hat{\xi}_R^2/n_2}}, \tag{9.6}$$

where $\hat{\xi}_T^2$ and $\hat{\xi}_R^2$ are the estimator of the variance of the test and reference group, ξ_T^2 and ξ_R^2, respectively. Without losing generality, assume that number of subjects in each group is n. BE can be concluded if and only if $T_1 \geq t_{\alpha,2n-2}$ and $T_2 \leq -t_{\alpha,2n-2}$. The power function is given by:

$$1 - \beta = Pr\left(T_1 > t_{\alpha,2n-2} \text{ and } T_2 < -t_{\alpha,2n-2} \mid \theta_1 < \theta < \theta_2, \sigma_T^2, \sigma_R^2, \rho\right), \tag{9.7}$$

where ρ is the correlation coefficient between T_1 and T_2. Note that in a T_1/T_2 test, two statistics T_1 and T_2 are correlated. The random vector (T_1, T_2) follows a bivariate non-central t-distribution with non-centrality parameters φ_1, φ_2, and correlation coefficient ρ, which are given by:

$$\varphi_1 = \frac{\pi_T - \theta_1 \pi_R}{\sqrt{\left(\xi_T^2 + \theta_1^2 \xi_R^2\right)/n}} \quad \text{and} \quad \varphi_2 = \frac{\pi_T - \theta_2 \pi_R}{\sqrt{\left(\xi_T^2 + \theta_2^2 \xi_R^2/n\right)}};$$

$$\rho(T_1, T_2) = \frac{\sigma_T^2 + \theta_1 \theta_2 \sigma_R^2}{\sqrt{\left(\sigma_T^2 + \theta_1^2 \sigma_R^2\right)\left(\sigma_T^2 + \theta_2^2 \sigma_R^2\right)}}. \tag{9.8}$$

In this way, for a specific power level, the sample size of each group n can be calculated numerically using Owen' Q function, as:

$$1 - \beta = Q\left(\infty, -t_{\alpha,2n-2}, \varphi_1, \varphi_2, \rho\right) - Q\left(t_{\alpha,v}, -t_{\alpha,2n-2}, \varphi_1, \varphi_2, \rho\right). \tag{9.9}$$

9.3.2 PD Bioequivalence Study Using the Dose-Scale Method

When PK or *in vitro* studies are not applicable for BE assessment of certain products, PD BE studies are very recommended. Comparing with clinical BE studies, PD BE studies are lower cost, shorter in study duration, and more flexible in study design. Therefore, when there exists a suitable PD measurement, a PD BE study can be given priority over clinical BE studies. Generally, PD BE studies are recommended when: (i) lack of suitable analytical methods, (ii) PK endpoints can not be used as surrogate endpoints for efficacy and safety, and (iii) PK endpoints are not available due to sampling difficulty or other limitations (Zou & Yu, 2014).

In PD BE studies, the nonlinear dose-PD response relationship is a complex issue. Generally, the dose-PD response may have a linear portion only around EC_{50}. Within this range, the observed PD response difference can proportionally reflect the dose difference, which is same as the case of dose-PK response, and therefore, BE can be tested using PD endpoints in the same way as using PK endpoints. On the other hand, when the dose is in the nonlinear range of the dose-PD response curve, the PD response difference between test and reference product may not directly reflect the differences in relative bioavailability of two products because of nonlinear dose-PD response relationship. Therefore, in such cases, a 90% CI of PD response ratio may not be appropriate for BE assessment. To address this issue, the FDA proposed a dose-scale method to establish BE using the relative bioavailability of the test product. In this method, PD responses are transformed into linear-scale dose measurements through the E_{max} model (Zhao et al., 2019).

9.3.2.1 Study Design Considerations

To date, the dose-scale method has been recommended in guidance for orlistat capsule (US FDA, 2010a) and albuterol sulfate inhaler (US FDA, 2020b). Multiple-dose crossover designs consisting of two doses of reference product and at least one dose of test product are recommended. In the cases of one dose of test product, a three-period, three-sequence, four-treatment Latin square design could be considered. When the study consists of two doses of test product, a four period, four sequences, four treatment Latin square design is recommended (US FDA, 2020b). Generally, the latter is more preferable because in this design, the relative bioavailability of test product can be estimated directly by fitting the E_{max} model based on both reference and test products, and the estimated value could be more precise. If necessary, a run-in period should be considered to obtain baseline PD response.

In PD BE studies, the PD endpoints are quite different for different categories of products. In studies of orlistat capsule for treatment of obesity, the amount of fat excretion in feces over a 24-h period are used as PD endpoints. While in studies of albuterol sulfate inhalers, the provocative concentrations of methacholine causing a 20% drop in forced expiratory volume in one second ($PC_{20}FEV_1$) are used as PD endpoints, which are tested through bronchoprovocation studies.

The BE limits are determined by the category of products and PD endpoints. For instance, the BE limits are 80.00% to 125.00% in studies for orlistat capsules. While in studies for albuterol sulfate inhalers, the BE could be concluded if the 90% CI of relative bioavailability lies within 67–150%.

9.3.2.2 Statistical Analysis

The dose-scale method consists of two steps. First, an E_{max} model is fitted to obtain a point estimate of the relative bioavailability, refer to as "F". Next, a bootstrap procedure is performed to estimate the 90%CI of relative bioavailability. Then the BE could be determined based on the relative bioavailability.

Point Estimate of Relative Bioavailability F

For studies with one dose of test product, the E_{max} model is fitted based on PD response of the reference product, which is given by:

$$E_R = \phi_R(D_R) = E_{0R} + \frac{E_{maxR} \times D_R}{ED_{50R} + D_R}, \tag{9.10}$$

where E_R is the PD response of the reference product, D_R is administered doses of reference product, E_{0R} is the baseline PD response, E_{maxR} is the fitted maximum PD response of the reference product, ED_{50R} is the dose of the reference product that produces 50% of the maximal response, and $\phi_R(\cdot)$ is a function of dose and PD response. Then, with the point estimate of E_{0R}, ED_{50R}, and E_{maxR}, the inverse of $\phi_R(\cdot)$ can be expressed as:

$$\phi_R^{-1}(x) = \frac{(x - E_{0R}) \times ED_{50R}}{E_{maxR} - (x - E_{0R})}. \tag{9.11}$$

The relative bioavailability F of the test product can be calculated by putting the mean of response data of the test product, refer to as E_T, into the equation:

$$F = \frac{\phi_R^{-1}(E_T)}{D_T},$$ (9.12)

where D_T is the administered doses of test product.

For studies with two dose of test product, the relative bioavailability F can be estimated directly by fitting the E_{max} model based on PD response data of both reference and test. Assuming that E_0 and E_{max} are same for reference and test products, the E_{max} model is modified as follow:

$$E = E_0 + \frac{E_{max} \times D \times F^i}{ED_{50R} + D \times F^i},$$ (9.13)

where E is PD response, D is administered doses, and i is the treatment indicator (0 for reference product and 1 for test product) that $F^0 = 1$ and F^1 is the relative bioavailability of interest. In addition, ED_{50} for test product can be calculated with the equation $ED_{50T} = ED_{50R}/F$.

Nonlinear Mixed Effect (NLME) modeling method is recommended for E_{max} model fitting. Comparing to approaches in which data from all individuals is pooled as one individual, both Between-Subject Variability (BSV) and Residual Unexplained Variability (RUV) are considered in NLME model. Therefore, the NLME approach is less biased when BSV is large and relatively less sensitive to aberrant observations. The NLME approach has been routinely used in PD BE assessment (Gong Xiajing, 2019).

Confidence Interval of Relative Bioavailability F

The interval estimation of relative bioavailability in the dose-scale method is performed using a bootstrap procedure. Since the dose-scale method based on crossover designs, the bootstrap sampling unit is should be the subject, i.e. all the data of an individual is resampled with replacement simultaneously, in order to preserve the intra-subject correlation of observations from different periods. A minimum of 1000 bootstrap replicates are typically needed. As recommended in the FDA guidance, the 90%CI of F is calculated using the Bias-Corrected and accelerated (BCa) method. The main advantage of the BCa method is that it corrects for bias and skewness in the distribution of bootstrap estimates. The BCa interval can be obtained by the following steps (DiCiccio & Efron, 1996; Hutchison et al., 2018):

Step 1: Bootstrapping n_j subjects in jth sequence with replacement, where n_j is the number of subjects in jth sequence repeatedly K times (K is typically at least 1000 times).

Step 2: For the kth bootstrap replicate, the E_{max} model is fitted on the resampled data and an estimate of relative bioavailability, $\hat{F}_k$ is obtained.

Step 3: Calculate the acceleration parameter based on the actual study data, using the jackknife approach, in which the acceleration parameter can be expressed as:

$$\hat{a} = \frac{\sum_{i=1}^{n} \left(\frac{1}{n} \sum_{i=1}^{n} \hat{F}_{(i)} - \hat{F}_{(i)} \right)^3}{6 \left[\sum_{i=1}^{n} \left(\frac{1}{n} \sum_{i=1}^{n} \hat{F}_{(i)} - \hat{F}_{(i)} \right)^2 \right]^{3/2}},$$ (9.14)

where n is the total number of subjects, $\hat{F}_{(i)}$ is estimate of F leaving out ith subject. The acceleration parameter $\hat{a}$ measures the rate of change of the standard error of $\hat{F}$ on the normalized scale, with respect to the true parameter F.

Step 4: Calculate the bias correction factor, which is given by:

$$\hat{z}_0 = \Phi^{-1}\left\{\frac{\sum_{k=1}^{K}\left[I\left(\hat{F}_k < \hat{F}\right)\right]}{K}\right\}, \tag{9.15}$$

where $I(\cdot)$ is the indicator function, $\Phi^{-1}(\cdot)$ is the inverse of the standard normal cumulative distribution function (CDF).

Step 5: Calculate 90% BCa confidence interval, $[\hat{F}_{\alpha_1}, \hat{F}_{\alpha_2}]$, which is comprised by $100 \times \alpha_1$th and $100 \times \alpha_2$th percentile of all bootstrap replicates. α_1 and α_2 are estimated by:

$$\alpha_1 = \Phi\left(\hat{z}_0 + \frac{\hat{z}_0 + z_\alpha}{1 - \hat{a} \times \left(\hat{z}_0 + z_{0.05}\right)}\right)$$

and

$$\alpha_2 = \Phi\left(\hat{z}_0 + \frac{\hat{z}_0 + z_{1-\alpha}}{1 - \hat{a} \times \left(\hat{z}_0 + z_{0.95}\right)}\right). \tag{9.16}$$

Then BE could be concluded if the interval $[\hat{F}_{\alpha_1}, \hat{F}_{\alpha_2}]$ lies within pre-specified BE limits.

9.3.2.3 Remarks

The dose-scale method is an appropriate approach for BE assessment with PD endpoint when establishing BE through ratios and corresponding confidence intervals on PD-response scale is not reliable due to the non-linearity of dose response. This method provides a general solution for BE studies for locally acting drugs, in which BE are often established based on PD endpoints.

Study designs and analysis of the dose-scale method can be more flexible. For instance, a five-way, five-treatment crossover design could be considered when placebo effect should be taken into account. Moreover, other PD models, such as inhibitory effect model and sigmoid E_{max} model can be incorporated into the dose-scale method to handle different type of dose-response relationships.

There are also some challenges in application of the dose-scale method. Since this method is based on nonlinear modeling and bootstrap procedure, sample size estimation could be a challenge issue. Although an optimal sample size could be determined through simulation studies, the simulation process is relatively cumbersome and time consuming. Pilot studies are generally needed to obtain necessary parameters for simulation studies. In addition, since the dose-scale method is based on crossover design, the analysis may be sensitive to missing data and estimation of F can be biased consequently. Statistical methods including Multiple Imputation (MI), complete-case analysis, as well as Expectation Maximization (EM) algorithm can be used for missing data handling. Sensitivity analysis should be conducted to evaluate the impact of missing data. Missing data handling strategies, as well as justifications should be prospectively stated in the protocol.

9.3.3 AH PK Bioequivalence Study for Topical Ophthalmic Corticosteroids

Topical corticosteroid eye drops are commonly used for ocular inflammation. The therapeutic effect of topical corticosteroid eye drops is determined by the drug concentration in the anterior segment tissues. Therefore, measurement of drug concentration in AH can provide the rate and extent of bioavailability for establishing the BE between generic and innovative products. Drug concentrations in AH can only be measured when the subject is undergoing cataract surgery. Therefore, for the products indicated for subjects undergoing cataract surgery, an AH PK BE study can be used for BE assessment.

9.3.3.1 Study Design Considerations

Due to the limitations that AH sample can only be obtained when the eye is undergoing cataract surgery, complete sampling data for each individual subject are unattainable in AH PK BE studies. In this case, a serial sampling regime could be applied, in which multiple subjects are randomly assigned to each of several prespecified sampling timepoints, and only one sample is obtained per subject at one of the prespecified timepoints. The concentration-time profile of the study drugs is obtained with multiple subjects sampled at different time points. Either a parallel or crossover design is recommended for establishing BE. In AH PK BE studies, sampling multiple times from a single eye is not practical. Instead, it is possible to perform a pseudo crossover design by sampling from each eye contingent upon cataract surgery being required for both eyes of the subject. The washout period between surgery for each eye should not exceed 35 days (Harigaya et al., 2019).

9.3.3.2 Statistical Analysis

In a BE study with serial sampling regime, mean concentration at each sampling time can be calculated, and AUC of each product can be obtained from the mean concentration-time profile. As recommended in the FDA guidance, the hypotheses for equivalence test are given as follows:

$$H_0: AUC_T / AUC_R < \theta_1 \quad \text{or} \quad AUC_T / AUC_R > \theta_2 \quad \text{versus} \quad H_a: \theta_1 \leq AUC_T / AUC_R \leq \theta_2,$$

Where θ_1 and θ_2 be the pre-specified BE limits.

Parallel Designs

The point estimate and variance of AUC can be calculated using Bailer's method (Nedelman et al., 1995). Consider a parallel design, let y_{ikq} denote the drug concentration of the *i*th subject ($i = 1, \ldots, n_q$) at the *q*th time point ($q = 1, \ldots, Q$) in group k ($k = T, R$). Then, using Bailer's algorithm, the estimate of the AUC from 0 to the last time point of group k is approximated by (Wolfsegger, 2007):

$$AUC_k = \sum_{q=1}^{Q} c_q \mu_{kq}, \tag{9.17}$$

where c_q is equal to:

$$c_1 = \frac{1}{2}\left(t_2 - t_1\right) \text{ for } q = 1,$$

$$c_q = \frac{1}{2}\left(t_{q+1} - t_{q-1}\right) \text{ for } q = 2, \ldots, Q-1,$$

$$c_Q = \frac{1}{2}\left(t_Q - t_{Q-1}\right) \text{ for } q = Q. \tag{9.18}$$

The AUC_k can be estimated by:

$$\widehat{AUC}_k = \sum_{q=1}^{Q} c_q \bar{y}_{kq}, \tag{9.19}$$

with $\bar{y}_{kq} = \frac{1}{n_q}\sum_{i=1}^{n_q} y_{ikq}$. Since subjects at different time points are independent, there are no covariance terms involved in the variance of $\widehat{AUC}_k$, which is estimated by:

$$\hat{s}^2\left(\widehat{AUC}_k\right) = \hat{\sigma}_k^2 = \sum_{q=1}^{Q} \frac{c_q^2 \hat{s}_{kq}^2}{n_q}, \tag{9.20}$$

with $\hat{s}_{kq}^2 = \frac{1}{n_q-1}\sum_{i=1}^{n_q}(y_{ikq} - \bar{y}_{kq})$. Confidence interval of AUC_T/AUC_R can be calculated using Fieller's method, as described in Section 9.3.1. In a parallel design, AUC_T and AUC_R are mutually independent. Therefore, the covariance of AUC_T and AUC_R, $\hat{\sigma}_{TR}$, is zero. Then, the test statistic T is given by:

$$T = \frac{\widehat{AUC}_T - \theta \widehat{AUC}_R}{\sqrt{\hat{\sigma}_T^2 + \theta^2 \hat{\sigma}_R^2}}. \tag{9.21}$$

The corresponding degree of freedom can be obtained using the Satterthwaite approximation, which gives:

$$df = \frac{\left(\hat{\sigma}_T^2 + \theta^2 \hat{\sigma}_R^2\right)^2}{\hat{\sigma}_R^4/\left(n_q - 1\right) + \theta^4 \hat{\sigma}_R^4/\left(n_q - 1\right)}. \tag{9.22}$$

The lower and upper limits of confidence interval θ_L and θ_U are given by:

$$\theta_L = \left[-B - \left(B^2 - AC\right)^{1/2}\right]/A$$

and

$$\theta_U = \left[-B + \left(B^2 - AC\right)^{1/2}\right]/A, \tag{9.23}$$

where

$$A = \widehat{AUC}_R^2 - t_{\alpha,df}^2 \hat{\sigma}_R^2,$$

$$B = -\widehat{AUC}_T \widehat{AUC}_R,$$

$$C = \widehat{AUC}_T^2 - t_{\alpha,df}^2 \hat{\sigma}_T^2. \tag{9.24}$$

To construct a Fieller confidence interval that contains no negative values, both AUC_T and AUC_R should be statistically significant compared to 0.

Crossover Designs

In crossover designs, each eye of a subject receives different products in separate study periods and between periods there is a sufficient long washout period. Therefore, carry-over effect in AH PK BE study can be excluded through suitable study design. The test statistic T for crossover design is given by:

$$T = \frac{\widehat{AUC}_T - \theta \widehat{AUC}_R}{\sqrt{\hat{\sigma}_T^2 + \theta^2 \hat{\sigma}_R^2 - 2\theta \hat{\sigma}_{T,R}}}. \tag{9.25}$$

Let y_{ijkq} denote the drug concentration of the ith subject at the qth time point ($q = 1,\ldots,Q$) of period j ($j = 1, 2$) in sequence k ($k = 1, 2$), AUC_{jk} and $\hat{\sigma}_{jk}^2$ denote the AUC and corresponding variance of jth period of kth sequence, which can be estimated through the following procedure. For simplicity, following notations are used for the AUCs in each sequence and period as listed in Table 9.1.

Then follow Locke's method, the estimators of AUC_T and AUC_R are given by:

$$\widehat{AUC}_T = \frac{\widehat{AUC}_{11} + \widehat{AUC}_{22}}{2}$$

and

$$\widehat{AUC}_R = \frac{\widehat{AUC}_{12} + \widehat{AUC}_{21}}{2}. \tag{9.26}$$

The standard errors are then given by:

$$s^2\left(\widehat{AUC}_T\right) = \hat{\sigma}_T^2 = \frac{1}{4}\left(\hat{\sigma}_{11}^2 + \hat{\sigma}_{22}^2\right)$$

TABLE 9.1

Notations of AUCs in Each Sequence and Period

Sequence	Period 1 ($j = 1$)	Period 2 ($j = 2$)
Sequence TR ($k = 1$)	$\widehat{AUC}_{11}$	$\widehat{AUC}_{21}$
Sequence RT ($k = 2$)	$\widehat{AUC}_{12}$	$\widehat{AUC}_{22}$

and

$$s^2\left(\widehat{AUC}_R\right) = \hat{\sigma}_R^2 = \frac{1}{4}\left(\hat{\sigma}_{12}^2 + \hat{\sigma}_{21}^2\right). \tag{9.27}$$

The covariance of $\widehat{AUC}_T$ and $\widehat{AUC}_R$ can be estimated as:

$$\hat{\sigma}_{T,R} = \frac{1}{4}\left(\hat{\sigma}_{11,12} + \hat{\sigma}_{12,21}\right). \tag{9.28}$$

where $\hat{\sigma}_{11,21}$ and $\hat{\sigma}_{12,22}$ are estimates of covariance between $\widehat{AUC}_{1k}$ and $\widehat{AUC}_{2k}$, as:

$$\hat{\sigma}_{1k,2k} = \frac{1}{n_q}\sum_{q=1}^{Q}\sum_{i=1}^{n_q}\frac{\left(y_{i1kq} - \bar{y}_{1kq}\right)\left(y_{i21q} - \bar{y}_{2kq}\right)}{n_q - 1}. \tag{9.29}$$

Then we can calculate

$$A = \widehat{AUC}_R^2 - t_{\alpha,df}^2 \hat{\sigma}_R^2,$$

$$B = t_{\alpha,df}^2 \hat{\sigma}_{T,R} - \widehat{AUC}_T \widehat{AUC}_R,$$

$$C = \widehat{AUC}_T^2 - t_{\alpha,df}^2 \hat{\sigma}_T^2, \tag{9.30}$$

to construct the Fieller-type confidence interval of AUC_T / AUC_R.

An alternative way for BE assessment with serial AH sampling data is bootstrap methods. Confidence interval of AUC_T / AUC_R can be obtained through the BCa method described in Section 9.3.3. Simulation studies show that the power and type I error of bootstrap methods are similar to the Fieller confidence interval.

9.3.3.3 Sample Size Considerations

As aforementioned in Section 9.3.1, sample size of the Fieller confidence interval can be calculated using the power function of the T_1/T_2 test. With minor modifications, the power function of the T_1/T_2 test, which is given by:

$$1 - \beta = Q\left(\infty, -t_{\alpha,df}, \varphi_1, \varphi_2, \rho\right) - Q\left(t_{\alpha,df}, -t_{\alpha,df}, \varphi_1, \varphi_2, \rho\right), \tag{9.31}$$

can be applied to address the case of AH PK studies using crossover design. The non-centrality parameters φ_1, φ_2, and correlation coefficient ρ are given by:

$$\varphi_l = \frac{\widehat{AUC}_T - \theta_l\widehat{AUC}_R}{\sqrt{\hat{\sigma}_T^2 + \theta_l^2\hat{\sigma}_R^2 - 2\theta_l\hat{\sigma}_{T,R}}}, \quad l = 1,2; \tag{9.32}$$

$$\rho = \frac{\hat{\sigma}_T^2 + \theta_1\theta_2\hat{\sigma}_R^2 - \hat{\sigma}_{T,R}\left(\theta_1 + \theta_2\right)}{\sqrt{\left(\hat{\sigma}_T^2 + \theta_1^2\hat{\sigma}_R^2 - 2\theta_1\hat{\sigma}_{T,R}\right)\left(\hat{\sigma}_T^2 + \theta_2^2\hat{\sigma}_R^2 - 2\theta_2\hat{\sigma}_{T,R}\right)}}. \tag{9.33}$$

The parameters $\hat{\sigma}_T^2$, $\hat{\sigma}_R^2$, $\hat{\sigma}_{T,R}$ and *df* are related to n_q, which is the number of subjects per timepoint of each sequence. In this way, for a specific power level, the sample size n_q can be calculated through numerical iteration with the power function.

9.3.4 Reference-Scaled Average Bioequivalence (RSABE) Study for NTI Drugs

Narrow Therapeutic Index (NTI) drugs are products that small changes in drug exposure could potentially cause serious therapeutic failures and/or serious adverse drug reactions in patients. Therefore, the one-size-fits-all approach in which BE is determined if the 90% confidence interval of geometric means of primary PK parameter lies within the BE criteria of (0.80,1.25) is not stringent enough for BE assessment of NIT drugs (Jiang & Yu, 2014). Although BE criteria and approval pathways vary in different regulatory authorities, approaches for NIT drugs can be generally categorized into two classes: (i) tightening BE limits directly and (ii) scaled average BE with variance of reference products.

In approaches that tighten BE limits directly, the criterion for the 90% confidence interval of PK parameters are tightened to a narrower range such as 90% to 111.11%, and BE is tested using TOST. For instance, Health Canada requires the acceptance interval for AUC of NTI drugs to be tightened to 90.00% to 111.11% and the European Medicines Evaluation Agency (EMEA) requires that the 90.00% to 111.11% acceptance interval should be applied for both AUC and C_{max} (European Medicines Agency, 2010; Health Canada, 2012). A drawback of the tightened, fixed acceptance interval, i.e. 90.00% to 111.11%, can be too strict for those NTI drugs with medium Within-Subject Variance (WSV), even though the generic product is actually equivalent with the reference product. FDA recommends a Reference-Scaled Average BE (RSABE) approach, in which BE limits are tightened based on WSV of reference product (US FDA, 2012b).

9.3.4.1 Study Design Considerations

The FDA BE criteria for NTI drugs consist of equivalence in both mean and WSV. Therefore, the study design should permit not only the comparison of the mean of the test and reference drug products but also the comparison of WSV. FDA recommends a four-way, fully replicated, crossover study design (TRTR and RTRT) to demonstrate BE for NTI drugs (US FDA, 2012b). Each subject receives both test and reference products twice, and therefore the WSV of the test and reference products can be estimated, respectively. Then the scaling of the BE limits based on the WSV of the reference product and the comparison of the WSV of the test and reference products can be performed (Chow & Liu, 1999).

9.3.4.2 Statistical Analysis

Equivalence Test for Means

The hypotheses for reference-scaled average BE test are given as follows:

$$H_0: \frac{(\mu_T - \mu_R)^2}{\sigma_{WR}^2} > \theta$$

versus

$$H_a: \frac{(\mu_T - \mu_R)^2}{\sigma_{WR}^2} \le \theta,$$

where μ_T and μ_R are the means of log-transformed PK parameters (C_{max} and AUC) respectively; σ_{WR}^2 is the WSV of reference product; and θ is the scaled BE limit, defined as:

$$\theta = \frac{[ln(\Delta)]^2}{\sigma_{W0}^2}, \tag{9.34}$$

where $\Delta = 1/0.9$ is the upper limit of ratio of geometric means, and $\sigma_{W0} = 0.10$. From the definition of θ, it can be seen that the initial baseline BE limits are 0.90–1.11 with the reference WSV of 10%, and then be scaled using the observed WSV of reference product, as:

$$\frac{ln(0.90)\sigma_{WR}}{\sigma_{W0}} \le \mu_T - \mu_R \le \frac{ln(1.11)\sigma_{WR}}{\sigma_{W0}}. \tag{9.35}$$

The parameter σ_{WR}^2 in the BE limits is a random variable, therefore the BE can't be tested directly using TOST procedure. Instead, the statistics of RSABE can be rewritten as $(\mu_T - \mu_R)^2 - \sigma_{WR}^2\theta$, BE can be determined if the corresponding 95% upper confidence bound less than zero. Confidence interval can be obtained using Howe's approximation(Howe, 1974).

The scaled-BE limits expand as the variability increases and, consequently, these limits may exceed 80.00–125.00%, which is not desirable for BE assessment of NTI products. Therefore, FDA further requires that besides the RSABE, NTI drugs should also pass the unscaled average BE test with the limits of 80.00–125.00%.

Comparison of Within-Subject Variabilities

Besides of equivalence in geometric means, the FDA standard for NIT drugs additionally requires that the WSV of test products should not greater than that of the reference drug product by a specific value. This is because a higher WSV may imply a higher likelihood of serious therapeutic failures and/or adverse events for NTI drugs. The comparison of WSV of the test and reference products can be performed using a one-sides F test. The test hypotheses of WSV comparison are given by:

$$H_0: \sigma_{WT}/\sigma_{WR} > \delta \quad \text{versus} \quad H_a: \sigma_{WT}/\sigma_{WR} \le \delta,$$

where δ is the regulatory limit, which is generally set to be 2.5. The confidence interval of σ_{WT}/σ_{WR} can be calculated through the F distribution with degrees of freedom v_1 and v_2, as:

$$\left(\frac{S_{WT}/S_{WR}}{\sqrt{F_{\alpha/2}(v_1, v_2)}}, \frac{S_{WT}/S_{WR}}{\sqrt{F_{1-\alpha/2}(v_1, v_2)}} \right), \tag{9.36}$$

where S_{WT} and S_{WR} are the estimates of σ_{WT} and σ_{WR}, respectively, and $\alpha = 0.1$ is the significant level. The equivalence in WSV can be concluded if the upper limit of the 90%CI is less than or equal to 2.5.

9.3.4.3 Remarks

Comparing with methods with fixed BE limits, the RSABE approach can not only tighten the BE limits to provide a stringent standard for approval of NTI drugs but can also avoid being too strict for NTI drugs with moderate WSVs. The RSABE approach can be applied for both HV drugs and NTI drugs. The BE criteria and study design of RSABE approach for HV drugs and NTI drugs are different. The details of RSABE for highly variable drugs are described in the last chapter.

In practice, sample size for the RSABE approach is often obtained through simulation studies. With the R package 'powerTOST', the sample size for RSABE assessment of NTI drugs can be simulated conveniently (Labes et al., 2016). The FDA guidance didn't provide a closed-form power function of RSABE approach. Since the criteria and statistic of RSABE is very similar to that of PBE and Individual BE (IBE), methods for sample size determination of the RSABE approach can be derived through the similar procedure as PBE and IBE, which is based on the Modified Large-Simple (MLS) method, as described by Chow et al.(Chow et al., 2003). To date, the studies for sample size of the RSABE approach are still limited.

9.4 In Vitro Studies

Although, a large number of complex generic drugs can be evaluated using *in vivo* BE studies, for some specific issues such as evaluation of particle size distribution of formulation and BE assessment for locally acting drugs, *in vivo* studies may not be sufficient or practicable. *In vitro* studies, on the other hand, are often less expensive and easier to conduct. In practice, *in vitro* studies can not only be used as supportive evidence of BE in addition to *in vivo* studies, but also be used as pivotal studies for cases when *in vivo* studies are not applicable. In this section, following *in vitro* studies are introduced: (i) *in vitro* population BE studies, (ii) IVRT-based BE study, (iii) IVPT-based BE study.

9.4.1 In Vitro Population Bioequivalence Studies

PBE is usually used to assess prescribability of drug products. Drug prescribability is referred to that physicians can prescribe either innovative drugs or its generic copies (Tóthfalusi et al., 2014). Furthermore, the PBE approach can also be applied to *in vitro* studies for establishing BE for delivery characteristics of drug products. For instance, the FDA guidance on bioavailability and BE studies for nasal aerosols and nasal sprays recommends that PBE approach can be applied to the evaluation of following characteristics: (i) single actuation content through container life, (ii) droplet size distribution, (iii) drug in small particles/droplets by cascade impactor, and (iv) spray pattern (US FDA, 2003).

For convenience of description, study design and analysis of PBE approach are introduced by taking PBE assessment of particle size distribution for metered nasal spray as an example. Other products, as well as characteristics can be evaluated in the same way.

9.4.1.1 Study Design Considerations

In practice, *in vitro* PBE evaluations are often based on parallel designs. Variance from batches, canister, and life stage of product should be considered for *in vitro* PBE studies. As recommended in the FDA guidance, *in vitro* PBE should be demonstrated based on at least ten canisters from each of three or more batches of test and reference products. Canisters are randomly drawn from each batch. Parameter of interest should be tested at beginning and end, or beginning, middle and end of life stage of each canister (US FDA, 2012a, 2019b).

9.4.1.2 Statistical Analysis

Similar to *in vivo* PBE assessment, the criterion of in vitro PBE is a mixed criterion on logarithmic scale, as:

$$\theta = \frac{(\mu_T - \mu_R)^2 + (\sigma_T^2 - \sigma_R^2)}{max(\sigma_0^2, \sigma_R^2)}, \tag{9.37}$$

where μ_T and μ_R are the means of log-transformed measurements of the test and reference products, respectively, σ_T^2 and σ_R^2 are the total variance, and σ_0^2 is the scaling variance. The PBE criterion is scaled depending on the variance of reference product. When σ_R^2 is larger than the scaling variance, σ_0^2, the limit is widened. As stated in the FDA guidance, the scaling variance should set to be at least 0.01. The hypotheses for *in vitro* PBE are given as follows:

$$H_0: \theta \geq \theta_0 \quad \text{versus} \quad H_a: \theta < \theta_0,$$

where θ_0 is the PBE limit, which is defined as:

$$\theta_0 = \frac{[ln(\Delta)]^2 + \epsilon}{\sigma_0^2}, \tag{9.38}$$

Where Δ is the ABE limit, ϵ is the variance terms offset. The ABE limit is tentatively recommended to be 1.11. The variance terms offset allows some acceptable difference between the total variances of test and reference products that may be inconsequential. Since the variance of measurements are generally low in *in vitro* studies, the variance terms offset is often set to be 0.01 (or 0 for some cases) for *in vitro* BE assessment. Therefore, the PBE limit becomes:

$$\theta_0 = \frac{[ln(1.11)]^2 + 0.01}{0.1^2} = 2.0891.$$

As suggested by Hyslop et al.(Hyslop et al., 2000), the PBE criterion can be expressed in terms of the following linearized criteria, as:

$$\eta = \delta^2 + \sigma_T^2 - \sigma_R^2 - \theta_0 max(\sigma_0^2, \sigma_R^2), \tag{9.39}$$

where $\theta_0 = \mu_T - \mu_R$. Then, the hypotheses for *in vitro* PBE becomes:

$$H_0: \eta \geq 0 \quad \text{versus} \quad H_a: \eta < 0.$$

In this way, PBE test can be performed by constructing a 95% upper one-sided confidence bound for η. Let Y_{ijks} denote the measurement at life stage s ($s = 1, \ldots, m$) of canister i ($i = 1, \ldots, n_k$) from batch j ($j = 1, \ldots, l_k$) for product k ($k = T, R$). As aforementioned in this section, most PSGs requires that canister should be randomly drawn from three batches of test and reference products, respectively. While three batches are not sufficient to estimate the between batch component of variance, the PBE method that recommended by a number of PSGs consider the three batches being combined as a "super-batch". The data can be described by the following model:

$$Y_{ijks} = \mu_k + b_{ijk} + \varepsilon_{ijks} \tag{9.40}$$

Where μ_k is the overall mean of product k, $b_{ijk} \sim N(0, \sigma^2_{k,C})$ is the random effect of canister i in batch j of product k, $\varepsilon_{ijks} \sim N(0, \sigma^2_{k,L})$ is the random effect of life stage s, and b_{ijk} and ε_{ijks} are independent. Define

$$\bar{Y}_{ijk\cdot} = \frac{\sum_{s=1}^{m} Y_{ijks}}{m},$$

$$\bar{Y}_{\cdot\cdot k\cdot} = \frac{\sum_{i=1}^{l_k} \sum_{j=1}^{n_k} \bar{Y}_{ijk\cdot}}{m},$$

$$SS_{k,e} = \sum_{i=1}^{l_k} \sum_{j=1}^{n_k} \sum_{s=1}^{m} \left(Y_{ijks} - \bar{Y}_{ijk\cdot}\right)^2 \text{ and}$$

$$SS_{k,b} = m \sum_{i=1}^{l_k} \sum_{j=1}^{n_k} \left(\bar{Y}_{ijk\cdot} - \bar{Y}_{\cdot\cdot k\cdot}\right)^2. \tag{9.41}$$

The corresponding mean squares for life stage (within-canister) and canister (between-canister) are given by:

$$MS_{k,e} = \frac{SS_{k,e}}{n_k l_k (m-1)} \quad \text{and} \quad MS_{k,b} = \frac{SS_{k,b}}{n_k l_k - 1}. \tag{9.42}$$

The variance components for life stage and canister can be estimated, as:

$$\hat{\sigma}^2_{k,C} = \frac{MS_{k,b} - MS_{k,e}}{m} \quad \text{and} \quad \hat{\sigma}^2_{k,L} = MS_{k,e}. \tag{9.43}$$

An unbiased estimator for the total variance of test and reference products can be calculated as:

$$\hat{\sigma}^2_k = \hat{\sigma}^2_{k,C} + \hat{\sigma}^2_{k,L} = \frac{MS_{k,b}}{m} + \frac{(m-1)MS_{k,e}}{m} \text{ for } k = T, R. \tag{9.44}$$

Then a 95% one-sided upper confidence bound for η can be calculated using the extension of the modified large sample (MLS) method (Lee et al., 2004), as:

$$\hat{\eta}_U = E + \sqrt{U} \tag{9.45}$$

where $E = \hat{\delta}^2 + \hat{\sigma}_T^2 - \hat{\sigma}_R^2 - \theta_0 max(\sigma_0^2, \hat{\sigma}_R^2)$, and U is the sum of the following quantities:

$$U_1 = \left[\left(\left| \hat{\delta} \right| + Z_{0.95} \sqrt{\frac{MS_{T,b}}{n_T l_T m} + \frac{MS_{R,b}}{n_R l_R m}} \right)^2 - \hat{\delta}^2 \right]^2,$$

$$U_2 = \frac{MS_{T,b}^2}{m^2} \left(\frac{n_T l_T - 1}{\chi_{n_T l_T - 1, 0.05}^2} - 1 \right)^2,$$

$$U_3 = \frac{(m-1)^2 \, MS_{T,e}^2}{m^2} \left[\frac{n_k l_k (m-1)}{\chi_{n_k l_k (m-1), 0.05}^2} - 1 \right]^2,$$

$$U_4 = \frac{(1 + c\theta_0)^2 \, MS_{R,b}^2}{m^2} \left(\frac{n_R l_R - 1}{\chi_{n_R l_R - 1, 0.05}^2} - 1 \right)^2,$$

and

$$U_5 = \frac{(1 + c\theta_0)^2 (m-1)^2 \, MS_{R,e}^2}{m^2} \left[\frac{n_R l_R (m-1)}{\chi_{n_R l_R (m-1), 0.05}^2} - 1 \right]^2, \quad (9.46)$$

where $c = 1$ if $\hat{\sigma}_R^2 > \hat{\sigma}_0^2$ and $c = 0$ if $\hat{\sigma}_R^2 < \hat{\sigma}_0^2$. PBE can be concluded if the 95% upper confidence bound, $\hat{\eta}_U$, is less than 0.

The test statistics $\hat{\eta}_U$ can also be modified to be one-sided with respect to mean comparison, such as PBE assessment for drug in small particles/droplets for fluticasone propionate nasal spray. If $\hat{\mu}_T > \hat{\mu}_R$, PBE assessment can be performed following the above standard procedure. If $\hat{\mu}_T < \hat{\mu}_R$, PBE would be determined by removing $\hat{\delta}^2$ and U_1 from $\hat{\eta}_U$.

9.4.1.3 Sample Size Considerations

Generally, *in vitro* PBE studies are recommended to include at least 30 canisters from three of more batches of test and reference, i.e. no fewer than ten canisters from each batch. However, whether BE is determined based on sufficient power is unknown if a study is conducted without sample size calculation. The 2001 FDA guidance (US FDA, 2001) did not provide a close-form formulation for sample size calculation. Instead, the guidance recommends using simulation studies to estimate the sample size.

An alternative method for sample size determination is Chow's MLS method (Chow et al., 2003). For sample size determination of *in vitro* PBE studies, the number of canisters for each batch, refer to as $n = n_T = n_R$, and the number of batches, refer to as $l = l_T = l_R$, are parameters of interest. Define U_β be the same as U but with 5% and 95% replaced by β and $1 - \beta$, respectively, where $1 - \beta$ is the target power. Since

$$Pr\left(\hat{\eta}_U < \eta + \sqrt{U} + \sqrt{U_\beta} \right) \approx 1 - \beta, \quad (9.47)$$

the power of PBE test, $Pr(\hat{\eta}_U < 0)$, is approximately larger than $1 - \beta$ if $\eta + \sqrt{U} + \sqrt{U_\beta} \leq 0$. Then, with some suitable assumed value for δ, $MS_{T,b}$, $MS_{T,e}$, $MS_{R,b}$, and $MS_{R,e}$ taking into the equation, a series of combination of the sample sizes n and l can be obtained through numerical iteration, and a preferable combination of n and l can be selected with respect to the most possible number of canisters per batch and number of batches.

9.4.2 Bioequivalence Assessment with *in Vitro* Release Test (IVRT)

Complexity of locally acting drugs often comes from difficulties in measuring drug exposure in acting location. Apart from clinical BE studies, *in vitro* studies including IVRT and/or IVPT studies provide a practical alternative way for establishing bioequivalence for locally acting dermatological drugs (Brown & Williams, 2019).

The procedure and apparatus of IVRT and IVPT are similar. Both methods require a diffusion cell, which is separated into a donor compartment and a receptor compartment by a membrane. The drug product is applied in donor compartment, and receptor compartment contains dissolution media. The concentrations of drug substance in the dissolution media at a series of pre-defined time points can be measured. If a synthetic membrane is used, the system would measure the release profile, and alternatively, if a biological origin membrane (human or pig) is used, the permeation profile can be obtained (Miranda et al., 2018).

IVRT is an effective method to quantify the rate of drug release from semisolid dosage forms. An *in vitro* release rate reflects the combined effect of a series of physical and chemical properties in both drug substance and formulation, and thereby highly related to the bioavailability of drug product. Therefore, IVRT are widely accepted as a component of evidence of BE for locally acting dermatological drugs.

9.4.2.1 Study Design Considerations

Since the characteristics of drug substance and formulations vary, it is difficult to devise a standard test system to quantify the drug release rate for every category of drug product. Instead, methodologies, including apparatus, procedures and analytical techniques should be developed and validated specifically to dosage form category, formulation type and individual product characteristics. In addition, studies (Tiffner et al., 2018; Yacobi et al., 2014) have shown that the IVRT results are vulnerable to changes in any of several parameters. Therefore, a series of validation tests of the IVRT method, including linearity, precision, reproducibility, sensitivity, specificity, selectivity, recovery and robustness should be performed prior to pivotal studies. Technical details for method development, validation, and corresponding statistical method for IVRT are provided in the United States Pharmacopeia (USP) general chapter <1724> (Miranda et al., 2018; USP, 2011).

To prevent underlying differential cointerventions or biased assessment of outcomes in the IVRT pivotal study, experimental operators should be blinded to the test and reference product. The blinding procedure should be described in the study protocol and final report. In addition, in order to control the bias due to the potential systematic difference between runs, the test and reference product should be dosed in an alternating sequence on successive diffusion cells. The sequence could be randomly selected from possible sequences, such as TRTRTR or RTRTRT (EMEA, 2018; US FDA, 2014a, 2016a).

9.4.2.2 Calculation of Release Rates

Based on measurements of drug concentration in the receptor medium, the release rates are estimated using the Higuchi model (Higuchi, 1961; Tiffner et al., 2018). Let C_n denote the drug concentrations in the receptor medium at sampling time n, and the amount of drug released per unit area, Q_n can be expressed as:

$$Q_n = C_n \frac{V_C}{A_C} + \frac{V_S}{A_C} \sum_{i=1}^{n} C_{i-1},$$

where V_C is the volume of the cell, A_C is the area of the orifice of the cell, and V_S is the volume of each sample. This equation takes the dilution of the receptor medium due to the replacement of sampling into account. According to Higuchi's square root approximations, Q_n has an approximate linear relation with square root of sampling time $\sqrt{t}$, given by:

$$Q = \sqrt{t\left(2ADC_s\right)}, \tag{9.48}$$

where Q is the amount of drug released per unit area of exposure, t is the time, D denotes the diffusion coefficient, C_s is the solubility of the drug in the formulation, and A is the initial drug concentration in the product. The release rate, which corresponds to the slope of regression line, can be obtained by fitting a linear regression model of Q_n versus $\sqrt{t}$.

9.4.2.3 Statistical Analysis

Generally, measurements of IVRT are not normally distributed due to testing artefacts, such as air bubbles and membrane defects. Subsequently, BE assessment based on IVRT should be performed using non-parametric statistical methods. The USP general chapter <1724> recommends using the Mann-Whitney U test to calculate the 90% confidence interval for the ratio of the release rates of the test and reference products (Habjanič et al., 2020; USP, 2011). The BE assessment can be performed in a two-stage manner. In the first stage, six samples for each product are tested. Then the ratio of release rate for each individual test-reference combination are calculated. A total of 36 T/R ratios are obtained and ordered from the lowest to highest. The 8th and 29th T/R ratios are corresponding to the lower and upper bounds of the 90% confidence interval. BE could be concluded if the 90% confidence interval lies within the range of 75.00–133.33%. Otherwise, the second stage would be performed, in which 12 additional sample of each products are tested. Based on all 18 release rate for the test and reference products, a total of 324 T/R ratios are calculated. The 110th and 215th represent the 90% confidence interval. BE can be determined using the criterion of 75.00–133.33% (Lusina Kregar et al., 2015). It should be notice that some regulatory agencies are now seeking to amend the BE criterion to 90–110%.

9.4.3 Bioequivalence Assessment with *in Vitro* Permeation Test (IVPT)

IVPT, which is a methodology to assess the skin permeation of a topical drug product, has been shown to be well-correlated with *in vivo* drug exposure, particularly when the IVPT and *in vivo* study designs are harmonized (Lehman et al., 2011; Shin et al., 2020). A typical IVPT study is based on open chamber diffusion cell systems, in which excised human skins are mounted and a donor compartment and a receptor compartment are therefore separated. Product being tested is placed on the upper side of the skin in the donor compartment (Miranda et al., 2018). The receptor compartment on the side of the skin is filled with dissolution media. Through a sequential sampling from the receptor, drug concentration at a series of time points can be obtained and permeation profiles are calculated correspondingly. To date, IVPT studies are recommended for BE assessment of many locally acting drugs (EMEA, 2018; US FDA, 2016a).

9.4.3.1 Study Design Considerations

Like IVRT, the outcomes of IVPT studies are sensitive to changes in study methodologies and experimental conditions. Therefore, a series of studies should be performed to develop and validate the methodology of IVPT. In addition, since products are often applied with a finite dose in an IVRT study, studies should be performed to justify the selection of the dose amount in method development stage, even if the dose is within the recommended range. These studies can also support the selection of an appropriate schedule and duration for the pivotal study.

Following the IVPT method development studies, a pilot study is recommended to estimate the number of donors required for the pivotal study. A minimum of four replicate skin sections per donor per treatment group as well as at least eight non-zero sampling time points is recommended (US FDA, 2016a, 2018a). In addition, as recommended by the FDA guidances, besides the test and reference product, a third product that is different from the reference product should be included to evaluate the performance of the IVPT method on discriminating differences in cutaneous PK.

A parallel, single-dose, multiple-replicate per treatment group design is recommended for the IVPT pivotal study. Same number of replicated skin sections from each donor are used in the pivotal study, and skin sections from each donor are evenly allocated into each group. As recommended by the FDA guidance, a minimum of four replicated skin sections from each donor should be included for each group. In addition, in order to ensure a balanced number of replicate skin sections per donor per group in the final analysis, skin sections that were discontinued from the study should be replaced by skin sections from the same donor. Skin sections from each donor are treated with the test or reference product in an alternating order, such as TRTRTR or RTRTRT. The donors could be randomly assigned to one of the two orders. Moreover, the pivotal IVRT study should be conducted in a blind manner to prevent potential bias due to differential cointerventions or biased assessment of outcomes (Shin et al., 2020).

The rate and extent of permeation are characterized by flux and total cumulative amount of the drug permeated into the receptor solution across the study duration, respectively. BE is established using the maximum flux (denote as J_{max}), which is analogous to C_{max} of *in vivo* plasma PK, and total cumulative penetration, which corresponds to the AUC of flux-time plots.

9.4.3.2 Statistical Analysis

In each IVPT run, a series of concentrations at pre-specified time-points for product applied to an individual excised skin section are tested. For IVPT studies using a vertical diffusion cell, in which case the entire receptor solution volume is removed and replaced at each time point, the flux can be calculated as:

$$J_k = (C_k \times V)/A/t_k, \tag{9.49}$$

where C_k is the concentration at time point k; V is the volume of the specific diffusion cell, which vary between different diffusion cells and is generally measured for each individual diffusion cells; A is the area of dosing; and t_k is the length of the kth sampling interval for which the receptor is accepting drugs. Both J_{max} and total cumulative penetration should be log-transformed prior to bioequivalence analysis.

BE with IVRT can be established using the RSABE approach (Grosser et al., 2015). In a typical IVPT study, each donor would contribute multiple observation of both test and reference products, therefore the study data can be treated in the similar manner with RSABE analysis in *in vivo* replicated crossover designs for Highly Variable Drugs (HVD). Denote T_{ij} and R_{ij} as penetration parameter (J_{max} or total cumulative penetration) of the *i*th replicate i ($i = 1, \ldots, r$) of the *j*th donor j ($j = 1, \ldots, n$) from the test and reference group, respectively. The estimate of within-reference variability of reference product, σ_{WR}^2, can be calculated as:

$$S_{WR}^2 = \frac{\sum_{j=1}^{n} \sum_{i=1}^{n} \left(R_{ij} - \bar{R}_{.j} \right)^2}{(r-1)n},$$ (9.50)

where $\bar{R}_{.J}$ is the average of observations of reference product for donor J. The mean difference for each donor can be calculated as:

$$I_j = \frac{1}{r} \sum_{i=1}^{r} \left(T_{ij} - R_{ij} \right),$$ (9.51)

and subsequently, the point estimate of geometric mean ratio (GMR):

$$\bar{I} = \frac{1}{n} \sum_{j=1}^{n} I_j \sim N \left(\mu_T - \mu_R, \frac{\sigma_I^2}{n} \right),$$ (9.52)

where σ_I^2 is the inter-donor variability, which can be estimated as:

$$S_I^2 = \frac{1}{(n-1)} \sum_{j=1}^{n} \left(I_j - \bar{I} \right)^2.$$ (9.53)

For the cases that $S_{WR} > 0.294$, the bioequivalence is tested using the RSABE criterion which is scaled with the within-reference variability, the corresponding hypotheses to be tested are

$$H_0: \frac{\left(\mu_T - \mu_R \right)^2}{\sigma_{WR}^2} > \theta$$

versus

$$H_a: \frac{\left(\mu_T - \mu_R \right)^2}{\sigma_{WR}^2} \leq \theta.$$

where μ_T and μ_R are the means of log-transformed penetration parameters, respectively; σ_{WR}^2 is the WSV of reference product; and $\theta = [ln(\Delta)]^2 / \sigma_{W0}^2$ is the scaled bioequivalence limit, where $\sigma_{W0} = 0.25$ and Δ is the bioequivalence 1.25. The confidence interval of the test statistic, $(\mu_T - \mu_R)^2 - \sigma_{WR}^2 \theta$, can be calculated using Howe's approach. The null hypothesis is rejected if the upper bound of the 95% confidence interval is lower than zero. In addition, the RSABE criterion includes a constraint that the point estimate of GMR, $\bar{I}$, has to fall within the limits $(0.80, 1.25)$.

If $S_{WR} \leq 0.294$, an ABE criterion is used. Bioequivalence can be determined is the 90% confidence interval of GMR, which is given by $\bar{I} \pm t_{(n-1),0.95} \sqrt{S_I^2/n}$, lies within the bioequivalence limits $(0.80, 1.25)$.

9.4.3.3 Sample Size Considerations

When designing an IVPT-based BE study, both number of donors and number of replicate skin sections per donor should be determined. Like *in vivo* RSABE assessment, sample size for IVPT-based BE study is usually obtained through simulation studies. Since a minimum of four replicated skin sections per donor per product is recommend, a series of simulation studies could be performed for each number of replicated skin sections per donor to determine the least adequate number of donors, and then find the optimal combination of the number of donors and the number of replicates per donor. A potential alternative way to determine the sample size of IVPT-based BE study is using Chow's MLS method (Chow et al., 2003). By taking assumed value for within-donor and between-donor variability for reference product into the MLS equations and power function of Equation (9.47), the number of donors and the number of replicates per donor can be obtained through numerical iteration. The performance of this method for IVPT-based BE study is yet to be evaluated.

9.5 Case Studies

As characteristics of complex generic drugs vary considerably, pathways for establishing BE for complex generics could be different. In this section, we are not trying to illustrate practical applications for all methodologies introduced previously in this chapter. Instead, we present three representative cases of BE assessment for complex generic drugs, as follows: (i) a PD equivalence analysis for two formulations of orlistat using the dose-scale method, (ii) an AH PK BE study for dexamethasone-tobramycin ophthalmic suspension based on serial sampling data, and (iii) an IVPT-based BE study for acyclovir cream using the RSABE approach. Although these three cases are BE assessment of difference formulations rather than evaluation of generic drugs, these studies are conducted following the recommendation in the corresponding PSGs.

9.5.1 Bioequivalence Assessment of Two Formulations of Orlistat

Orlistat is a locally acting gastrointestinal lipase inhibitor for anti-obesity, acting by inhibiting the absorption of dietary fats. The acting location of orlistat is the lumen of the stomach and small intestine. Orlistat acts by binding gastric and pancreatic lipases, which are key enzymes involved in the digestion of dietary fat, and inhibits the hydrolysis of triglycerides, thereby reducing systemic fat absorption and resulting in a reduction in body weight. In 1999, the FDA approved a 120 mg orlistat capsule, named Xenical®, as a prescription product for obesity management in conjunction with a reduced-calorie diet. In February 2007, a 60 mg orlistat capsule, Alli®, was approved as an Over-The-Counter (OTC) product (Johnson & Schwartz, 2018).

According to the label of Xenical®, systemic absorption of orlistat is minimal (<2% of the dose), and consequently, it is inadequate for pharmacokinetic analysis due to the low concentrations in plasma. Complexity for BE assessment of orlistat is that the systemic drug exposure is minimal and not relevant to the efficacy and safety in the acting location. Instead, a PD endpoint, Percentage Fecal Fat excretion (PFF), is used for establishing BE (Jiang et al., 2014). As aforementioned in Section 9.3.2, when the administrated dose is not close to EC_{50}, the regular TOST approach is not suitable for PD BE assessment due to nonlinear dose-PD response relationship. Instead, the FDA recommended the dose-scale method, which is introduced in Section 9.3.3, to establishing BE of generic orlistat to the reference product (US FDA, 2010b).

Johnson and Schwartz (Johnson & Schwartz, 2018) reported two BE studies, sponsored by GlaxoSmithKline (GSK), for comparison of orlistat chewable tablet and capsule formulation. Though these two studies are not for development of generic drugs, the study design and statistical method are consistent with the BE study for generic drugs. Both studies are designed following the recommendation of PSG for orlistat. A randomized, 3-period, 3-treatment (Latin square) crossover design is employed. Healthy males and non-pregnant females are recruited and then experience a run-in period of controlled diet and no drug for six days. Following the run-in period, subjects were randomly allocated into three sequences and received orlistat 27-mg chewable tablet, orlistat 60-mg capsule, or orlistat 120 mg (2 60-mg capsules) in each treatment period. Standardized daily diet containing a total of 70 g of fat and 2200 calories was provided during the study period. Each of the three treatment periods lasted nine days and was separated by a washout period of two days. It should be noted that the FDA PSG recommends that the washout should be at least four days.

The primary pharmacodynamic variable in each study was PFF excretion. Both studies performed bioequivalence assessment using the dose-scale method. In the first study (refer to as study 1), the dose-scale method was used as a secondary analysis for BE. The primary analysis was based on TOST and 90% CI of the ratio of geometric means for the orlistat 27-mg chewable tablet over 60-mg capsule using log-transformed PFF. And there was an additional secondary analysis, Fieller 90%CI of the ratio of original scale means of PFF. Study 2 was a confirmative study based on the results of study 1, in which the sample size was increased to provide adequate power for the dose-scale method to demonstrate bioequivalence of orlistat 27-mg chewable tablet to 60-mg capsule. The primary analysis of study 2 was the dose-scale method using original data. Secondary analyses included TOST and Fieller CI based on log-transformed and original scale PFF, respectively.

A total of 48 subjects were included in the analysis of study 1, and 144 subjects were included study 2. Results for bioequivalence analysis are shown in Table 9.2. Although the 90%CI of the relative bioavailability (F) of study 1, 0.73–1.28, was wider than the BE limits of 0.80–1.25, the point estimate of F, 0.996, still shown a very similar PD activity between orlistat 27-mg chewable tablet and 60-mg capsule. Study 2 increased the sample size and yield a relative bioavailability of 1.094 and 90%CI of 0.978–1.215 using dose-scale method, which fell within the bioequivalence limits. Therefore, it could be concluded that 27-mg orlistat chewable tablet is bioequivalent to 60-mg capsule based on the results of these two studies.

TABLE 9.2

BE Assessment of Orlistat Chewable Tablet and Capsule Formulation

	Study 1	Study 2
Dose-scale method BCa (90%CI)	0.996(0.73,1.28)	1.094(0.978,1.215)
TOST (90%CI)	0.96(0.87,1.06)	1.02(0.98,1.07)
Fieller's method (90%CI)	0.96(0.87,1.06)	1.04(1.00,1.09)

9.5.2 An AH PK Bioequivalence Study for Dexamethasone-Tobramycin Ophthalmic Suspension

Tobramycin–dexamethasone ophthalmic suspension is an antibiotic-steroid combination product indicated for steroid responsive inflammatory ocular conditions for which a corti-costeroid is indicated and where superficial bacterial ocular infection or a risk of bacterial ocular infection exists (Andrew et al., 2012). As one of the primary indications of tobramycin–dexamethasone ophthalmic suspension is to control inflammation after cataract surgery, concentrations of dexamethasone in AH can be obtained through sampling during opera-tion procedure. Therefore, BE for tobramycin–dexamethasone ophthalmic suspension can be evaluated based on AH PK data.

In 1988, the FDA approved TOBRADEX® (tobramycin 0.3%, dexamethasone 0.1%) manu-factured by Alcon Inc. In 2007, Alcon Inc. submitted an application for Tobradex® ST, which contains the same API and has a lower concentration of dexamethasone (tobramycin 0.3%, dexamethasone 0.05%). With the application of a retention-enhancing vehicle (xanthan gum), Tobradex® ST was theorized to provide similar efficacy as TOBRADEX®. Tobradex® ST was approved in February 2009.

The pivotal study for approval of Tobradex® ST was a randomized, double-masked, parallel group, single-dose BE study (Shen & Machado, 2017; US FDA Center for Drug Evaluation and Research, 2008). Although Tobradex® ST is an enhanced formulation rather than a generic of TOBRADEX®, the technical details of AH PK BE study for both scenarios are in common. In this study, male and female patients 18 years of age and older, of any race, who required cataract surgery would be enrolled. Subjects were randomized into test group (Tobradex® ST, referred to as T) and reference group (TOBRADEX®, referred to as R) and then randomly allocated to each of 5 post-dose sampling time points: 0.5, 1, 2, 3, and 5 hours. AH sample of each subject was obtained during the cataract surgery, at pre-specified time point after dosing.

The primary PK parameter was AUC up to five hours after dosing (AUC_{0-5}). The point estimate of AUC_{0-5} was calculated using Bailer's method (Nedelman et al., 1995). Based on the estimate of the mean concentration of each time point, bioequivalence was tested using Fieller's method, which is described in section 9.3.3. In addition, a bootstrap confidence interval was calculated as a supportive analysis.

A total of 987 subjects were enrolled into the study, 957 and 886 subjects were included into the ITT and PP population. PP population was the primary population for bio-equivalence test. The Fieller 90%CI for AUC_T/AUC_R was 0.983–1.16 and bootstrap CI was 0.996–1.19, both lies within the prespecified bioequivalence limits of 0.80–1.25. When the application of Tobradex® ST was under review, the FDA reviewer verified the results. The Fieller's methods yielded identical result with the sponsor's calculation, the 90%CI was 0.983–1.158. In addition to unstratified bootstrap CI, 0.983–1.159, the reviewer calculated a stratified bootstrap CI of 0.981–1.153. All these outcomes supported that Tobradex® ST is bioequivalent to TOBRADEX®. Tobradex® ST was approved by FDA in February 2009.

TABLE 9.3

Bioequivalence Assessment of Tobradex® ST and TOBRADEX®

AUC_T/AUC_R	Sponsor's Analysis	FDA Reviewer's Analysis
Fieller's method (90%CI)	1.07(0.983,1.16)	1.067(0.983,1.158)
Unstratified Bootstrap (90%CI)	1.07(0.996,1.19)	1.069(0.983,1.159)
Stratified Bootstrap (90%CI)		1.065(0.981,1.153)

9.5.3 An IVPT-Based Bioequivalence Study for Acyclovir Cream

Acyclovir cream, known as an antiviral product, is indicated for treatment of recurrent herpes labialis (cold sores). The API, acyclovir, is a synthetic purine nucleoside analogue, which exerts its pharmacologic activity by inhibiting replication of herpes viral DNA. In December 2002, the first acyclovir cream in US, ZOVIRAX® (5%), was approved by FDA.

Since acyclovir cream, 5% is a product with modest efficacy, comparative studies with clinical endpoints would be resource-consuming and not feasible to perform. The FDA PSG for acyclovir cream recommends an IVPT-based BE study (US FDA, 2016a). Although a novel technique, dermal open flow microperfusion (dOFM), can provide a direct *in vivo* measurement of drug concentration at or near the site of action in the skin and thereby characterize the rate and extent of drug exposure (Bodenlenz et al., 2017), this method may not as feasible and economical as IVPT. Furthermore, dOFM devices are still yet to be approved for utilization in human in some country up to date. Currently, IVPT have been used in a number of pre-clinical studies and bioavailability studies.

Shin et al. (Shin et al., 2020) conducted an IVPT-based BE study for comparison of two Zovirax® creams registered in the United States (refer to as US Zovirax®) and in the United Kingdom (refer to as UK Zovirax®), respectively. A replicated design was used in this study. In the pivotal study, six skin sections from each of six donors who experienced an abdomino-plasty surgery was used. All these abdominoplasty surgical waste skin pieces were obtained from the Cooperative Human Tissue Network (CHTN). Skin samples were dermatomed to a thickness of 260 ± 40 µm, removing subcutaneous fat and keeping the outer layers of skin containing Stratum Corneum (SC), viable epidermis, and some dermis. A PermeGear flow-through In-Line diffusion system (PermeGear, Inc.; Hellertown, PA) with an automated fraction collector was used for IVPT experiments. The permeation area of diffusion cells was 0.95 cm^2, where a single dose of 15 mg/cm^2 of acyclovir cream was applied. The flow rate of the receptor solution was approximately 0.22 mL/h (pump setting at 0.5 rpm). Duration for each IVPT run was 48 hours, with continuous sampling every four hours.

The primary endpoints were J_{max} and total cumulative penetration (total AUC). BE was tested using the RSABE procedure introduced in Section 9.4.3. In the analysis, the US Zovirax® was used as reference product. The results of equivalence test are shown in Table 9.4. The S_{WR} of J_{max} and total AUC, 0.4238 and 0.4457, respectively, both larger than 0.294. Subsequently, the bioequivalence would be determined using the RSABE criterion. The upper bound of the 95% confidence interval of J_{max} and total AUC were both larger than zero, and the point estimate of GMR were not included in the limits of 0.80–1.25.

Simulation studies were performed to evaluate whether the number of donors was adequate for BE assessment. The results of simulation studies shown that for true GMR inside the interval [0.80,1.25], a sample size of six and 14 donors can achieve 80% power for equivalence test of total AUC and J_{max}. Therefore, the equivalence total AUC was tested with adequate statistical power. In summary, the current result of Shin et al.'s study cannot support the conclusion that the U.K. Zovirax® is equivalent to the US Zovirax®.

TABLE 9.4

IVPT-Based Bioequivalence Assessment of U.S. Zovirax® and U.K. Zovirax®

	T/R	S_{WR}	RSABE 95% Upper Bound	ABE 90%CI
J_{max}	0.4926	0.4238	0.9859	(0.3459,0.6711)
Total AUC	0.5314	0.4457	0.5957	(0.4208,0.6711)

9.6 Concluding Remarks

In development of complex generic drugs, the typical one-size-fits-all approach may not be adequate. Instead, it is necessary to choose appropriate methodologies for BE assessment according to the complexities the different products. In this context, PSGs are essential to reduce the uncertainty in development of complex generic drugs by regulating studies that need to be conducted, framework of study design, technical requirement of analytical methods, and statistical methods for establishing BE. Since 2007, FDA has issued more than 1650 PSGs.

In this chapter, we summarize statistical designs and methodologies for bioequivalence assessment utilized in *in vivo* and *in vitro* studies, which are recommended by PSGs. Generally speaking, besides of TOST, statistical methods in BE study of complex generic drugs mainly include the following: (i) Fieller's method can be used for equivalence test for clinical endpoints, PD endpoints, and sparse sampling data; (ii) model-based methods, which can be fitted using bootstrap or NLME modeling, are often utilized in BE studies with PD endpoints or sparse sampling data; (iii) RSABE procedures are used for bioequivalence assessment of HVD, NIT, and some *in vitro* experimental data with high variability; (iv) PBE procedure are often recommended for *in vitro* BE assessment of formulation/device-related characteristics, such as liposome size distribution for liposome drugs and spray pattern for nasal sprays; (v) non-parametrical methods such as Mann-Whitney U test are often used in *in vitro* studies in which observation are not normally distributed.

For *in vivo* BE studies, the endpoints are generally limited to PK parameters, PD parameters, and a few clinical endpoints. For *in vitro* studies, on the other hand, there could be various endpoints as the characters being compared are various. Moreover, a number of new measurements have been introduced into evaluation of generic drugs for some specific challenges. A representative example is the Earth Mover's Distance (EMD) for comparison of globule size distribution in BE studies for cyclosporine emulsion, in which case the globule size distribution is bi-peak and conventional D50/SPAN method is not suitable for the description of the globule size distribution profile (Hu et al., 2018).

New sampling as well as analytical techniques promote the development of the methodology of BE study for complex generic drugs. For instance, the application of the dOFM technique can provide a direct *in-vivo* measurement of drug concentration at or near the site of action in the skin and thereby make it possible to establish BE for dermal-topical drug products through *in vivo* PK studies. Correspondingly, appropriate study designs and statistical methods should be applied with respect to the requirement and characteristics of the new sampling/analytical methods.

References

Andrew, R., Luecke, G., Dozier, S., & Diven, D. G. (2012). A Pilot Study to Investigate the Efficacy of Tobramycin–Dexamethasone Ointment in Promoting Wound Healing. *Dermatology and Therapy*, 2(1), 12. https://doi.org/10.1007/s13555-012-0012-8

Bell, C., Anderson, J., Ganguly, T., Prescott, J., Capila, I., Lansing, J. C., Sachleben, R., Iyer, M., Fier, I., Roach, J., Storey, K., Miller, P., Hall, S., Kantor, D., Greenberg, B. M., Nair, K., & Glajch, J. (2017). Development of Glatopa® (Glatiramer Acetate): The First FDA-Approved Generic Disease-Modifying Therapy for Relapsing Forms of Multiple Sclerosis. *Journal of Pharmacy Practice*, 31(5), 481–488. https://doi.org/10.1177/0897190017725984

Berger, R. L. (1989). Uniformly More Powerful Tests for Hypotheses Concerning Linear Inequalities and Normal Means. *Journal of the American Statistical Association, 84*(405), 192–199. https://doi.org/10.2307/2289863

Berger, R. L., & Hsu, J. C. (1996). Bioequivalence Trials, Intersection-Union Tests and Equivalence Confidence Sets. *Statistical Science, 11*(4), 283–302. http://www.jstor.org/stable/2246021

Bodenlenz, M., Tiffner, K. I., Raml, R., Augustin, T., Dragatin, C., Birngruber, T., Schimek, D., Schwagerle, G., Pieber, T. R., Raney, S. G., Kanfer, I., & Sinner, F. (2017). Open Flow Microperfusion as a Dermal Pharmacokinetic Approach to Evaluate Topical Bioequivalence. *Clinical Pharmacokinetics, 56*(1), 91–98. https://doi.org/10.1007/s40262-016-0442-z

Braddy, A. C., & Conner, D. P. (2014). Bioequivalence for Topical Drug Products. In L. X. Yu & B. V. Li (Eds.), *FDA Bioequivalence Standards* (pp. 335–367). Springer New York. https://doi.org/10.1007/978-1-4939-1252-0_13

Braddy, A. C., Davit, B. M., Stier, E. M., & Conner, D. P. (2015). Survey of International Regulatory Bioequivalence Recommendations for Approval of Generic Topical Dermatological Drug Products. *The AAPS Journal, 17*(1), 121–133. https://doi.org/10.1208/s12248-014-9679-3

Brown, M. B., & Williams, A. C. (2019). *The Art and Science of Dermal Formulation Development.* CRC Press.

Chen, M.-L. (2014). Fundamentals of Bioequivalence. In L. X. Yu & B. V. Li (Eds.), *FDA Bioequivalence Standards* (pp. 29–53). Springer New York. https://doi.org/10.1007/978-1-4939-1252-0_2

Choi, S. H., Wang, Y., Conti, D. S., Raney, S. G., Delvadia, R., Leboeuf, A. A., & Witzmann, K. (2018). Generic Drug Device Combination Products: Regulatory and Scientific Considerations. *International Journal of Pharmaceutics, 544*(2), 443–454. https://doi.org/10.1016/j.ijpharm.2017.11.038

Chow, S.-C. (2014). Bioavailability and Bioequivalence in Drug Development. *WIREs Computational Statistics, 6*(4), 304–312. https://doi.org/10.1002/wics.1310

Chow, S.-C., & Liu, J.-P. (1999). *Design and analysis of bioavailability and bioequivalence studies.* CRC press.

Chow, S.-C., Shao, J., & Wang, H. (2003). In Vitro Bioequivalence Testing [https://doi.org/10.1002/sim.1345]. *Statistics in Medicine, 22*(1), 55–68. https://doi.org/10.1002/sim.1345

Cox, C. (1990). Fieller's Theorem, the Likelihood and the Delta Method. *Biometrics, 46*(3), 709–718. https://doi.org/10.2307/2532090

DiCiccio, T. J., & Efron, B. (1996). Bootstrap Confidence Intervals. *Statistical Science, 11*(3), 189–212. http://www.jstor.org/stable/2246110

EMEA. (2018). *Draft guideline on quality and equivalence of topical products.* Retrieved from https://www.ema.europa.eu/en/quality-equivalence-topical-products

European Medicines Agency. (2010). *Guideline on the investigation of bioequivalence.* Retrieved from https://www.ema.europa.eu/en/documents/scientific-guideline/guideline-investigation-bioequivalence-rev1_en.pdf

GDUFA. (2016). *GDUFA Reauthorization Performance Goals and Program Enhancements Fiscal Years 2018-2022 (GDUFA II Commitment Lette).*

Gong, X.-J. (2019). Regulatory Considerations on Dose-Scale Analysis in Assessing Pharmacodynamic Equivalence. Regulatory Education for Industry: 2019 Complex Generic Drug Product Development Workshop: Quantitative Methods and Modeling-Informed Regulatory Descision Making, the University of Maryland, United States.

Grosser, S., Park, M., Raney, S. G., & Rantou, E. (2015). Determining Equivalence for Generic Locally Acting Drug Products. *Statistics in Biopharmaceutical Research, 7*(4), 337–345. https://doi.org/10.1080/19466315.2015.1093541

Habjanič, N., Kerec Kos, M., & Kristan, K. (2020). Sensitivity of Different In Vitro Performance Tests and Their In Vivo Relevance for Calcipotriol/Betamethasone Ointment. *Pharmaceutical Research, 37*(3), 52. https://doi.org/10.1007/s11095-020-2766-5

Harigaya, Y., Jiang, X., Zhang, H., Chandaroy, P., Stier, E. M., & Pan, Y. (2018). Bioequivalence Study Methods with Pharmacokinetic Endpoints for Topical Ophthalmic Corticosteroid Suspensions and Effects of Subject Demographics. *Pharmaceutical Research, 36*(1), 13. https://doi.org/10.1007/s11095-018-2537-8

Harigaya, Y., Jiang, X., Zhang, H., Chandaroy, P., Stier, E. M., & Pan, Y. (2019). Bioequivalence Study Methods with Pharmacokinetic Endpoints for Topical Ophthalmic Corticosteroid Suspensions and effects of Subject Demographics. *Pharmaceutical Research, 36*(1), 1–8.

Hauschke, D., Kieser, M., Diletti, E., & Burke, M. (1999). Sample Size Determination for Proving Equivalence based on the Ratio of Two means for Normally Distributed Data [https://doi.org/10.1002/(SICI)1097-0258(19990115)18:1<93::AID-SIM992>3.0.CO;2-8]. *Statistics in Medicine, 18*(1), 93–105. https://doi.org/10.1002/(SICI)1097-0258(19990115)18:1<93::AID-SIM992>3.0.CO;2-8

Health Canada. (2012). *Comparative bioavailability standards: formulations used for systemic effects.* Retrieved from https://www.hc-sc.gc.ca/dhp-mps/alt_formats/pdf/prodpharma/applic-demande/guide-ld/bio/gd_standards_ld_normes-eng.pdf

Higuchi, T. (1961). Rate of Release of Medicaments from Ointment Bases Containing Drugs in Suspension. *Journal of Pharmaceutical Sciences, 50*(10), 874–875. https://doi.org/10.1002/jps.2600501018

Howe, W. G. (1974). Approximate Confidence Limits on the Mean of X + Y Where X and Y Are Two Tabled Independent Random Variables. *Journal of the American Statistical Association, 69*(347), 789–794. https://doi.org/10.1080/01621459.1974.10480206

Hu, M., Jiang, X., Absar, M., Choi, S., Kozak, D., Shen, M., Weng, Y.-T., Zhao, L., & Lionberger, R. (2018). Equivalence Testing of Complex Particle Size Distribution Profiles Based on Earth Mover's Distance. *The AAPS Journal, 20*(3), 62. https://doi.org/10.1208/s12248-018-0212-y

Hutchison, A. L., Allada, R., & Dinner, A. R. (2018). Bootstrapping and Empirical Bayes Methods Improve Rhythm Detection in Sparsely Sampled Data. *Journal of Biological Rhythms, 33*(4), 339–349. https://doi.org/10.1177/0748730418789536

Hyslop, T., Hsuan, F., & Holder, D. J. (2000). A small sample confidence interval approach to assess individual bioequivalence [https://doi.org/10.1002/1097-0258(20001030)19:20<2885::AID-SIM553>3.0.CO;2-H]. *Statistics in Medicine, 19*(20), 2885–2897. https://doi.org/10.1002/1097-0258(20001030)19:20<2885::AID-SIM553>3.0.CO;2-H

Jiang, W., & Yu, L. X. (2014). Bioequivalence for Narrow Therapeutic Index Drugs. In L. X. Yu & B. V. Li (Eds.), *FDA Bioequivalence Standards* (pp. 191–216). Springer New York. https://doi.org/10.1007/978-1-4939-1252-0_8

Jiang, X., Yang, Y., & Stier, E. (2014). Bioequivalence for Drug Products Acting Locally Within Gastrointestinal Tract. In L. X. Yu & B. V. Li (Eds.), *FDA Bioequivalence Standards* (pp. 297–334). Springer New York. https://doi.org/10.1007/978-1-4939-1252-0_12

Johnson, S., & Schwartz, S. M. (2018). Pharmacologic and Pharmacodynamic Equivalence of 2 Formulations of Orlistat [https://doi.org/10.1002/cpdd.457]. *Clinical Pharmacology in Drug Development, 7*(7), 773–780. https://doi.org/https://doi.org/10.1002/cpdd.457

Kanfer, I., & Shargel, L. (2007). *Generic Drug Product Development: Bioequivalence Issues.* CRC Press.

Labes, D., Schuetz, H., & Lang, B. (2016). PowerTOST: Power and Sample Size Based on Two One-Sided *t*-Tests (TOST) for (Bio) equivalence studies. *R Package Version, 3*(3).

Lee, C.-Y., Chen, X., Romanelli, R. J., & Segal, J. B. (2016). Forces Influencing Generic Drug Development in the United States: A Narrative Review. *Journal of Pharmaceutical Policy and Practice, 9*(1), 26. https://doi.org/10.1186/s40545-016-0079-1

Lee, Y., Shao, J., & Chow, S.C. (2004). Modified Large-Sample Confidence Intervals for Linear Combinations of Variance Components: Extension, Theory, and Application. *Journal of the American Statistical Association, 99*(466), 467–478. http://www.jstor.org/stable/27590402

Lehman, P. A., Raney, S. G., & Franz, T. J. (2011). Percutaneous Absorption in Man: In vitro-in vivo Correlation. *Skin Pharmacology and Physiology, 24*(4), 224–230. https://doi.org/10.1159/000324884

Lunawat, S., & Bhat, K. (2020). Complex Generic Products: Insight of Current Regulatory Frameworks in US, EU and Canada and the Need of Harmonisation. *Therapeutic Innovation & Regulatory Science.* https://doi.org/10.1007/s43441-020-00114-6

Lusina Kregar, M., Dürrigl, M., Rožman, A., Jelčić, Ž., Cetina-Čižmek, B., & Filipović-Grčić, J. (2015). Development and Validation of an In Vitro Release Method for Topical Particulate Delivery Systems. *International Journal of Pharmaceutics, 485*(1), 202–214. https://doi.org/10.1016/https://doi.org/10.1016/j.ijpharm.2015.03.018

Miranda, M., Sousa, J. J., Veiga, F., Cardoso, C., & Vitorino, C. (2018). Bioequivalence of Topical Generic Products. Part 2. Paving the Way to a Tailored Regulatory System. *European Journal of Pharmaceutical Sciences, 122,* 264–272. https://doi.org/10.1016/j.ejps.2018.07.011

Nedelman, J. R., Gibiansky, E., & Lau, D. T. W. (1995). Applying Bailer's Method for AUC Confidence Intervals to Sparse Sampling. *Pharmaceutical Research, 12*(1), 124–128. https://doi.org/10.1023/A:1016255124336

Peters, J. R. (2014). Clinical Endpoint Bioequivalence Study. In L. X. Yu & B. V. Li (Eds.), *FDA Bioequivalence Standards* (pp. 243–274). Springer New York. https://doi.org/10.1007/978-1-4939-1252-0_10

Saluja, B., Li, B. V., & Lee, S. L. (2014). Bioequivalence for Orally Inhaled and Nasal Drug Products. In L. X. Yu & B. V. Li (Eds.), *FDA Bioequivalence Standards* (pp. 369-394). Springer New York. https://doi.org/10.1007/978-1-4939-1252-0_14

Shen, M., & Machado, S. G. (2017). Bioequivalence Evaluation of Sparse Sampling Pharmacokinetics Data using Bootstrap Resampling Method. *Journal of Biopharmaceutical Statistics, 27*(2), 257–264. https://doi.org/10.1080/10543406.2016.1265543

Shin, S. H., Rantou, E., Raney, S. G., Ghosh, P., Hassan, H., & Stinchcomb, A. (2020). Cutaneous Pharmacokinetics of Acyclovir Cream 5% Products: Evaluating Bioequivalence with an In Vitro Permeation Test and an Adaptation of Scaled Average Bioequivalence. *Pharmaceutical Research, 37*(10), 210. https://doi.org/10.1007/s11095-020-02821-z

Smith, E. W., Meyer, E., & Haigh, J. M. (1993). The Human Skin Blanching Assay for Topical Corticosteroid Bioavailability Assessment. In V. P. Shah & H. I. Maibach (Eds.), *Topical Drug Bioavailability, Bioequivalence, and Penetration* (pp. 155–162). Springer US. https://doi.org/10.1007/978-1-4899-1262-6_8

Sun, W., Grosser, S., Kim, C., & Raney, S. G. (2019). Statistical Considerations and impact of the FDA Draft Guidance for Assessing Adhesion with Transdermal Delivery Systems and Topical Patches for ANDAs. *Journal of Biopharmaceutical Statistics, 29*(5), 952–970. https://doi.org/10.1080/10543406.2019.1657440

Sykes, A. M. (2000). Ratio Estimates and Fieller's Theorem in Regression Modelling. *Communications in Statistics - Theory and Methods, 29*(9–10), 2055–2063. https://doi.org/10.1080/03610920008832595

Tiffner, K. I., Kanfer, I., Augustin, T., Raml, R., Raney, S. G., & Sinner, F. (2018). A comprehensive Approach to Qualify and Validate the Essential Parameters of an In vitro Release Test (IVRT) Method for Acyclovir Cream, 5%. *International Journal of Pharmaceutics, 535*(1), 217–227. https://doi.org/10.1016/j.ijpharm.2017.09.049

Tóthfalusi, L., Endrényi, L., & Chow, S.C. (2014). Statistical and Regulatory Considerations in Assessments of Interchangeability of Biological Drug Products. *The European Journal of Health Economics: HEPAC: Health Economics in Prevention and Care, 15*(Suppl 1), S5–11. https://doi.org/10.1007/s10198-014-0589-1

US FDA. (2001). *Guidance for Industry: Statistical Approaches to Establishing Bioequivalence.* Retrieved from https://www.fda.gov/regulatory-information/search-fda-guidance-documents/statistical-approaches-establishing-bioequivalence

US FDA. (2003). *Guidance for Industry: bioavailability and bioequivalence studies for nasal aerosols and nasal sprays for local action.* Retrieved from https://www.fda.gov/regulatory-information/search-fda-guidance-documents/bioavailability-and-bioequivalence-studies-nasal-aerosols-and-nasal-sprays-local-action

US FDA. (2010a). *Draft Guidance on Orlistat.*

US FDA. (2011). *Draft Guidance on Ciclopirox.*

US FDA. (2012a). *Draft Guidance on Budesonide.*

US FDA. (2012b). *Draft Guidance on Warfarin Sodium.* Retrieved from https://www.accessdata.fda.gov/drugsatfda_docs/psg/Warfarin_Sodium_tab_09218_RC12-12.pdf

US FDA. (2014a). *Draft Guidance on Benzyl Alcohol.*

US FDA. (2014b). *Draft Guidance on Conjugated Estrogens.*

US FDA. (2016a). *Draft Guidance on Acyclovir.*

US FDA. (2016b). *Draft Guidance on Colesevelam Hydrochloride.*

US FDA. (2016c). Draft Guidance on Mometasone Furoate.

US FDA. (2016d). Draft Guidance on Nepafenac

US FDA. (2016e). Draft Guidance on Risperidone.

US FDA. (2018a). *Draft Guidance on Dapsone.*

US FDA. (2018b). *Draft Guidance on Doxorubicin Hydrochloride.*

US FDA. (2018c). *Draft Guidance on Glatiramer Acetate.*

US FDA. (2018d). *Draft Guidance on Loteprednol Etabonate.*

US FDA. (2018e). *Draft Guidance on Selegiline.*

US FDA. (2018f). DRAFT GUIDANCE: Assessing Adhesion With Transdermal and Topical Delivery Systems for ANDAs Guidance for Industry.

US FDA. (2018g). *Guidance for Industry: Assessing the Irritation and Sensitization Potential of Transdermal and Topical Delivery Systems for ANDAs.*

US FDA. (2019a). *Draft Guidance on Adapalene; Benzoyl Peroxide.*

US FDA. (2019b). *Draft Guidance on Fluticasone Propionate.*

US FDA. (2019c). *Draft Guidance on Fluticasone Propionate; Salmeterol Xinafoate.*

US FDA. (2020a). CFR-code of federal regulations title 21. In.

US FDA. (2020b). *Draft Guidance on Albuterol Sulfate.*

US FDA. (2020c). *Draft Guidance on Triamcinolone Acetonide.*

US FDA Center for Drug Evaluation and Research. (2008). Statistical review for application number 50818. In.

USP. (2011). *United States Pharmacopeia (USP) general chapter <1724> Semisolid durg prodcuts – performance tests.*

Wolfsegger, M. J. (2007). Establishing Bioequivalence in Serial Sacrifice Designs. *Journal of Pharmacokinetics and Pharmacodynamics, 34*(1), 103-113. https://doi.org/10.1007/s10928-006-9037-x

Yacobi, A., Shah, V. P., Bashaw, E. D., Benfeldt, E., Davit, B., Ganes, D., Ghosh, T., Kanfer, I., Kasting, G. B., Katz, L., Lionberger, R., Lu, G. W., Maibach, H. I., Pershing, L. K., Rackley, R. J., Raw, A., Shukla, C. G., Thakker, K., Wagner, N., Zovko, E., & Lane, M. E. (2014). Current Challenges in Bioequivalence, Quality, and Novel Assessment Technologies for Topical Products. *Pharmaceutical Research, 31*(4), 837–846. https://doi.org/10.1007/s11095-013-1259-1

Zhao, L., Kim, M.-J., Zhang, L., & Lionberger, R. (2019). Generating Model Integrated Evidence for Generic Drug Development and Assessment [https://doi.org/10.1002/cpt.1282]. *Clinical Pharmacology & Therapeutics, 105*(2), 338–349. https://doi.org/https://doi.org/10.1002/cpt.1282

Zheng, N., Jiang, W., Lionberger, R., & Yu, L. X. (2014). Bioequivalence for Liposomal Drug Products. In L. X. Yu & B. V. Li (Eds.), *FDA Bioequivalence Standards* (pp. 275–296). Springer New York. https://doi.org/10.1007/978-1-4939-1252-0_11

Zou, P., & Yu, L. X. (2014). Pharmacodynamic Endpoint Bioequivalence Studies. In L. X. Yu & B. V. Li (Eds.), *FDA Bioequivalence Standards* (pp. 217–241). Springer New York. https://doi.org/10.1007/978-1-4939-1252-0_9

10

Rare Diseases Drug Development

Shein-Chung Chow[1], Shutian Zhang[2], and Wei Zhang[3]

[1]*Duke University School of Medicine, Durham, NC, USA*

[2]*National Clinical Research Center for Digestive Disease, Beijing Friendship Hospital, Beijing, China*

[3]*AffaMed Therapeutics, New York, NY, USA*

CONTENTS

DOI: 10.1201/9781003107323-10

10.1 What is Rare Disease?

In the United States, a rare disease is defined as a condition that affects fewer than 200,000 people (ODA, 1983). Under this definition, there may be as many as 7,000 rare diseases in the United States. The total number of Americans living with a rare disease is estimated at between 25–30 million. This estimate has been used by the rare disease community for several decades to highlight that while individual diseases may be rare, the total number of people with a rare disease is large. In the United States, however, only a few types of rare diseases are tracked when a person is diagnosed. These include certain infectious diseases, birth defects, and cancers. It also includes the diseases on state newborn screening tests. Because most rare diseases are not tracked, it is hard to determine the exact number of rare diseases or how many people are affected. Rare diseases are also known as orphan diseases because drug companies were not interested in developing treatments under economic (or return of investment) consideration. To overcome this dilemma, in 1983, the United States Congress passed the Orphan Drug Act which created several financial incentives to encourage pharmaceutical companies to develop new drugs for rare diseases (ODA, 1983).

Other countries have their own official definitions of a rare disease. For example, in the European Union (EU), a disease or disorder is defined as rare in Europe when it affects fewer than 1 in 2,000 people. Under this definition, there are more than 6,000 rare diseases. On the whole, rare diseases may affect 30 million European Union citizens. 80% of rare diseases are of genetic origin, and are often chronic and life-threatening. On the other hand, in Japan, according to the National Programme on Rare and Intractable Diseases launched in 1972, rare diseases are defined as those with a prevalence of less than 50,000, or one in 2500, and with no known cause or cure. Under this definition, 123 diseases have been identified/specified by an Expert Advisory Board on the basis of research priorities. which include Behçet disease, multiple sclerosis, and amyotrophic lateral sclerosis. In China, thus far, rare diseases have not been officially defined. The definition that is commonly considered is based on a consensus of experts reached by the Genetics Branch of the Chinese Medical Association in May 2010. According to this definition, a rare disease is a disease with a prevalence of less than 1/500,000 or a neonatal morbidity of less than 1/10,000. Since epidemiological data on rare diseases are lacking in China, the current list of rare diseases is based on actual conditions, and the list is mainly derived from the professional opinions of the Expert Committee on the Diagnosis, Treatment, and Care for Rare Diseases established by the Medical Administration Bureau of the former National Health and Family Planning Commission.

For orphan drug designation, FDA considers using the Mechanism Of Action (MOA) of the drug to determine what distinct disease or condition the drug is intended to treat, diagnose or prevent. Whether a given medical condition constitutes a distinct disease or condition for the purpose of orphan-drug designation depends on a number of factors, assessed cumulatively, including: pathogenesis of the disease or condition; course of the disease or condition; prognosis of the disease or condition; and resistance to treatment. These factors are analyzed in the context of the specific drug for which designation is requested. During the course of reviewing a request for orphan drug designation, equipped with the most current scientific literature about a particular disease or condition, FDA may come to a new understanding about the nature of that disease or condition. Table 10.1 provides a list of some diseases or conditions for which FDA's views on how it categorizes or otherwise understands the disease or condition has evolved. This is not a comprehensive list of orphan disease determinations, but reflective of some of the more common questions we receive. FDA will update this list as appropriate when it makes orphan drug designation determinations that change how we approach the disease or condition in question. For a complete list of orphan drug designations and approvals see the searchable Orphan Products Designation Database.

As most rare diseases may affect far fewer persons, one of the major concerns of rare disease clinical trials are that often there are only a small number of subjects available. However, FDA does not have the intention to create a statutory standard for approval of orphan drugs that is different from the standard for approval of drugs in common conditions. Thus, in rare disease clinical trials, power calculation for required sample size may not be feasible. In this case, innovative thinking and approach are necessary for achieving same standard with limited number of patients available. In this chapter, some innovative

TABLE 10.1

List of Orphan Disease Determination

Disease or Condition	FDA's Perspectives
Ovarian, Fallopian Tube, and Primary Peritoneal Cancer	FDA considers ovarian cancer, fallopian tube cancer, and primary peritoneal cancer to be one distinct disease or condition.
Metastatic Brain Cancer	FDA considers any primary tumor type that has metastasized to the brain to be its own distinct disease or condition. For example, breast cancer that has metastasized to the brain is a distinct disease from breast cancer.
Pulmonary Hypertension	FDA recognizes the five WHO classifications of pulmonary hypertension as distinct diseases or conditions.
Scleroderma	FDA considers systemic sclerosis to be a different disease or condition than localized scleroderma.
Lymphoma	FDA recognizes the WHO classifications of lymphoma as distinct diseases or conditions.
Familial Adenomatous Polyposis	FDA recognizes Familial Adenomatous Polyposis as a distinct disease or condition from sporadic adenomatous polyps
Medication-induced Dyskinesia in Parkinson's Disease	FDA recognizes Medication-induced Dyskinesia in Parkinson's Disease (PD) as the disease or condition. Levodopa-induced dyskinesia in PD is considered to be a subset of Medication induced Dyskinesia in PD.

thinking for rare diseases drug development such as (i) probability monitoring procedure for justification of the selected small sample size, (ii) the concept of demonstrating not-ineffectiveness (non-inferiority) rather than demonstrating effectiveness (superiority) with limited number of patients available, (iii) the combined use of data from randomized clinical trial (RCT) and RWD and real-world evidence (RWE) in support of rare diseases drug development, and (iv) innovative two-stage adaptive seamless clinical trial design are proposed.

In the next section, regulatory perspectives (including regulatory incentives and regulatory guidance) regarding rare disease drug development are outlined. Some innovative thinking for rare diseases drug development is described in Section 10.3. Section 10.4 discusses some complex innovative designs and analyses of rare diseases clinical trials. Section 10.5 discusses sponsors' strategy and perspectives regarding rare disease drug development. Also included in the section is a case study about the unique and remarkable story of Velcade® drug development. Some concluding remarks are given in the last section of this chapter.

10.2 Regulatory Perspectives

10.2.1 Regulatory Incentives

As indicated in FDA (2015, 2019a), most rare diseases are genetic related, and thus are present throughout the person's entire life, even if symptoms do not immediately appear. Many rare diseases appear early in life, and about 30% of children with rare diseases will die before reaching their fifth birthday. FDA is to advance the evaluation and development of products including drugs, biologics, and devices that demonstrate promise for the diagnosis and/or treatment of rare diseases or conditions. Along this line, FDA evaluates scientific and clinical data submissions from sponsors to identify and designate products as promising for rare diseases and to further advance scientific development of such promising medical products. To encourage the development of rare disease drug products, FDA provides several incentive (expedited) programs including (i) fast track designation, (ii) breakthrough therapy designation, (iii) priority review designation, and (iv) accelerated approval for approval of rare disease drug products, which are briefly described below.

10.2.1.1 Fast Track Designation

Fast track is a designation of an investigational drug for expedited review to facilitate development of drugs which (i) treat a serious or life-threatening condition and (ii) fill an unmet medical need. Fast Track designation must be requested by the sponsors. The request can be initiated at any time during the drug development process. FDA will review the request and make a decision within 60 days.

Fast track designation is designed to aid in the development and expedite the review of drugs which show promise in treating a serious or life-threatening disease and address an unmet medical need. Serious condition is referred to as the determination of the seriousness of a disease. The determination is a matter of judgment, but generally is based on whether the drug will affect the factors such as survival, day-to-day functioning, or the likelihood that the disease (if left untreated) will progress from a less severe condition to a more serious one. For a drug to address an unmet medical need, the drug must be developed as a treatment or preventative measure for a disease that exists no current therapy. If there are existing therapies, a fast track eligible drug must show some advantage over available treatment. For example, (i) showing superior effectiveness, (ii) avoiding serious side effects of an available treatment, (iii) improving the diagnosis of a serious disease where early diagnosis results in an improved outcome, (iv) decreasing a clinically significant toxicity of an available treatment, and (v) addressing an expected public health need.

Once a drug receives Fast Track designation, early and frequent communication between the FDA and a drug sponsor is encouraged throughout the entire drug development and review process. The frequency of communication assures that questions and issues are resolved quickly, often leading to earlier drug approval and access by patients. Note that the drug sponsor may appeal to the division responsible for reviewing the application within the Center for Drug Evaluation and Research (CDER) at the FDA if its request for Fast Track designation is not granted or any other general dispute. The drug sponsor can subsequently utilize the Agency's procedures for internal review or dispute resolution if necessary.

10.2.1.2 Breakthrough Therapy Designation

Breakthrough Therapy designation is a process designed to expedite the development and review of drugs that are intended to treat a serious condition and preliminary clinical evidence indicates that the drug may demonstrate substantial improvement over available therapy on a clinically significant endpoint(s). To determine whether the improvement over available therapy is substantial is a matter of judgment and depends on both the magnitude of the treatment effect, which could include the duration of the effect and the importance of the observed clinical outcome. In general, the preliminary clinical evidence should show a clear advantage over available therapy.

For purposes of Breakthrough Therapy designation, clinically significant endpoint generally refers to an endpoint that measures an effect on Irreversible Morbidity or Mortality (IMM) or on symptoms that represent serious consequences of the disease. A clinically significant endpoint can also refer to findings that suggest an effect on IMM or serious symptoms, which includes, but are limited to, (i) an effect on an established surrogate endpoint, (ii) an effect on a surrogate endpoint or intermediate clinical endpoint considered reasonably likely to predict a clinical benefit (i.e., the accelerated approval standard), (iii) an effect on a pharmacodynamic biomarker(s) that does not meet criteria for an acceptable surrogate endpoint, but strongly suggests the potential for a clinically meaningful effect on the underlying disease, and (iv) a significantly improved safety profile compared to available therapy (e.g., less dose-limiting toxicity for an oncology agent), with evidence of similar efficacy.

A drug that receives Breakthrough Therapy designation is eligible for the following: (i) all Fast Track designation features, (ii) intensive guidance on an efficient drug development program, beginning as early as phase 1, and (iii) organizational commitment involving senior managers. Similar to Fast Track designation, Breakthrough Therapy designation is requested by the drug sponsor. If a sponsor has not requested breakthrough therapy designation, FDA may suggest that the sponsor consider submitting a request provided that (i) after reviewing submitted data and information (including preliminary clinical evidence), the Agency thinks the drug development program may meet the criteria for Breakthrough Therapy designation and (ii) the remaining drug development program can benefit from the designation. It should be noted that FDA does not anticipate that Breakthrough Therapy designation requests will be made after the submission of an original Biologic License Application (BLA) or New Drug Application (NDA) or a supplement. FDA will respond to Breakthrough Therapy designation requests within 60 days of receipt of the request.

10.2.1.3 Priority Review

Prior to approval, each drug marketed in the United States must go through a detailed FDA review process. In 1992, under the Prescription Drug User Act (PDUFA), FDA agreed to specific goals for improving the drug review time and created a two-tiered system of review times – *Standard Review* and *Priority Review*. A Priority Review designation means FDA's goal is to take action on an application within 6 months (compared to ten months under standard review).

A *Priority Review* designation will direct overall attention and resources to the evaluation of applications for drugs that, if approved, would be significant improvements in the safety or effectiveness of the treatment, diagnosis, or prevention of serious conditions when compared to standard applications. Significant improvement may be demonstrated by the following: (i) evidence of increased effectiveness in treatment, prevention, or diagnosis of condition, (ii) elimination or substantial reduction of a treatment-limiting drug reaction, (iii) documented enhancement of patient compliance that is expected to lead to an improvement in serious outcomes, or (iv) evidence of safety and effectiveness in a new subpopulation.

FDA decides on the review designation for every application. However, an applicant may expressly request priority review as described in the Guidance for Industry Expedited Programs for Serious Conditions – Drugs and Biologics. It does not affect the length of the clinical trial period. FDA informs the applicant of a Priority Review designation within 60 days of the receipt of the original BLA, NDA, or efficacy supplement. Designation of a drug as "Priority" does not alter the scientific/medical standard for approval or the quality of evidence necessary.

10.2.1.4 Accelerated Approval

In 1992, FDA initiated the FDA Accelerated Approval Program to allow faster approval of drugs for serious conditions that fill an unmet medical need. The faster approval relies on use of surrogate endpoints. Drug approval typically requires clinical trials with endpoints that demonstrate a clinical benefit, such as increased survival for cancer patients. Drugs with accelerated approval can initially be tested in clinical trials that use a surrogate endpoint, or something that is thought to predict clinical benefit. Surrogate endpoints typically require less time, and in the case of a cancer patient, it is much faster to measure a reduction in tumor size, for example, than overall patient survival.

10.2.2 Regulatory Guidance

In January 2019, FDA published a draft guidance on *Rare Diseases: Common Issues in Drug Development* to assist sponsors of drug and biological products for the treatment or prevention of rare diseases (FDA, 2019a). The purpose of this draft guidance is to assist sponsors in conducting more efficient and successful drug development programs. As indicated in the draft guidance, the statutory requirements for marketing approval for drugs to treat rare and common diseases are the *same*. FDA does not have the intention to create a statutory standard for approval of orphan drugs that is different from the standard for approval of drugs in common conditions. For approval of drug products, FDA requires that substantial evidence regarding effectiveness and safety of the drug products be provided. Substantial evidence is based on the results of adequate and well-controlled investigations (21 CFR 314.126(a)).

FDA recognized that issues that are encountered in rare disease drug development are frequently more difficult to be addressed because there is often limited medical and scientific knowledge, natural history data, and drug development experience. This draft guidance addresses the importance of the following elements in development programs for rare diseases: (i) adequate description and understanding of the disease's natural history, (ii) adequate understanding of the pathophysiology of the disease and the drug's mechanism of action, (iii) nonclinical pharmacotoxicology and human toxicology considerations to support the proposed clinical investigation or investigations, (iv) selection or development of outcome assessments and endpoints, (v) evidence to establish safety and effectiveness, (vi) drug manufacturing considerations during drug development (e.g., pharmaceutical quality system considerations), (vii) participation of patients, caretakers, and advocates in development programs, and most importantly, (viii) interactions with the Agency (FDA, 2015, 2019). As FDA pointed out, early consideration of these issues gives sponsors the opportunity to efficiently and effectively address the issues and to have productive meetings with FDA.

10.2.2.1 Natural History Studies

Since the natural history of rare diseases is often poorly understood, there is a need for prospectively designed, protocol-driven natural history studies initiated in the earliest drug development planning stages. Although it is not required, FDA encourages sponsors to evaluate early the depth and quality of existing natural history knowledge to determine if it is sufficient to inform their drug development programs (FDA, 2019a). A natural history study initiated early may run in parallel with early stages of drug development and may allow updating of drug development strategies as new learning emerges. In general, natural history study designs can be characterized as (i) retrospective or prospective and (ii) cross-sectional or longitudinal. Retrospective and prospective studies differ with respect to when patient data are collected. The information to be collected in the study is typically set forth in a protocol or procedure manual. On the other hand, cross-sectional and longitudinal natural history studies collect data from cohorts of patients. Note that cross-sectional and longitudinal studies may be retrospective or prospective.

As the draft guidance pointed out, each type of natural history study has advantages and disadvantages (FDA, 2019a). In general, retrospective studies may be conducted more quickly than prospective studies. However, retrospective studies are limited in that they can only obtain data elements available in existing records. Retrospective studies are also limited by many factors including but not limited to inconsistent measurement procedures, irregular time intervals, and unclear use of terms that may limit the completeness and generalizability of the information. These limitations often preclude the use of such studies as an external control group for drug trials if it is not possible to match characteristics of patients in the drug trial with the historical controls. Prospective studies provide systematically and comprehensively captured data using consistent medical terms and methodologies relevant to future clinical trials. For a prospective design, a cross-sectional study may be conducted more quickly than a longitudinal study. However, cross-sectional studies are unable to provide a comprehensive description of the course of progressive or recurrent disease. Cross-sectional studies may be helpful to inform the design of a longitudinal natural history study. Longitudinal studies typically yield the most comprehensive information about a disease, can characterize the course of disease within patients and can help distinguish different phenotypes.

10.2.2.2 Endpoint Selection

For many rare diseases, well-established efficacy endpoints for the disease may not be available. Thus, FDA suggested that a sponsor should define a trial endpoint by selecting a patient assessment to be used as an outcome measure and define when in the trial the patient would be assessed (FDA, 2019a). As indicated in the draft guidance, endpoint selection in a clinical trial involves the knowledge and understanding of the following: (i) the range and course of clinical manifestations associated with the disease, (ii) the clinical characteristics of the specific target population, which may be a subset of the total population with a disease, (iii) the aspects of the disease that are meaningful to the patient and that could be assessed to evaluate the drug's effectiveness, (iv) the possibility of using the accelerated approval pathway. Despite continuing efforts to develop novel surrogate endpoints, FDA emphasized that only the usual clinical endpoints for the adequate and well-controlled trials can provide the substantial evidence of effectiveness supporting marketing approval of the drug (FDA, 2019a). Thus, it is suggested that sponsors should select endpoints considering the objectives of each trial in the context of the overall clinical development program.

More details and discussions regarding study endpoint selection are provided in Chapter 3 of this book.

10.2.2.3 Remarks

This draft guidance has addressed some important issues that are commonly encountered in rare disease drug development such as the use of natural history data and endpoint selection. In addition, this draft also indicated that (i) exploratory evidence from earlier phase trials helps inform the choice of dose and timing of endpoints, and (ii) the use of adaptive seamless trial design may allow early evidence to be used later in a study, especially helpful when there are limited numbers of patients to study. If an adaptive design is under consideration, a thorough statistical analysis plan including the key features of the trial design and preplanned analyses should be discussed with the review division before trial initiation. This draft guidance, however, has little discussion of the general issues of sample size requirement and statistical analysis, which play important roles for the success of rare diseases drug development.

10.3 Innovative Thinking for Rare Diseases Drug Development

For rare disease drug development, one of the major challenges is that there are only limited subjects available for clinical trials. FDA (2019a), however, indicated that the Agency does not have intention to create a statutory standard for rare diseases drug development. In this case, some out-of-the-box innovative thinking is necessarily applied for obtaining substantial evidence for approval of rare disease drug product (Chow, 2020). The out-of-the-box innovative thinking includes (i) probability monitoring procedure for sample size requirement, (ii) the concept of demonstrating not-ineffectiveness rather than demonstrating effectiveness, (iii) borrowing RWD in support of regulatory approval of rare diseases drug products, and (iv) the use of complex innovative design to shorten the process of drug development. Along this line, Chow and Chang (2019) and Chow (2020) proposed an innovative approach for rare diseases drug development by first demonstrating not-ineffectiveness with limited subjects available and then utilizing (borrowing) RWD to rule out the probability of inconclusiveness for demonstration of effectiveness under a two-stage adaptive seamless trial design. The proposed innovative approach cannot only overcome the problem of small patient population for rare diseases, but also achieve the same standard for evaluation of drug products with common conditions.

10.3.1 Probability Monitoring Procedure for Sample Size

For rare disease clinical development, it is recognized that a pre-study power analysis for sample size calculation is not feasible due to the fact that there are only limited number of subjects available for the intended trial, especially when the anticipated treatment effect is relatively small and/or the variability is relatively large. In this case, alternative methods such as precision analysis (or confidence interval approach), reproducibility analysis, and probability monitoring approach may be considered for providing substantial evidence with certain statistical assurance (Chow et al., 2017). It, however, should be noted that the resultant sample sizes from these different analyses could be very different with different levels of statistical assurance achieved. Thus, for rare disease clinical trials, it is suggested that an appropriate sample size should be selected for achieving certain statistical assurance under a valid trial design. To overcome the problem, Huang and Chow (2019) proposed a probability monitoring procedure for sample size calculation/justification, which can substantially reduce the required sample size for achieving certain statistical assurance.

As an example, an appropriate sample size may be selected based on a probability monitoring approach such that the probability of crossing safety boundaries is controlled at a pre-specified level of significance. Suppose an investigator plans to monitor the safety of a rare disease clinical trial sequentially at several times t_i, $i = 1, \ldots, K$. Let n_i and P_i be the sample size and the probability of observing an event at time t_i. Thus, an appropriate sample size can be selected such that the following probability of crossing safety stopping boundary is less than a pre-specified level of significance

$$p_k = P\{\text{across safety stopping boundry} \mid n_k, P_k\} < \alpha, k = 1, \ldots, K. \tag{10.1}$$

Note that the concept of the probability monitoring approach should not be mixed up the concepts with those based on power analysis, precision analysis, and reproducibility analysis. Statistical methods for data analysis should reflect the desired statistical assurance under the trial design.

10.3.2 Demonstrating Not-Ineffectiveness Versus Demonstrating Effectiveness

For approval of a new drug product, the sponsor is required to provide substantial evidence regarding the safety and efficacy of the drug product under investigation. In practice, a typical approach is to conduct adequate and well-controlled (placebo-controlled) clinical studies and test the following point hypotheses:

$$H_0: \text{ineffectiveness} \quad \text{versus} \quad H_a: \text{effectiveness}. \tag{10.2}$$

The rejection of the null hypothesis of *in*effectiveness is in favor of the alternative hypothesis of effectiveness. Most researchers interpret the rejection of the null hypothesis is the demonstration of the alternative hypothesis of effectiveness. It, however, should be noted that "in favor of effectiveness" does not imply "the demonstration of effectiveness". In practice, hypotheses (10.2) should be

$$H_0: \text{ineffectiveness} \quad \text{versus} \quad H_a: \text{not-ineffectiveness}. \tag{10.3}$$

In other words, the rejection of H_0 would lead to the conclusion of "*not H_0*", which is H_a, i.e., "not-ineffectiveness" as given in (10.3). As can be seen from H_a in (10.2) and (10.3), the concept of *effectiveness* (10.2) and the concept of *not ineffectiveness* (10.3) are not the same. Not ineffectiveness does not imply effectiveness in general. Thus, the traditional approach for clinical evaluation of the drug product under investigation can only demonstrate "*not-ineffectiveness*" but not "*effectiveness*". The relationship between demonstrating "effectiveness" (10.2) and demonstrating "not-ineffectiveness" (10.3) is illustrated in Figure 10.1. As it can be seen from Figure 10.1, in a placebo-controlled study, "not-ineffectiveness" consists of two parts, namely, the portion of "inconclusiveness" and the portion of "effectiveness". As a result, the rejection of the null hypothesis of ineffectiveness cannot directly imply that the drug product is effective unless the probability of inconclusiveness, denoted by p_{IC}, is negligible, i.e.,

$$p_{IC} = P\{\text{inconclusiveness}\} < \varepsilon, \tag{10.4}$$

where ε is a pre-specific number which is agreed upon between clinician and regulatory reviewer (Chow and Huang, 2019a).

Note that in active-controlled studies, the concept of demonstrating "not ineffectiveness" is similar to that of establishing non-inferiority of the test treatment as compared

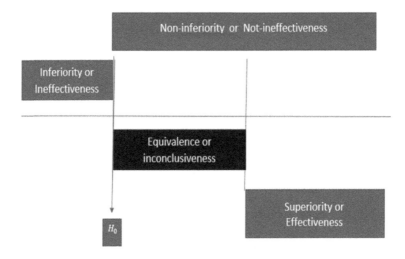

FIGURE 10.1
Demonstrating not-ineffectiveness or effectiveness in active-controlled (top line) and placebo-controlled (bottom line) studies.

to the active control agent. One can test for superiority (i.e., effectiveness) once the non-inferiority has been established without paying any statistical penalties.

10.3.3 The Use of RWD/RWE

The 21st Century Cures Act passed by the United States Congress in December 2016 requires that the FDA shall establish a program to evaluate the potential use of (RWE which is derived from RWD to (i) support approval of new indication for a drug approved under Section 505 (c) and (ii) satisfy post-approval study requirements. RWD refers to data relating to patient health status and/or the delivery of health care routinely collected from a variety of sources. RWD sources include, but are not limited to, Electronic Health Record (EHR), administrative claims and enrollment, personal digital health applications, public health databases, and emerging sources (FDA, 2017, 2019b). Although RWE offers the opportunities to develop robust evidence using high quality data and sophisticated methods for producing causal-effect estimates regardless of randomization is feasible. In this chapter, we have demonstrated that the assessment of treatment effect (RWE) based on RWD could be biased due to the potential selection and information biases of RWD. Although fit-for-purpose RWE may meet regulatory standards under certain assumptions, it is not the same as substantial evidence (current regulatory standard). In practice, it is then suggested that when there are gaps between fit-for-purpose RWE and substantial evidence, we should make efforts to fill the gaps for an accurate and reliable assessment of the treatment effect.

In order to map RWE to substantial evidence (current regulatory standard), we need to have a good understanding of the RWD in terms of data relevancy/quality and its relationship with substantial evidence so that a fit-for-regulatory purpose RWE can be derived to map to regulatory standard.

Although RWE offers the opportunities to develop robust evidence using high quality data and sophisticated methods for producing causal-effect estimates regardless of randomization is feasible. In this chapter, we have demonstrated that the assessment of treatment effect (RWE) based on RWD could be biased due to potential selection and information biases of RWD. Although fit-for-purpose RWE may meet regulatory standards under certain assumptions, it is not the same as substantial evidence (current regulatory standard). In practice, it is then suggested that when there are gaps between fit-for-purpose RWE and substantial evidence, we should make efforts to fill the gaps for an accurate and reliable assessment of the treatment effect.

As indicated by Corrigan-Curay (2018), there is a value in using RWE to support regulatory decisions in drug review and approval process. However, incorporating RWE into evidence generation, many factors must be considered at the same time before we can map RWE to substantial evidence (current regulatory standard) for regulatory review and approval. These factors include, but are not limited to, (i) efficacy or safety, (ii) relationship to available evidence, (iii) clinical context, e.g., rare, severe, life-threatening, or unmet medical need, and (iv) natural of endpoint/concerns about bias. In addition, leveraging RWE to support new indications and label revisions can help accelerate high quality RWE earlier in the product lifecycle, providing more relevant evidence to support higher quality and higher value care for patients. Incorporating RWE into product labeling can lead to better-informed patient and provider decisions with more relevant information. For this purpose, it is suggested characterizing RWD quality and relevancy for regulatory purposes. Ultimate regulatory acceptability, however, will depend upon how robust these studies can be. That is, how well they minimize the potential for bias and confounding.

10.4 Complex Innovative Trial Design and Analysis

Small patient population in rare diseases drug development is a challenge to rare disease clinical trials. Thus, there is a need for innovative trial designs in order to obtain substantial evidence with small number of subjects available for achieving the same standard for regulatory approval. In this section, several innovative trial designs including n-of-1 trial design, an adaptive trial design, master protocols, and a Bayesian design are discussed.

10.4.1 Adaptive Seamless Design and Analysis

Another useful innovative trial design for rare disease clinical trials is an adaptive trial design. In its draft guidance on adaptive clinical trial design, FDA defines an adaptive design as a study that includes a *prospectively* planned opportunity for modification of one or more specified aspects of the study design and hypotheses based on analysis of (usually interim) data from subjects in the study (FDA 2010, 2019c). The FDA guidance has been served as an official document describing the potential use of adaptive designs in clinical trials since it was published in 2019. It, however, should be noted that the FDA draft guidance on adaptive clinical trial design is currently being revised in order to reflect pharmaceutical practice and FDA's current thinking.

10.4.1.1 Adaptive Seamless Design

As indicated by Chow (2011), a seamless trial design is defined as a trial design that combines two independent trials into a single study that can address study objectives from individual studies. An adaptive seamless design is referred to as a seamless trial design that would use data collected before and after the adaptation in the final analysis. In practice, a two-stage seamless adaptive design typically consists of two stages (phases): a learning (or exploratory) phase (stage 1) and a confirmatory phase (stage 2). The objective of the learning phase is not only to obtain information regarding the uncertainty of the test treatment under investigation but also to provide the investigator with the opportunity to stop the trial early due to safety and/or futility/efficacy based on accrued data or to apply some adaptations such as adaptive randomization at the end of Stage 1. The objective of the second stage is to confirm the findings observed from the first stage. A two-stage seamless adaptive trial design has the following advantages that (i) it may reduce the lead time between studies (the traditional approach); (ii) it provides the investigator with the second chance to re-design the trial after the review of accumulated data at the end of Stage 1. Most importantly, data collected from both stages are combined for a final analysis in order to fully utilize all data collected from the trial for a more accurate and reliable assessment of the test treatment under investigation.

As indicated in Chow and Tu (2008) and Chow (2011), in practice, two-stage seamless adaptive trial designs can be classified into the following four categories depending upon study objectives and study endpoints at different stages.

Table 10.2 indicates that there are four different types of two-stage seamless adaptive designs depending upon whether study objectives and/or study endpoints at different stages are the same. For example, Category I designs (i.e., SS designs) include those designs with the same study objectives and same study endpoints, while Category II and Category III designs (i.e., SD and DS designs) are referred to those designs with the same study objectives but different study endpoints and different study objectives but same study

TABLE 10.2

Types of Two-Stage Seamless Adaptive Designs

Study Objectives	Study Same (S)	Endpoint Different (D)
Same (S)	I=SS	II=SD
Different (D)	III=DS	IV=DD

Source: Chow (2011).

endpoints, respectively. Category IV designs (i.e., DD designs) are the study designs with different study objectives and different study endpoints. In practice, different study objectives could be treatment selection for Stage 1 and efficacy confirmation for Stage 2. On the other hand, different study endpoints could be biomarker, surrogate endpoints, or a clinical endpoint with a shorter duration at the first stage versus a clinical endpoint at the second stage. Note that a group sequential design with one planned interim analysis is often considered an SS design.

In practice, typical examples for a two-stage adaptive seamless design include a two-stage adaptive seamless phase 1/2 design and a two-stage adaptive seamless phase 2/3 design. For the two-stage adaptive seamless phase 1/2 design, the objective at the first stage may be for biomarker development and the study objective for the second stage is usually to establish early efficacy. For a two-stage adaptive seamless phase 2/3 design, the study objective is often for treatment selection (or dose finding) while the study objective at the second stage is for efficacy confirmation. In this article, our focus will be placed on Category II designs. The results can be similarly applied to Category III and Category IV designs.

It should be noted that the terms seamless and phase 2/3 were not used in the FDA draft guidance as they have sometimes been adopted to describe various design features (FDA 2010, 2019c). In this chapter, a two-stage adaptive seamless phase 2/3 design only refers to a study containing stage 1 (an exploratory phase for phase 2 trial) and stage 2 (a confirmatory phase for phase 3 study) while data collected at both stages (phases) will be used for final analysis.

One of the questions that are commonly asked when applying a two-stage adaptive seamless design in clinical trials is sample size calculation/allocation. For the first kind (i.e. Category I, SS) of two-stage seamless designs, the methods based on individual p-values as described in Chow and Chang (2011) can be applied. However, for other kinds (i.e. Category II to Category IV) of two-stage seamless trial designs, standard statistical methods for group sequential design are not appropriate and hence should not be applied directly. For Category II-IV trial designs, power analysis and/or statistical methods for data analysis are challenging to the biostatistician. For example, a commonly asked question is "How do we control the overall type I error rate at a pre-specified level of significance?" In the interest of stopping trial early, "How to determine stopping boundaries?" is a challenge to the investigator and the biostatistician. In practice, it is often of interest to determine whether the typical O'Brien-Fleming type of boundaries is feasible. Another challenge is "How to perform a valid analysis that combines data collected from different stages?" To address these questions, Chow (2011) discussed the concept of a multiple-stage transitional seamless adaptive design which takes into consideration of different study objectives and study endpoints.

A two-stage seamless adaptive trial design has the following advantages. First, it may help in reducing lead time between studies for the traditional approach. In practice, the lead time between the end of the phase II trial and kick-off the phase 3 study is estimated at about 6-12 months. This is because usually the phase 3 study will not be initiated until the final clinical report of the phase II trial is completed. After the completion of a clinical study, it will usually take about 4-6 months to clean and lock the database, programming and data analysis, and final report. Besides, before we kick-off the phase 3 trial, protocol development, site selection/initiation, and IRB review/approval will also take some time. Thus, the use of a two-stage phase 2/3 adaptive trial design will definitely reduce the lead time between studies. In addition, the nature of adaptive trial design will also allow the investigator to make a go/no-go decision early (i.e., at the end of the first stage). In terms of the sample size required, a two-stage phase 2/3 adaptive design may require a smaller sample size as compared to the traditional approach. Most importantly, a two-stage phase 2/3 adaptive trial design allows us to fully utilize data collected from both stages for a combined analysis which will provide a more accurate and reliable assessment of the test treatment under investigation.

In what follows, an overview of statistical methods for analysis of different types (i.e. Category I to IV) of two-stage designs is provided (see also Chow and Lin, 2015). In addition, a case study concerning the evaluation of a test treatment for treating the patient with hepatitis C infection of a clinical study utilizing a Category IV adaptive design is presented.

10.4.1.2 *Analysis for Two-Stage Adaptive Seamless Designs*

Category I design with the same study objectives and same study endpoints at different stages is considered similar to a typical group sequential design with one planned interim analysis. Thus, standard statistical methods for group sequential design are often employed. It, however, should be noted that with various adaptations that applied, these standard statistical methods may not be appropriate. In practice, many interesting methods for Category I designs are available in the literature. These methods include (i) Fisher's criterion for combining independent p-values (Bauer and Kohne, 1994; Bauer and Rohmel, 1995; Posch and Bauer, 2000), (ii) weighted test statistics (Cui, Hung, and Wang, 1999), (iii) the conditional error function approach (Liu and Chi, 2001; Proschan and Hunsberger, 1995), and (iv) conditional power approaches (Li, Shih, and Wang, 2005).

Among these methods, Fisher's method for combining p-values provides great flexibility in selecting statistical tests for individual hypotheses based on sub-samples. Fisher's method, however, lacks flexibility in the choice of boundaries Muller and Schafer (2001). For Category I adaptive designs, many related issues have been studied. For example, Rosenberger and Lachin (2003) explored the potential use of response-adaptive randomization. Chow, Chang, and Pong (2005) examined the impact of population shift due to protocol amendments. Li, Shih, and Wang (2005) studied a two-stage adaptive design with a survival endpoint, while Hommel, Lindig, and Faldum (2005) studied a two-stage adaptive design with correlated data. An adaptive design with a bivariate-endpoint was studied by Todd (2003). Tsiatis and Mehta (2003) showed that there exists a more powerful group sequential design for any adaptive design with sample size adjustment,

For illustration purposes, in what follows, we will introduce the method based on sum of the p-values (MSP) by Chang (2007) and Chow and Chang (2011). The MSP follows the idea of considering a linear combination of the p-values from different stages.

As indicated earlier, a small patient population is a challenge to rare disease clinical trials. Thus, there is a need for innovative trial designs in order to obtain substantial evidence with small number of subjects available for achieving the same standard for regulatory approval. In this sub-section, several innovative trial designs including n-of-1 trial design, an adaptive trial design, master protocols, and a Bayesian design are discussed.

One of the major dilemmas for rare diseases clinical trials is the in-availability of patients with the rare diseases under study. In addition, it is unethical to consider a placebo control in the intended clinical trial. Thus, it is suggested an n-of-1 crossover design be considered. An n-of-1 trial design is to apply n treatments (including placebo) in an individual at different dosing periods with sufficient washout in between dosing periods. A complete n-of-1 trial design is a crossover design that consists of all possible combinations of treatment assignments at different dosing periods.

10.4.2 Complete n-of-1 Trial Design and Analysis

In recent years, the n-of-1 trial design has become a very population design for evaluation of the difference in treatment effect within the same individual when n treatments are administered at different dosing periods. Thus, n-of-1 trial design is in fact a crossover design. Following similar ideas of switching designs with a single switch and/or multiple switches, Chow et al. (2017) proposed the use of so-called complete n-of-1 trial design for assessment of relative risk between switching/alternation and without switching/alternation.

10.4.2.1 Complete n-of-1 Trial Design

The construction of a complete n-of-1 trial design depends upon m, the number of switches. For example, if $m = 1$ (single switch), the complete n-of-1 trial design will consist of $m + 1 = 2$ periods. At each dosing period, there are two choices (i.e., either R or T). Thus, there are a total of $2^{m+1} = 2^2 = 4$ sequences (i.e., combinations of R and T). This results in a 4×2 Balaam design, i.e., (RR, TT, RT, TR). When $m = 2$ (two switches), the complete n-of-1 trial design will consist of $m + 1 = 3$ periods. At each dosing period, there are two choices (i.e., either R or T). Thus, there are a total of $2^{m+1} = 2^3 = 8$ sequences. This results in an 8×3 crossover design. Similarly, where there are three switches (i.e., $m = 3$), the complete n-of-1 trial design will consist of $m + 1 = 4$ periods. At each dosing period, there are two choices (i.e., either R or T). Thus, there are a total of $2^{m+1} = 2^4 = 16$ sequences (i.e., combinations of R and T). This results in a 16×4 crossover design. To provide a better understanding, Table 10.3 lists complete n-of-1 trial design with $m = 1$ (single switch), $m = 2$ (two switches), and $m = 3$ (three switches) that maybe useful for biosimilar switching studies.

As it can be seen from Table 10.3, the switching designs with single switch, i.e., (RT, RR), with two switches, i.e., (RTR, RRR), and three switches, i.e., (RTRT, RRRR) are partial designs of the n-of-1 trial designs with single switch (two periods), two switches (three periods), and three switches (four periods), respectively.

10.4.2.2 Statistical Model and Analysis

The switching designs discussed in the previous section can be generally described as a $K \times J$ crossover design. For example, for FDA recommended switching designs with two switches, $K = 2$ and $J = 3$, while for the complete n-of-1 trial design with two switches, $K = 8$ and $J = 3$, Thus, the switching designs discussed in the previous section can be described in a statistical model under a general $K \times J$ (K-sequence and J-period) crossover design comparing two treatments (i.e., R and T).

TABLE 10.3

Complete n-of-1 Trial Design with $m = 1, 2$, and 3

Group	Period I	Period II	Period III	Period IV
1	R	R	R	R
2	R	T	R	R
3	T	T	R	R
4	T	R	R	R
5	R	R	T	R
6	R	T	T	T
7	T	R	T	R
8	T	T	T	T
9	R	R	R	T
10	R	R	T	T
11	R	T	R	T
12	R	T	T	R
13	T	R	R	T
14	T	R	T	T
15	T	T	R	T
16	T	T	T	R

Note: $m = 1$ (single switch with 2 periods); $m = 2$ (two switches with 3 periods) $m = 3$ (three switches with 4 periods)

Let Y_{ijk} be the response of the ith subject in the kth sequence at the jth period. Thus, Y_{ijk} can be described in the following model:

$$Y_{ijk} = \mu + G_k + S_{ik} + P_j + D_{d(j,k)} + C_{d(j-1,k)} + e_{ijk} \tag{10.5}$$

$$i = 1, 2, \cdots, n_k; j = 1, 2, \cdots, J; k = 1, 2, \cdots, K; d = T \quad \text{or} \quad R$$

where μ is the overall mean, G_k is the fixed kth sequence effect, S_{ik} is random effect for the ith subject within the kth sequence with mean 0 and variance σ_S^2, P_j is the fixed effect for the jth period, $D_{d(j,k)}$ is the drug effect for the drug at the kth sequence in the jth period, $C_{d(j-1,k)}$ is the carry-over effect, where $C_{d(0,k)} = 0$, and e_{ijk} is the random error with mean 0 and variance σ_e^2. Under the model, it is assumed that S_{ik} and e_{ijk} are mutually independent.

Under Model (10.5), denote β as a parameter vector,

$$(\mu, G_1, G_2, \ldots, G_K, P_1, P_2, \ldots, P_J \ D_T, D_R, C_T, C_R)',$$

which contains all unknown parameters in the model. Let X be the design matrix of the $K \times J$ crossover design. Thus, $\hat{\beta}$ can be estimated by $\hat{\beta} = (X'X)^{-1}X'\bar{Y}$, where $\bar{Y}$ is the vector of observed cell means. Thus, Statistical inference of the treatment effect after switch can then be assessed simply by the following steps:

Step 1 Set up the design matrix for the $K \times J$ crossover design;

Step 2 Find $(X'X)^{-1}X'$, where X is the $K \times J$ crossover design matrix. We then obtain $\hat{D}_R$ and $\hat{D}_T$;

Step 3 The estimates of $\theta_{ij} = D_i - D_j$ can be obtained by the difference of the corresponding coefficients between $\hat{D}_i$ and $\hat{D}_j$;

Step 4 The estimates of carryover effects $\lambda_{ij} = C_i - C_j$, $i \neq j$ can be similarly obtained.

10.4.3 Master Protocol Design

Woodcock and LaVange (2017) introduced the concept of master protocol for studying multiple therapies, multiple diseases, or both in order to answer more questions in a more efficient and timely fashion. Master protocols include the following types of trials: umbrella, basket and platform. The type of umbrella trial is to study multiple targeted therapies in the context of a single disease, while the type of basket trial is to study a single therapy in the context of multiple diseases or disease subtypes. The platform is to study multiple targeted therapies in the context of a single disease in a perpetual manner, with therapies allowed to enter or leave the platform on the basis of a decision algorithm. As indicated by Woodcock and LaVange (2017), if designed correctly, master protocols offer a number of benefits include streamlined logistics, improved data quality, collection and sharing, as well as the potential to use innovative statistical approaches to study design and analysis. Master protocols may be a collection of sub-studies or a complex statistical design or platform for rapid learning and decision-making.

Under the assumption that historical data (e.g., previous studies or experience) are available, Bayesian methods for borrowing information from different data sources may be useful. These data sources could include, but are not limited to, natural history studies and expert's opinion regarding prior distribution about the relationship between endpoints and clinical outcomes. The impact of borrowing on results can be assessed through the conduct of sensitivity analysis. One of the key questions of particular interest to the investigator and regulatory reviewer is that how much to borrow in order to (i) achieve desired statistical assurance for substantial evidence, and (ii) maintain the quality, validity, and integrity of the study.

The FDA draft guidance on master protocols defines a master protocol as a protocol designed with multiple sub-studies, which may have different objectives and involves coordinated efforts to evaluate one or more investigational drugs in one or more disease subtypes within the overall trial structure (FDA, 2018c). In practice, there are several types of master protocols depending upon the study designs and objectives. The commonly considered master protocols are basket trials and umbrella trials, which are briefly described below.

10.4.3.1 Basket Trials

A master protocol designed to test a single investigational drug or drug combination in different populations defined by disease stage, histology, number of prior therapies, genetic or other biomarkers, or demographic characteristics is commonly referred to as a basket trial. A typical basket trial design is illustrated in Figure 10.2.

A basket trial involves multiple diseases or histologic features (i.e., in cancer). After participants are screened for the presence of a target, target-positive participants are entered into the trial; as a result, the trial may involve many different diseases or histologic features. A master protocol for a basket trial could contain multiple strata that test various biomarker-drug pairs.

As it can be seen from Figure 10.2, the sub-studies within basket trials are usually designed as single-arm activity-estimating trials with Overall Response Rate (ORR) as the

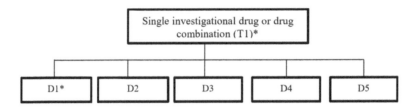

FIGURE 10.2
Schematic representation of a master protocol with basket trial design. * T = investigational drug; D = protocol defined subpopulation in multiple disease subtypes.

primary endpoint. A strong response signal seen in a sub-study may allow for expansion of the sub-study to generate data that could potentially support a marketing approval. Each sub-study should include specific objectives, the scientific rationale for inclusion of each population, and a detailed Statistical Analysis Plan (SAP) that includes sample size justification and stopping rules for futility.

An example of a master protocol with basket trial design is the phase II trial evaluating vemurafenib in multiple nonmelanoma cancers with BRAF V600 mutations (see Figure 10.3).

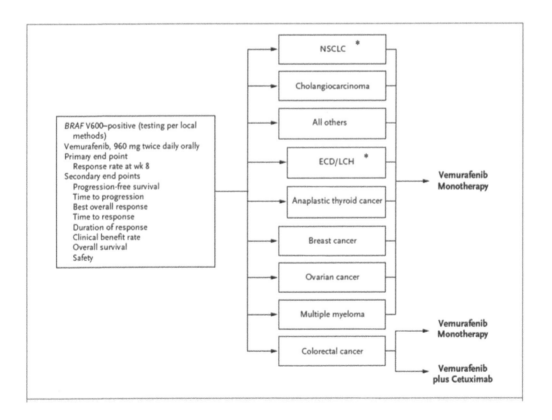

FIGURE 10.3
Vemurafenib in nonmelanoma cancers harboring BRAF V600 mutations. * NSCLC = Non-small cell lung cancer; ECD = Erdheim-Chester disease; LCH = Langerhans cell histiocytosis. *Source:* Hyman et al. (2015). N Engl J Med, 373(8): 726–736.

10.4.3.2 Umbrella Trials

A master protocol designed to evaluate multiple investigational drugs administered as single drugs or as drug combinations in a single disease population are commonly referred to as umbrella trials. A typical umbrella trial is illustrated in Figure 10.4.

An umbrella trial evaluates various (often biomarker-defined) subgroups within a conventionally defined disease. Patients with the disease are screened for the presence of a biomarker or other characteristic and then assigned to a stratum on the basis of the results. Multiple drugs are studied in the various strata, and the design may be randomized or use external controls depending on the disease (Woodcock and LaVange, 2017).

As indicated in the FDA draft guidance, umbrella trials can employ randomized controlled designs to compare the activity of the investigational drug(s) with a common control arm. The drug chosen as the control arm for the randomized sub-study or sub-studies should be the Standard of Care (SOC) for the target population, and this may change over time if newer drugs replace the SOC.

An example of a master protocol with umbrella trial design is the original version of the LUNG- MAP trial (Herbst et al., 2015), a multidrug, multi-sub-study, biomarker-driven trial in patients with advanced/metastatic squamous cell carcinoma of the lung. Eligible patients were assigned to sub-studies based on their biomarkers or to a nonmatch therapy sub-study for patients not eligible for the biomarker-specific sub-studies. Within the sub-studies, patients were randomized to a biomarker-driven target or to SOC therapy (see Figure 10.5)

10.4.3.3 Other Trial Designs

Master protocol designs may also incorporate design features common to both basket and umbrella trials and may evaluate multiple investigational drugs and/or drug combination regimens across multiple tumor types. A typical example of a master protocol with a complex trial design is the NCI-MATCH trial, which aims to establish whether patients with one or more tumor mutations, amplifications, or translocations in a genetic pathway of interest identified in solid tumors or hematologic malignancies derive clinical benefit if treated with drugs targeting that specific pathway in a single-arm design (see Figure 10.6).

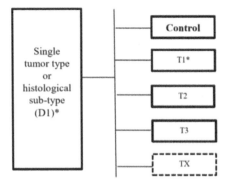

FIGURE 10.4
Schematic representation of a master protocol with umbrella trial design. * T = investigational drug; D = protocol defined subpopulation in single disease subtypes; TX = dotted border depicts future treatment arm.

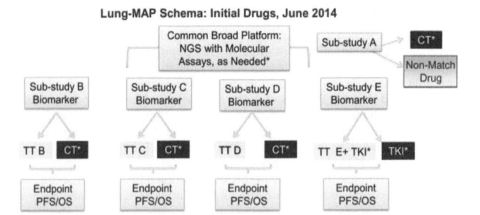

FIGURE 10.5
LUNG-MAP Trial in patients with squamous cell carcinoma of the lung. *Source:* Herbst et al. (2015). Clin Cancer Res, 21(7): 1514-1524.

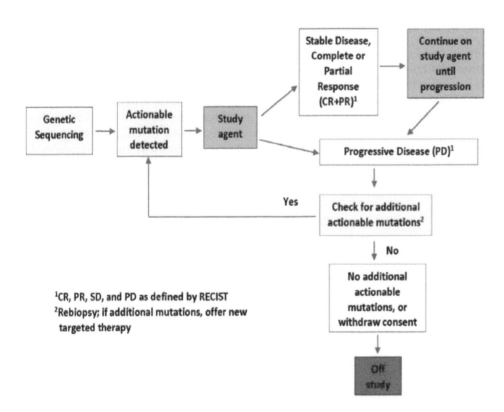

FIGURE 10.6
National cancer institute match trial scheme. *Source:* Abrams et al. (2014). Am Soc Clin Oncol Educ Book: 71-76, doi:10.14694/EdBook_AM.2014.34.71.

10.4.4 Bayesian Approach

Under the assumption that historical data (e.g., previous studies or experience) are available, Bayesian methods for borrowing information from different data sources may be useful. These data sources could include, but are not limited to, natural history studies and expert's opinion regarding prior distribution about the relationship between endpoints and clinical outcomes. The impact of borrowing on results can be assessed through the conduct of sensitivity analysis. One of the key questions of particular interest to the investigator and regulatory reviewer is that how much to borrow in order to (i) achieve desired statistical assurance for substantial evidence, and (ii) maintain the quality, validity, and integrity of the study.

Let D_0 and D be the historical data available from similar previous studies and data from the current randomized clinical trial, respectively. Also, let $\pi(\theta)$ be the prior distribution of θ, where θ is the parameter of interest. In this case, we may update the prior $\pi(\theta)$ by incorporate the information obtained from the historical data or relevant real-world data (RWD) as follows

$$\pi(\theta \mid D, D_0) \propto L(\theta \mid D)\pi(\theta \mid D_0), \tag{10.6}$$

where $L(\theta \mid D)$ is the likelihood function given D. Under (10.6), Ibrahim and Chen (2000) proposed the concept of power prior (PP) distribution to raising the likelihood function of the historical data to a desired power under four commonly used classes of regression models. These regression models include (i) generalized liner model, (ii) generalized linear mixed model, (iii) semi-parametric proportional hazards model, and (iv) cure rate model for survival data.

Let $\pi_0(\theta)$ be the prior distribution of θ based on D_0. The idea is to update the prior based on D_0. Then, use the posterior as the new prior for obtaining statistical inference for θ, which incorporate information D_0 into D. In other words, we have

$$\pi(\theta \mid D_0, \delta) \propto L(\theta \mid D_0)^\delta \pi_0(\theta),$$

where $L(\theta \mid D_0)$ is the likelihood function of θ given D_0 and $\delta \in [0,1]$ is a parameter that determines the amount of information D_0 that will be incorporated into D. Note that when $\delta = 1$, D_0 is fully utilized. When $\delta = 0$, no information from D_0 was borrowed. Thus, we have

$$\pi(\theta \mid D, D_0, \delta) \propto L(\theta \mid D)\pi(\theta \mid D_0, \delta) \propto L(\theta \mid D)L(\theta \mid D_0)^\delta \pi_0(\theta). \tag{10.7}$$

One of the major disadvantages of (10.7) is that δ is unknown in practice. To overcome the problem, alternatively, Duan, Ye, and Smith (2006) suggested the use of a Modified Power Prior (MPP) by treating δ as a random variable following a distribution $\pi(\delta)$. This gives

$$\pi(\theta, \delta \mid D_0) = \frac{L(\theta \mid D_0)^\delta \pi_0(\theta)\pi(\delta)}{C(\delta)},$$

where $C(\delta) = \int_\theta L(\theta \mid D_0)^\delta \pi_0(\theta)d\theta$ given D_0. Thus, the posterior distribution of θ and δ is given by

$$\pi(\theta, \delta \mid D, D_0) \propto L(\theta \mid D)\pi(\theta, \delta \mid D_0). \tag{10.8}$$

Since there exists no data to support the method of modified prior, Pan, Yuan, and Xia (2017) proposed a method using Kolmogorov-Smirnov (KS) statistic to measure and calibrate the difference between current data and historical data. This method is referred to as the method of Calibrated Power Prior (CPP). Let $D = (y_1, \cdots, y_n)$ be the historical data, $D_0 = (x_1, \cdots, x_m)$ be the current data, and $Z_{(1)} \leq \cdots Z_{(N)}$ be the ordered combined sample of D_0 and D with sample size of $N = n + m$. Thus, KS can be obtained as follows

$$S_{KS} = \max_{i=1,\cdots,N} \left\{ \left| F(Z_{(i)}) - G(Z_{(i)}) \right| \right\}$$

where

$$F_m(t) = \sum I(x_j \leq t)/m \text{ and } G(t) = \sum I(y_i \leq t)/n$$

are the distribution functions of D_0 and D, respectively.

Since KS measures the difference between distributions of D_0 and D, a larger value of S_{KS} is an indication that the distribution of D_0 is inconsistent with that of D. If we define

$$S = \max(m, n)^{1/4} S_{KS},$$

the relationship between δ and S can then be described as follows:

$$\delta = g(S; \phi) = \frac{1}{1 + \exp\{a + b \log(S)\}}, \tag{10.9}$$

where $\phi = (a, b)$ is a parameter that controls δ and S correlation, $b > 0$. As it can be seen, a relatively smaller value of δ corresponds that the distribution of D_0 is significantly inconsistent with that of D.

Under the assumptions that D_0 and D are normally distribute, i.e., $x_i \sim N(\mu_0, \sigma_0^2)$ and $y_j \sim N(\mu_0 + \gamma, \sigma_0^2)$, $i = 1, \cdots, m$ and $j = 1, \cdots, n$, parameters a and b in (3) can be determined by the following steps.

Step 1. Obtain estimates of population mean and population variance of D_0. That is, $\hat{\mu}_0 = \bar{x}$, where $\bar{x} = \sum_{i=1}^{m} x_i/m$ and $\hat{\sigma}_0^2 = \sum_{i=1}^{m}(x_i - \bar{x})/(m - 1)$;

Step 2. Let γ be the difference in mean between D_0 and D. Denote by γ_c the mean difference which is negligible (in other words, D_0 and D are consistent). Then, obtain the minimum mean difference, denote by $\gamma_{\bar{c}}$, that will lead to the conclusion of inconsistence between the distributions of D_0 and D.

Step 3. Simulate M samples $(y_1, \cdots, y_n)$ from $N(\hat{\mu}_0 + \gamma, \hat{\sigma}_0^2)$. Then, for each sample, calculate KS between D_0 and D. Let $S^*(\gamma_c)$ be the median of the M KS statistics. Replace $\gamma_{\bar{c}}$ with γ_c and repeat step 3;

Step 4. Let $S^*(\gamma_c)$ be the median of the M KS statistics. Parameters can be solved from the following equations:

$$\delta_c = g\{S^*(\gamma_c); \phi\}$$

$$\delta_{\bar{c}} = g\{S^*(\gamma_{\bar{c}}); \phi\}$$

If we choose δ_c close to 1 (say 0.98), $\delta_{\bar{c}}$ is constant close to 0 (say 0.01), a and b can be obtained as follows:

$$a = \log\left(\frac{1-\delta_c}{\delta_c}\right) - \frac{\log\left\{\dfrac{(1-\delta_c)\delta_{\bar{c}}}{(1-\delta_{\bar{c}})\delta_c}\right\}\log\left\{S^*(r_c)\right\}}{\log\left\{\dfrac{S^*(r_c)}{S^*(r_{\bar{c}})}\right\}}$$

$$b = \frac{\log\left\{\dfrac{(1-\delta_c)\delta_{\bar{c}}}{(1-\delta_{\bar{c}})\delta_c}\right\}}{\log\left\{\dfrac{S^*(r_c)}{S^*(r_{\bar{c}})}\right\}}$$

Once a and b have been determined, θ's calibrated power prior is given by

$$\pi(\theta \mid D_0, a, b) = L(\theta \mid D_0)^{\left[1+\exp\{a+b\log(S)\}\right]^{-1}} \pi_0(\theta). \tag{10.10}$$

Viele et al. (2014) proposed a method which is referred to as a test-then-pool approach to examine the difference between the current data (e.g., data collected from RCT) and historical data (e.g., real-world data) by testing the following hypotheses

$$H_0: p_h = p_c \quad \text{vs} \quad H_a: p_h \neq p_c, \tag{10.11}$$

where p_h and p_c are response rates of the historical data and current data, respectively. If we fail to reject the null hypothesis, historical data and current data can be combined for final analysis. It should be noted that the above method can only determine whether the historical data can be combined for a final analysis. This method is not useful to determine how much information can be borrowed for further analysis. To overcome the problem, Liu (2017) proposed the method of p-value based power prior (PVPP) by testing the following hypotheses

$$H_0: |\theta_h - \theta| > \eta \quad \text{vs} \quad H_1: |\theta_h - \theta| < \eta. \tag{10.12}$$

Alternatively, Gravestock et al. (2017) proposed adaptive power priors with empirical Bayes (EBPP) by considering the estimate of δ

$$\hat{\delta}(D_0, D) = \arg \max_{\delta \in [0,1]} L(\delta; D_0, D)$$

where

$$L(\delta; D_0, D) = \int L(\delta; D)\pi(\theta \mid \delta, D_0)d\theta = \frac{\int L(\delta; D)L(\theta; D_0)^\delta \pi(\theta)d\theta}{\int L(\theta; D_0)^\delta \pi(\theta)d\theta}$$

in which $\eta > 0$ is pre-specified constant. Let p be the maximum of the two one-sided test p-values. Since under the test-then-pool approach, we can only take 0 or 1 for δ, Gravestock et al. (2017) suggested considering the following continuous function of p

$$\delta = exp\left[\frac{k}{1-p}ln(1-p)\right],$$

where k is a pre-specified constant. A small p-value suggests that more information from the historical data or relevant RWD can be borrowed.

10.4.5 Innovative Approach for Rare Diseases Drug Development

Combining the out-of-the-box innovative thinking regarding rare disease drug development described in the previous section, Chow and Huang (2019b) and Chow (2020) proposed the following innovative approach utilizing a two-stage adaptive approach in conjunction with the use of RWD/RWE for rare diseases drug development. This innovative approach is briefly summarized below.

Step 1. Select a small sample size n_1 at Stage 1 as deemed appropriate by the principal investigator (PI) based on both medical and non-medical considerations. Note that n_1 may be selected based on the probability monitoring procedure.

Step 2. Test hypotheses (3) for not-ineffectiveness at the α_1 level, a pre-specified level of significance. If fails to reject the null hypothesis of ineffectiveness, then stop the trial due to futility. Otherwise proceed to the next stage.

Note that an appropriate value of α_1 can be determined based on the evaluation of the trade-off with the selection of α_2 for controlling the overall type I error rate at the significance level of α. The goal of this step is to establish non-inferiority (i.e., not-ineffectiveness) of the test treatment with limited number of subjects available at the α_1 level of significance based on the concept of probability monitoring procedure for sample size justification and performing a non-inferiority (not-ineffectiveness) test with a significance level of α_1.

Step 3a. Recruit additional n_2 subjects at Stage 2. Note that n_2 may be selected based on the probability monitoring procedure. Once the non-inferiority (not ineffectiveness) has been established at Stage 1, sample size re-estimation may be performed for achieving the desirable statistical assurance (say 80% power) for establishment of effectiveness of the test treatment under investigation at the second stage (say N_2, sample size required at Stage 2).

Step 3b. Obtain (borrow) $N_2 - n_2$ data from previous studies (real-world data) if the sample size of n_2 subjects are not enough for achieving desirable statistical assurance (say 80% power) at Stage 2. Note that data obtained from the n_2 subjects are from randomized clinical trial (RCT), while data obtained from the other $N_2 - n_2$ are from RWD.

Step 4. Combined data from both Step 3a (data obtained from RCT) and Step 3b (data obtained from RWD) at Stage 2, perform a statistical test to eliminate the probability of inconclusiveness. That is, perform a statistical test to determine whether the probability of inconclusiveness has become negligible at the α_2 level of significance. For example, if the probability of inconclusiveness is less than a pre-specified value (say 5%), we can then conclude the test treatment is effective.

In summary, for review and approval of rare diseases drug products, Chow and Huang (2020) proposed first to demonstrate not-ineffectiveness with limited information (patients) available at a pre-specified level of significance of α_1. Then, after the not-ineffectiveness of the test treatment has been established, collect additional information (real-world data) to rule out the probability of *inconclusiveness* for demonstration of effectiveness at a pre-specified level of significance of α_2 under the two-stage adaptive seamless trial design.

10.4.5.1 Remarks

In this article, some out-of-the-box innovative thinking regarding rare disease drug development is described. These innovative thinking include (i) probability monitoring procedure for sample size calculation/justification for certain statistical assurance, (ii) the concept of testing non-inferiority (i.e., demonstrating not-ineffectiveness) with limited number of subjects available, (iii) utilizing (borrowing) RWD from various of data sources in support of regulatory approval of rare diseases drug products, and (iv) the use of a two-stage adaptive seamless trial design to shorten the process of drug development. Combining these innovative thinking, under a two-stage adaptive seamless trial design, Chow and Huang (2019b) and Chow (2020) proposed an innovative approach for rare diseases drug development by first demonstrating not-ineffectiveness based on limited subjects available and then utilizing (borrowing) real-world data to rule out the probability of inconclusiveness for demonstration of effectiveness. Chow and Huang's proposed innovative approach cannot only overcome the problem of small patient population for rare diseases but also achieve the same standard for evaluation of drug products with common conditions.

10.5 Case Studies

10.5.1 Sponsor's Strategy and Perspectives

Despite regulatory incentives for rare diseases drug development, it is of great interest to the sponsors regarding how to increase the probability of success with a limited number of subjects available and at the same time fulfill with the regulatory requirement for review and approval of rare diseases regulatory submissions.

10.5.1.1 Practical Difficulties and Challenges

For rare diseases drug development, despite FDA's incentive programs, some practical difficulties and challenges are evitably encountered at the planning stage of rare diseases clinical trials. These practical difficulties and challenges include, but are not limited to, (i) insufficient power due to small sample size available, (ii) little or no prior information regarding dose finding, (iii) the potential use of AI machine learning, and (iv) inflexibility in study design, which have an impact on the probability of success of the intended clinical trials.

10.5.1.2 *Insufficient Power*

In practice, for rare diseases drug development, it is expected that the intended clinical trial may not have the desired power (i.e., the probability of correctly detecting a clinically meaningful difference or treatment effect when such a difference truly exists) for confirming efficacy of the test treatment under investigation at the 5% level of significance due to small sample available. Thus, the commonly considered power calculation for sample size is not feasible for rare diseases clinical trials. In this case, the sponsor must seek for alternative methods for sample size calculation for achieving certain statistical assurance for the intended rare diseases clinical trials.

As indicated in Chow et al. (2017), in addition to power analysis, other methods such as precision analysis, reproducibility analysis, and probability monitoring procedure could be used for sample size calculation for achieving certain statistical assurance in clinical trials. The precision analysis is to select a sample size that controls type I error rate within a desired precision, while the reproducibility analysis is to select a sample size that will achieve a desired probability of reproducibility. The probability monitoring procedure is to justify a selected sample size based on the probability across efficacy/safety boundaries.

10.5.1.3 *Inefficient Dose Finding*

Regarding dose finding for Maximum Tolerable Dose (MTD), a traditional "3+3" dose escalation design is often considered. The traditional "3+3" escalation design is to enter three patients at a new dose level and then enter another three patients when a Dose Limiting Toxicity (DLT) is observed. The assessment of the six patients is then performed to determine whether the trial should be stopped at the level or to escalate to the next dose level. Note that DLT is referred to as unacceptable or unmanageable safety profile which is pre-defined by some criteria such as Grade 3 or greater hematological toxicity according to the US National Cancer Institute's Common Toxicity Criteria (CTC). This dose finding design, however, suffers the following disadvantages: (i) inefficient, (ii) often underestimate the MTD especially when the starting dose is too low, (iii) depending upon the DLT rate at MTD, and (iv) the probability of correctly identifying the MTD is low.

Alternatively, it is suggested that a Continued Re-Assessment Method (CRM) should be considered (Song and Chow, 2015). For the method of CRM, the dose-response relationship is continually reassessed based on accumulative data collected from the trial. The next patient who enters the trial is then assigned to the potential MTD level. Thus, the CRM involves (i) dose toxicity modeling, (ii) dose level selection, (iii) re-assessment of model parameters and (iv) assignment of next patient. Chang and Chow (2005) considered the CRM method in conjunction with a Bayesian approach for dose response trials which substantially improve the CRM for dose finding.

To select a more efficient dose finding design between the "3+3" escalation design and the CRM Design, FDA recommends the following criteria for design selection: (i) number of patients expected, (ii) number of DLT expected, (iii) toxicity rate, (iv) probability of observing DLT prior to MTD, (v) probability of correctly achieving the MTD, and (vi) probability of overdosing. Song and Chow (2015) compared the "3+3" dose escalation design and the CRM design in conjunction with a Bayesian approach for a radiation therapy dose finding trial based on a clinical trial simulation study. The results indicated that (i) CRM has an acceptable probability of correctly reaching the MTD, (ii) the "3+3" dose escalation design is always under estimate the MTD, and (iii) CRM generally performs better than that of the "3+3" dose escalation design.

10.5.1.4 Inflexible Study Design

Under the restriction of only a small sample available, the usual parallel-group design is considered not flexible. Instead, it is suggested that some Complex Innovative Designs (CID) such as n-of-1 trial design, adaptive trial design, master protocol, and Bayesian sequential design should be considered.

In recent years, the n-of-1 trial design has become a very popular design for evaluation of the difference in treatment effect within the same individual when n treatments are administered at different dosing periods. In general, as compared to parallel-group design, n-of-1 trial design requires less subjects for evaluation of the test treatment under investigation. On the other hand, adaptive trial design has the flexibility for modifying the study protocol as it continues after the review of interim data. Clinical trials utilizing adaptive design methods cannot only increase the probability of success of drug development but also shorten the development process.

In addition, the concept of master protocol and the use of Bayesian sequential design have received much attention lately, which also provide some flexibility for evaluation of treatment effects in rare diseases drug development. More details and discussions regarding the application of master protocol in clinical development are given in Chapter 2 of this book.

10.5.2 The Remarkable Story of the Development of Velcade®

10.5.2.1 Fast-Track Destination

Velcade® (Bortezomib) is an antineoplastic agent (a proteasome inhibitor) indicated for the treatment of multiple myeloma and mantle cell lymphoma (see Table 1.1). Multiple myeloma is the second most common cancer (an incurable cancer) of the blood, representing approximately 1% of all cancers and 2% of all cancer deaths. It is estimated that approximately 45,000 Americans have multiple myeloma with about 15,000 new cases diagnosed each year. Only about percent of multiple myeloma patients survive longer than five years with the disease. Although the disease is predominantly a cancer of the elderly (the average age at diagnosis is 70 years of age) recent statistics indicate both increased incidence and younger age of onset. Thus, multiple myeloma is considered a rare disease and meet the requirement for Fast-Track designation for expedited review.

Velcade® was co-developed by Millennium Pharmaceuticals, Inc. and Johnson & Johnson Pharmaceutical Research & Development. On 13 May 2003, the FDA approved Velcade® under Fast-Track Application for the treatment of multiple myeloma. As indicated by Sánchez-Serrano (2006), the success story behind the development of this drug is quite unique and remarkable and primarily due to the adaption of Core Model. The Core Model, as epitomized by the success story of bortezomib, emphasizes the potential power of maximizing collaborative approaches and is useful in providing insights to policy makers, scientists, investors and the public on how the process of drug development can be optimized, which should eventually lead to lower drug discovery and development costs, the creation of better, safer and more effective medicines, and affordable access to the best drugs, including those for neglected and orphan diseases, not only in the developed countries but also worldwide. Only then will we be able to build a better global system of health care, one which is not only more egalitarian but also more humane.

10.5.2.2 Innovative Science

Under the Core Model, adaptive methods were frequently developed and used in clinical trials not only to (i) increase the probability of success of the intended clinical trials, but also (ii) to shorten the development process. The adaptive design methods gave the PI the flexibility to identify any sign, signal, and trend/pattern of clinical benefits for the test treatment under investigation. The adaptive design methods used during the development of Velcade® include, but are not limited to, (i) adaptive-randomization, (ii) adaptive-hypotheses (i.e., switch from a superiority hypothesis to a non-inferiority hypothesis), (iii) adaptive-endpoint selection (e.g., change single primary endpoint such as response rate to a co-primary endpoint of response rate and time to disease progression), (iv) biomarker-adaptive such as enrichment design and targeted clinical trials, (v) flexible sample size re-estimation, (vi) adaptive dose finding, and (vii) two-stage adaptive seamless trial design. The use of these adaptive design methods has increased the probability of success and shorten the development process. As a result, Velcade® was granted FDA approval a little more than four and a half years after the initiation of the first clinical trial.

10.5.2.3 Priority Review

The FDA approval of Velcade® is based primarily upon the results of a major multicenter phase II open-label, single-arm trial, which included 202 patients with relapsed and refractory multiple myeloma receiving at least two prior therapies (median of six). Patients had advanced disease, with 91% refractory to their most recent therapy prior to study entry. Response rates were independent of the number or type of previous therapies. Key findings for the 188 patients evaluable for response showed: (i) overall, the response rate for complete and partial responders was 27.7% with 95% CI of (21, 35), (ii) significantly, 17.6% or almost one out of every five patients experienced a clinical remission with 95% CI of (10, 24), (iii) the median survival for all patients was 16 months (range was less than one to greater than 18 months), (iv) the median duration of response for complete and partial responders was 12 months with 95% CI of (224 days; NE), and (v) side effects were generally predictable and manageable. For safety assessment, in 228 patients who were treated with Velcade® in two phase II studies of multiple myeloma, the most commonly reported adverse events were asthenic conditions (including fatigue, malaise and weakness) (65%), nausea (64%), diarrhea (51%), appetite decreased (including anorexia) (43%), constipation (43%), thrombocytopenia (43%), peripheral neuropathy (including peripheral sensory neuropathy and peripheral neuropathy aggravated) (37%), pyrexia (36%), vomiting (36%), and anemia (32%). Fourteen percent of patients experienced at least one episode of grade four toxicity, with the most common toxicity being thrombocytopenia (3%) and neutropenia (3%).

In May 2003 Velcade® was launched for the treatment of relapsed and refractory multiple myeloma – a cancer of the blood. At the time, the FDA granted approval for the treatment of multiple myeloma for patients who had not responded to at least two other therapies for the disease. Velcade®, the first FDA-approved proteasome inhibitor, reached the market in record time and represented the first treatment in more than a decade to be approved for patients with multiple myeloma. In late December 2007, Millennium successfully submitted a supplemental New Drug Application (sNDA) to the FDA for Velcade® for previously untreated multiple myeloma. The sNDA submitted to the FDA for this indication included data from a phase III study, a large, well-controlled international clinical trial, comparing a Velcade®-based regimen to a traditional standard of care. Priority review was granted by the FDA in January 2008. On 20 June 2008, the FDA approved Velcade® in combination for patients with previously untreated multiple myeloma. This means that Millennium can market Velcade® to patients who have not had any prior therapies for multiple myeloma (a first-line therapy).

10.5.2.4 Lessons Learn

Millennium used innovative science to develop novel products that would address the unmet medical needs of patients. Millennium's success in bringing Velcade® to patients so rapidly reflects the high level of collaboration among many partners, both internally and externally. Moving forward, the sponsors of rare diseases drug development should adopt the innovative science in developing breakthrough products that make a difference in patients' lives. The FDA priority review and rapid approval of Velcade® represents a major advance in our fight against rare diseases. With its new and unique mechanism of action of inhibiting the proteasome, Velcade® is different from traditional chemotherapies and represents a new treatment option for patients. Thus, innovative thinking and approach such as complex innovative designs are necessarily implemented for rare disease drug development.

10.6 Concluding Remarks

As discussed, for rare disease drug development, power analysis for sample size calculation may not be feasible due to the fact that there is a small patient population. FDA draft guidance emphasizes that the same standards for regulatory approval will be applied to rare diseases drug development despite small patient population. Thus, often there is insufficient power for rare disease drug clinical investigation. In this case, alternatively, it is suggested that sample size calculation or justification should be performed based on precision analysis, reproducibility analysis, or probability monitoring approach for achieving certain statistical assurance.

In practice, it is a dilemma for having the same standard with less subjects in rare disease drug development. Thus, it is suggested that innovative design and statistical methods should be considered and implemented for obtaining substantial evidence regarding effectiveness and safety in support of regulatory approval of rare disease drug products. In this article, several innovative trial designs such as complete n-of-1 trial design, adaptive seamless trial design, trial design utilizing the concept of master protocols, and Bayesian trial design are introduced. The corresponding statistical methods and sample size requirements under respective study designs are derived. These study designs are useful in speeding up rare disease development process and identifying any signal, pattern or trend, and/or optimal clinical benefits of the rare disease drug products under investigation.

Due to the small patient population in rare disease clinical development, the concept of generalizability probability can be used to determine whether the clinical results can be generalized from the targeted patient population (e.g., adults) to a different but similar patient population (e.g., pediatrics or elderly) with the same rare disease. In practice, the generalizability probability can be evaluated through the assessment of sensitivity index between the targeted patient population and the different patient populations (Lu et al., 2017). The degree of generalizability probability can then be used to judge whether the intended trial has provided substantial evidence regarding the effectiveness and safety for the different patient populations (e.g., pediatrics or elderly).

In practice, although an innovative and yet complex trial design may be useful in rare disease drug development, it may introduce operational bias to the trial and consequently increase the probability of making errors. It is then suggested that the quality, validity, and integrity of the intended trial utilizing an innovative trial design should be maintained.

References

Abrams J., Conley B., Mooney M., Zwiebel J., Chen A., Welch J.J., Takebe N., Malik S., McShane L., Korn E., Williams M., Staudt L., Doroshow J. (2014) National Cancer Institute's Precision Medicine Initiatives for the new National Clinical Trials Network, *Am Soc Clin Oncol Educ Book*, 71–6

Bauer, P. and Kohne, K. (1994). Evaluation of experiments with adaptive interim analysis. *Biometrics*, 50, 1029–1041.

Bauer, P. and Rohmel, J. (1995). An adaptive method for etablishing a dose-response relationship. *Statistics in Medicine*, 14, 1595–1607.

Chang, M. (2007). Adaptive design method based on sum of p-values. *Statistics in Medicine*, 26, 2772–2784.

Chang, M. and Chow, S.C. (2005). A Hybrid Bayesian adaptive design for dose response trials. *Journal of Biopharmaceutical Statistics*, 15, 677–691.

Chow, S.C. (2011). *Controversial Issues in Clinical Trials*. Chapman and Hall/CRC, Taylor & Francis, New York, New York.

Chow, S.C. (2020). Innovative thinking for rare disease drug development. *American Journal of Biomedical Science & Research*. 7(3). DOI: 10.34297/AJBSR.2020.07.001159

Chow, S.C. and Chang, M. (2011). *Adaptive Design Methods in Clinical Trials*. Second Edition, Chapman and Hall/CRC Press, Taylor & Francis, New York, New York.

Chow, S.C., Chang, M., and Pong, A. (2005). Statistical consideration of adaptive methods in clinical development. *Journal of Biopharmaceutical Statatistics*, 15, 575–591.

Chow, S.C. and Chang, Y.W. (2019). Statistical considerations for rare diseases drug development. *Journal of Biopharmaceutical Statistics*. 29, 874–886.

Chow, S.C. and Huang, Z. (2019a). Demonstrating effectiveness or demonstrating not ineffectiveness – A potential solution for rare disease drug development. *Journal of Biopharmaceutical Statistics*, 29, 897–907.

Chow, S.C. and Huang, Z. (2019b). Innovative thinking on endpoint selection in clinical trials. *Journal of Biopharmaceutical Statistics*, 29, 941–951.

Chow, S.C. and Huang, Z. (2020). Innovative design and analysis for rare disease drug development. *Journal of Biopharmaceutical Statistics*, 30(3):537–549.

Chow, S.C. and Lin, M (2015). Analysis of two-stage adaptive seamless trial design. *Pharmaceutica Analytica Acta*, 6(3), 1–10. http://dx.doi.org/10.4172/2153-2435.1000341

Chow, S.C., Shao, J., Wang, H., and Lokhnygina, Y. (2017). *Sample Size Calculations in Clinical Research*. Third Edition, Chapman and Hall/CRC Press, Taylor & Francis, New York, New York.

Chow, S.C., Song, F.Y., and Cui, C. (2017). On hybrid parallel-crossover designs for assessing drug interchangeability of biosimilar products. *Journal of Biopharmaceutical Statistics*, 27, 265–271.

Chow, S.C. and Tu, Y.H. (2008). On two-stage seamless adaptive design in clinical trials. *Journal of Formosa Medical Association*, 107, S52–S60.

Corrigan-Curay, J. (2018). Real-world evidence – FDA update. Presented at RWE Collaborative Advisory Group Meeting, Duke-Margolis Center, Washington DC, October 1, 2018.

Cui, L., Hung, H.M.J., and Wang, S.J. (1999). Modification of sample size in group sequential clinical trials. *Biometrics*, 55, 853–857.

Duan, Y., Ye, K. and Smith, E.P. (2006). Evaluating water quality using power priors to incorporate historical information. *Environmetrics*, 17, 95–106.

FDA (2010). *Guidance for Industry - Adaptive Design Clinical Trials*. Center for Drug Evaluation and Research, the United States Food and Drug Administration, Rockville, Maryland

FDA (2015). *Guidance for Industry - Rare Diseases: Common Issues in Drug Development*. Center for Drug Evaluation and Research, the United States Food and Drug Administration, Silver Spring, Maryland.

FDA (2017). Use of Real-World Evidence to Support Regulatory Decision-Making for Medical Device. Guidance for Industry and Food and Drug Administration staff, US Food and Drug Administration, Silver Spring, Maryland.

FDA (2018c). Guidance for Industry – *Master Protocols: Efficient Clinical Trial Design Strategies to Expedite Development of Oncology Drugs and Biologics*. The United States Food and Drug Administration, Silver Spring, Maryland.

FDA (2019a). *Guidance for Industry – Rare Diseases: Common Issues in Drug Development*. The United States Food and Drug Administration, Silver Spring, Maryland.

FDA (2019b). Framework for FDA's Real-World Evidence Program. The United States Food and Drug Administration, Silver Spring, Maryland.

FDA (2019c). *Guidance for Industry – Adaptive Designs for Clinical Trials of Drugs and Biologics*. The United States Food and Drug Administration, Silver Spring, Maryland, November 2019.

Gravestock, I. and Held, L. on behalf of the COMACTE-Net consortium (2017). Adaptive power priors with empirical Bayes for clinical trials. *Pharmaceutical Statistics*, 16, 349–360.

Herbst, R.S., et al. (2015). Lung master protocol (Lung-MAP) - a biomarker-driven protocol for accelerating development of therapies for squamous cell lung cancer: SWOG S1400, *Clin Cancer Res*, 21(7), 1514–1524.

Hommel, G., Lindig, V., and Faldum, A. (2005). Two-stage adaptive designs with correlated test statistics. *Journal of Biopharmaceutical Statistics*, 15, 613–623.

Huang, Z. and Chow, S.C. (2019). Probability monitoring procedure for sample size determination. *Journal of Biopharmaceutical Statistics*, 29, 887–896.

Hyman D.M., Puzanov I., Subbiah V., Faris J.E., Chau I., Blay J.Y., Wolf J., Raje N.S., Diamond E.L., Hollebecque A., Gervais R., Elez-Fernandez M.E., Italiano A., Hofheinz R.D., Hidalgo M., Chan E., Schuler M., Lasserre S.F., Makrutzki M., Sirzen F., Veronese M.L., Tabernero J., Baselga J. (2015). Vemurafenib in Multiple Nonmelanoma Cancers with BRAF V600 Mutations. *New England Journal of Medicine*, 373(8):726–36.

Ibrahim, J.G. and Chen, M.H. (2000). Power prior distributions for regression models. *Statistical Science*, 15, 46–60.

Li, G., Shih, W.C.J., and Wang, Y.N. (2005). Two-stage adaptive design for clinical trials with survival data. *Journal of Biopharmaceutical Statistics*, 15, 707–718.

Liu, Q. and Chi, G.Y.H. (2001). On sample size and inference for two-stage adaptive designs. *Biometrics*, 57, 172–177.

Liu, G.F. (2017). A dynamic power prior for borrowing historical data in noninferiority trials with binary endpoint. *Pharmaceutical Statistics*, 17, 61–73

Lu Y., Kong Y.Y., Chow, S.C. (2017). Analysis of sensitivity index for assessing generalizability in clinical research. *Jacobs J Biostat*. 2(1):009

Muller, H.H. and Schafer, H. (2001). Adaptive group sequential designs for clinical trials: Combining the advantages of adaptive and of classical group sequential approaches. *Biometrics*, 57, 886–891.

ODA (1983). Orphan Drug Act of 1983. Pub L. No. 97-414, 96 Stat. 2049.

Pan, H., Yuan, Y., and Xia, J. (2017). A calibrated power prior approach to borrow information from historical data with application to biosimilar clinical trials. *Applied Statistics*, 66 (5), 979–996.

Posch, M. and Bauer, P. (2000). Interim analysis and sample size reassessment. *Biometrics*, 56, 1170–1176.

Proschan, M.A. and Hunsberger, S.A. (1995). Designed extension of studies based on conditional power. *Biometrics*, 51, 1315–1324.

Rosenberger, W.F. and Lachin, J.M. (2003). Randomization in Clinical Trials. John Wiley & Sons, Inc., New York.

Sánchez-Serrano I. (2006). Success in translational research: lessons from the development of bortezomib. *Nature Reviews Drug Discovery*. 107–14.

Song, F.Y. and Chow, S.C. (2015). A case study for radiation therapy dose finding utilizing Bayesian sequential trial design. *Journal of Case Studies*, 4(6), 78–83.

Todd, S. (2003). An adaptive approach to implementing bivariate group sequential clinical trial designs. *Journal of Biopharmaceutical Statistics*, 13, 605–619.

Tsiatis, A.A. and Mehta, C. (2003). On the inefficiency of the adaptive design for monitoring clinical trials. *Biometrika*, 90, 367–378.

Viele, K., Berry, S., Neuenschwancler, B., et al. (2014). Use of historical control data for assessing treatment effects in clinical trials. *Pharmaceutical Statistics*, 13 (1), 41–54.

Woodcock, J. and LaVange, L.M. (2017). Master protocols to study multiple therapies, multiple diseases, or both. *The New England Journal of Medicine*, 377, 62–70.

Index

Note: Locators in *italics* represent figures and **bold** indicate tables in the text.